# Living with COLON CANCER

The information contained in this book is not intended to be a substitute for professional medical advice. Please seek the advice of your physician or nurse practitioner with any questions you may have regarding a medical condition. Nothing contained herein is intended to be offered as medical advice or suggestion for treatment.

# Living with COLON CANCER

## beating the odds

*Eliza Wood Livingston, CNM, PMHNP*
*Foreword by David Spiegel, MD*

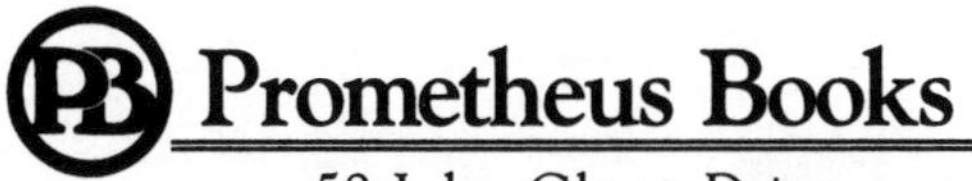

59 John Glenn Drive
Amherst, New York 14228-2197

Published 2005 by Prometheus Books



Inquiries should be addressed to
Prometheus Books
59 John Glenn Drive
Amherst, New York 14228–2197
VOICE: 716–691–0133, ext. 207
FAX: 716–564–2711
WWW.PROMETHEUSBOOKS.COM

09 08 07 06 05 5 4 3 2 1

Library of Congress Cataloging-in-Publication Data

Livingston, Eliza Wood.
Living with colon cancer : beating the odds / by Eliza Wood Livingston.
p. cm.
Includes bibliographical references and index.
ISBN 1-59102-347-5 (pbk. : alk. paper)
1. Livingston, Eliza Wood—Health. 2. Colon (Anatomy)—Cancer—Patients—Biography. I. Title. [DNLM: 1. Colonic Neoplasms—Personal Narratives. WI 529 L787L 2005]

RC280.C6L58 2005
362.196'994347'0092—dc22
[B]

2005014005

Printed in the United States of America on acid-free paper

*For Nicholas and Jessica*

# Contents

# Acknowledgments

There are many people to thank—people who were essential in helping me scale the many peaks to healing. Please, reader, forgive my omissions; there are surely people whose names I have not mentioned but who have been loving and helpful to me throughout this illness.

With a few notable exceptions (easily detectable by the reader), the doctors, nurses, and aides who cared for me did so with compassion, respect, and skill. Without question, Drs. Bhoyrul and Tsang saved my life with their skilled and rapid surgical intervention on the night of my admission. I will be forever grateful to them and to Dr. Yu, my gentle and wise oncologist. At a time when many might have allowed me to surrender to a bleak prognosis, Drs. Bhoyrul, Tsang, and Yu were my champions and cheerleaders, as well as my angels of mercy.

And my thanks to Drs. Kato, Hung, and Fischetti, who, although not involved during the initial onset of my disease, cared generously for me when the cancer metastasized in 1998, after Drs. Tsang and Yu had retired and Dr. Bhoyrul had relocated. And my thanks to Drs. Ready and Steck, masters of intestinal navigation, and to the interns and residents, especially Dr. Eghtesady, who were later called into the circle of my care. For the kindness of support staff, including radiology and lab technicians, aides, housekeepers, and orderlies, my gratitude. My thanks to my friend Anne Ankrom, an oncology nurse practitioner who told me about, among other things, "pink tape."

My thanks to the Kaiser Santa Teresa Medical Center labor and delivery staff for the support, encouragement, and generosity of the nurses, midwives, doctors, and support team and for their generous gifts of vacation time. Their belief in my capacity to heal never flagged.

For the keen skill of Dr. Anane-Sefah, who opted for surgery rather than discharge home on that February day in 2002, I am forever indebted. And for the generosity and cheer of Dr. Shapiro, who supported and respected my efforts to heal, and who could always bring a smile to my face, I am truly thankful. (It is with deep sadness that I note that Dr. Shapiro passed away just days before this book went to press. At only forty-one years old, this wonderful man suffered a heart attack while working out at his gym.)

My profound thanks to Dr. Mengke Kou, whose support continues to be essential to my health and healing. And thanks to Heiner Fruehof, who brought him from China to the United States, and to Connie Burns, who introduced us.

My thanks to the women in both the Cancer Club and the WomenCARE support group, who have been my friends, my colleagues, and my fellow travelers. In those circles of shared experiences, sympathetic ears and voices are generously given. My thanks to body workers and practitioners who have helped me at various stages of my illness, including Judith Barr, Mary Huse, Roz Crew, Shelley Patton, Gary Dolowich, Coeleen Kiebert, Amineh Raheem, Fritz Smith, and Michael Tierra.

My thanks to the people who have facilitated the writing of this book, from those who understood my need for uninterrupted hours of writing to those who were directly involved. Numerous writing workshops led by both Carolyn Foster and Patrice Vecchione have provided rich soil for planting the seeds of *Living with Colon Cancer*.

From the autumn of 2000 until October 2003, when I began spending more and more time in British Columbia, I have been part of a writing group that meets every week to read and talk about its work. Two members, Joan Safajek and Lorna Kohler, although no longer participating, were invaluable in helping me nurture the book's conception as it was initially taking form. The remaining members, Connie Batten, Sara Friedlander, Marcy Alancraig, and I (when I am in town) critique and analyze each other's writings, offering encouragement, praise, and validation as well. Although none of the others has had cancer, they have, in listening to hours and hours of my story, become "surrogate sufferers." I believe that without them, *Living with Colon Cancer* would still be waiting in the wings and might never have come on to the stage at all. When my energy flagged, and when I was sick to death of writing about colon cancer, they urged me on. I felt like a runner at the last lap; when I was eager to plop under a tree and forget the race, they were there with their cheers and their water bottles and their insistence that I could do it and that there are so many people who need this book.

My gratitude to my cousin Sara for her valuable input in editing the self-help aspects of this book, and to Cliff and Caroline Bliss-Isberg for their detailed copyediting. And thanks to my patient readers, including Robert Hamburger, Anne Ankrom, Mabsie Walters, Stan and Christina Grof, Karen Herbster, Sara Caldwell, Pat Smith, Katherine Livingston, and Jan Adrian, whose reflections and criticisms have been encouraging and helpful. And to Billie Harris, whose invitations to read from the manuscript on her weekly KUSP radio show, *From the Bookshelf*, provided test waters for the project.

My family and large extended family have been the backbone of my recovery. My husband, Clarke, has faithfully stood by me, helping me with the most unpleasant tasks, caring for me patiently and lovingly, never complaining, seldomly expressing exhaustion, rarely expressing frustration, and tolerating my absences while writing this book. My son, Matthew, whose frenzied phone call that night on July 2 aborted an untimely discharge and steered me into the hands of the surgeons; he spent hours and days at my bedside, gently enfolding me into the steady peace of his being even as the crisis around me grew, and has been unfailingly available, attentive, and loving. The little children, Nicholas and Jessica, now growing up, who continued to love me and believe in me regardless of my vanished hair, burnt face, blistered lips, or recurrent weariness. And Mattie, who even in adolescence, unashamedly and lovingly accepted my changed body and mind with utmost grace. My brother, Bruce, the consummate jokester, gleefully prodded me to recovery even when the future looked grim. My thanks also to his wife, Bethany, writer of droll notes on comical cards, and to her big-hearted children and generous parents, Muzz and George. And my thanks to Rachel, who, as well as supporting me lovingly, nurtured my relationship with the children with frequent visits and daily telephone calls. And my love and gratitude to my mother, Tash, who, generously skilled in the gentle art of motherhood, tenderly soothed and comforted me through this illness. For my aunt and uncle, Lal and Pat, and their daughters Cynthia, Sara, and Laura, who throughout this siege have gardened, cooked, played Scrabble, visited me in hospitals, cleaned my garage, and cheered me to wellness, I am forever grateful.

For the many more cousins and members of my extended family, including Carolyn, Lisa, and Mardi, my appreciation knows no bounds. My thanks also to loving and generous friends, including Betsy, Becky, Carolyn, Helen, Jaleh, Karen, Lizzie, Mabsie, Minou, Susan, Ziba, and many many others who cared for me and supported me at various times of this siege. And thanks to the many children of friends and relatives who sent their brief dictated notes and painstakingly drawn artwork to cheer me on the way to wellness.

Never flagging in their support, family members have cared for me with utmost grace, generosity, and love. Supporting me throughout this journey, they have also had the wisdom to step aside when I have had to find my own way through this landscape of puzzlement and discovery.

And my thanks to my agent, Nancy Rosenfeld, whose enthusiastic embrace of this book has not flagged, nor has her drive to get it to print. And to Don Ellis, who kindly connected us. My thanks also to my editor, Jeremy Sauer, who has patiently worked with me to fine-tune the story and has politely and patiently waited as edits and reedits shoot from coast to coast, invariably missing deadlines on the eastward trajectory. My thanks also to Steven L. Mitchell of Prometheus Books, who gambled on a book that will neither grace coffee tables nor break sales records, but hopefully will be helpful to those who read it.

# Foreword

Dreams turn into nightmares and back again to dreams in this book—an open, clearly written, and honest description of the journey Eliza Livingston and her body went through at the behest of colon cancer. Each chapter is ushered in with a dream—some terrifying, some comforting—but the reader is quickly anchored in the painfully clear details of seeking and receiving medical treatment. From having to convince ER doctors that she was more than a lady with a stomachache to playfully naming her stoma "Stella" and making it one of the characters from *A Streetcar Named Desire*, Eliza Livingston makes it clear why the word *living* is part of her name. She shares her real emotions, her fears of rejection by medical staff, and her worries about distressed family and friends.

People are social creatures, more like ants than eagles, needing social contact for our very survival in addition to our well-being. Yet the diagnosis (and treatment) of cancer often brings with it social isolation, pulling us from our friends, family, and work, making us feel like pariahs, unwelcome among people who live the fantasy that they are immune to disease and death. Add to that the burden of having a colostomy, with worry that at any moment it could reveal itself through odor or leakage, and social withdrawal is a natural response. By writing this book, Eliza makes it clear to us that she is not ashamed of her cancer, her fear, or her stoma named Stella. And she sends a clear message to other cancer patients that they should not be ashamed either. She transforms this cancer experience from the awful to the everyday by taking us through her everyday experiences.

I have been conducting research on the provision of emotional support for cancer patients for twenty-five years, running groups for most of those years, and listening to cancer patients help one another. It is clear to me that a kind of "social glue" quickly develops. Patients in the same boat speak one another's language; help one another through difficult times; find ways, as Eliza does, to joke about the grimmest things; and find new meaning in their lives as they face their own mortality. One might think that facing such fears of pain, dying, even death would be demoralizing. But we have found it to be *re*moralizing, helping cancer patients to put their illness into perspective by seeing their lives in a different way, with meaning given by the relationships they make and sustain. This book is written in that spirit and will be helpful to those facing cancer, as well as their families and friends. Smiles of recognition will cross your face as you read this book, as will pangs of fear and sadness. It will remind you that cancer is a human experience, not just a physical one.

David Spiegel, MD
Willson Professor in the School of Medicine
Associate Chair of Psychiatry and Behavioral Sciences
Medical Director, Center for Integrative Medicine
Stanford University
Author of *Living Beyond Limits*
and *Group Therapy for Cancer Patients*

# Introduction

In the last decade, as women have raised public awareness of breast cancer, it is being discussed more openly than ever before. That discussion and dissemination of information has been the genesis of cancer support communities, especially among women. This attention and insistence on blunt disclosure of the epidemiology, morbidity, and mortality rates of breast cancer has undoubtedly been responsible, in some measure, for the dramatic increase in funding for research and the release of new chemotherapies.

In contrast, colon cancer still remains a disease of secrecy and shame. Colorectal cancer—cancer located in either the colon or rectal tissue—is the third-most-common malignancy in the world, and second only to lung cancer, causing more deaths than any other. American Cancer Society statistics reveal that in 2004, there were 146,940 new cases of colorectal cancer diagnosed in the United States,[1] and 19,200 Canadians were diagnosed with colorectal cancers.[2] In both countries, colorectal cancer is the second-leading cause of death from cancers, killing more people than AIDS and breast cancer combined.[3]

When a woman learns that she has breast cancer, she is unfailingly welcomed into a sisterhood. There is direct support offered individually or through support groups, there are books for her and for her family and caregivers, and there are events such as Breast Cancer Awareness Week and Race for the Cure.

When a person learns that he or she has colon cancer, neither the support nor the networks of information that might mitigate and soften the impact of the disease are forthcoming. Many people remain in hiding with their disease, and adequate literature geared to the lay public is not easily available. An exception is Mark Pochapin's informative and useful 2004 book, *What Your Doctor May Not Tell You about Colorectal Cancer.*

In obituaries, the deceased is often listed as having died from complications of breast cancer, lymphoma, leukemia, or brain cancer. It is only in the last few years, especially since Katie Couric's courageous crusade to expose colon cancers to public scrutiny, that the deceased might be listed as having died of *colon* cancer. Has it become more acceptable to die from a disease suffered by a young, strong, good-looking man such as Ms. Couric's late husband? What are the cultural values that consign mention of this disease to hushed conversations in hallways?

When asked, I am very open about the nature of my cancer. Not infrequently, I have been told of a person's colon cancer *only after* my disclosure. Her type of cancer might have been identified as another kind—stomach cancer is a popular one. Only when it is known that I have colon cancer does the person feel "safe" in acknowledging the true nature of her disease.

The secrecy and shame associated with colorectal cancer is also evident when we note that people are commonly advised, in both public-relations campaigns and HMO patient-information literature, to have a simple screening procedure, a flexible sigmoidoscopy, or preferably a colonoscopy.[4] Yet the number of people who actually do so is relatively small: fewer than 40 percent in the over-fifty age bracket, when the incidence increases markedly. Many of the same women who faithfully go to their doctors for yearly Papinocoleau smears, a cervical cancer screening test, avoid screening for colon cancer.

Why do we prefer to take the risk that we may be growing a tumor of the GI tract rather than call attention to it by either requesting a screening test or bringing to the provider's attention symptoms that might herald an early cancer? Why is it that people who actually have colon cancer tend often to identify it falsely, seemingly embarrassed to have a cancer affecting the organs of elimination?

We as a society seem to have an endless tolerance for the vulgar vernacular that describes bodily functions. These terms are uttered with snickers (look at that ass!), in rage (you flaming asshole!), and in frustration (oh, shit!). We routinely hear and read these and other obscenities in the popular media.

Yet when the reality of someone's GI function comes into question, we generally have difficulty speaking of the anatomy and physiology of the elimination of waste. There are terms that accurately describe the organs associated with this function: colon, bowel, intestine, viscera, rectum, anus, and feces. Typically, these words are spoken with reluctance and unease.

When the subject of colon cancer comes out of the darkness and into the light, people struggling with the disease will be relieved of the added burden of shame and secrecy. And those not afflicted will feel more comfortable asking their doctors for referrals to get appropriate screening tests before symptoms arise.

There is no denying that being visited with colon cancer has been devastating in its effect on my life. It is also the case that having this disease has been a catalyst for personal transformation. I have learned new ways of being, thinking, and living that I attribute directly to this experience.

This is *not* to say that I *wanted* or that I *needed* this experience. Such a theory flies in the face of both reality and compassion. To blame the victim who is already struggling with cancer, claiming that he or she needed it or wanted it, is to add an unwarranted burden to an already heavy load. In reality, colon cancer strikes randomly and often without warning.

I write this book in the hope that it will be helpful to those living with cancer, especially colon cancer, and to their family, friends, and care providers. It is only one story, however, and in no way a prescription for how things should or should not be. *Living with Colon Cancer* is not a documentation of "the Truth." Rather, it is the telling of my story, and there are as many stories, each different in the filtering of perceived truths, as there are people in the book. Although I use my own name in this book, others are identified by pseudonyms to protect their privacy.

# *Chapter 1*
# Role Shift

## *Becoming a Patient*

### DREAMING THE SACRIFICE

#### *June 1996*

*Spread-eagled over the surface of a rectangular stone altar, my ankles and wrists are bound to the four corners of the slab with rough leather thongs. A tunnel-like opening above me admits narrow shafts of weak light. A square of deep blue sky at the end of the aperture is cloudless.*

*I am wearing wide linen pants and a loose tunic of the same cloth. An enormous hooded figure, a celebrant, perhaps a priest, looms above me. Dressed entirely in black, his face is obscured by a cowl thrown over his head.*

*In his raised hands, he holds long knives that arc into shimmering crescent moons. I am horrified to see him carve a huge X into my belly, ripping it open and pulling the skin back on itself. He reaches in and pulls out loops of thick blackish cording, throwing it down in disgust. I, too, am repelled.*

*Raising his knives once more, he again cuts the mark of an X deep into my flesh, this time in the middle of my chest. Pulling roughly at my ribs with one hand, he uses the other to scoop out my beating heart.*

The waiter sets down a plate on which is artfully arranged a fillet of wild salmon, a hillock of wild rice, a bundle of bright spring asparagus, and two orange nasturtiums with purple streaks blazing from their centers. The enticing arrangement of the food strikes a starkly dissenting note with the growing turmoil in my belly. Earlier I sampled the fried calamari with skordalia sauce. Perhaps the richness has thrown my bowels into this chaos. Yet, contrary to expectation, the cramping has not been relieved by a trip to the bathroom.

Listlessly pushing the food around my plate, I sip San Pellegrino in the hope that it might magically calm my stomach. Before the waiter can remark on my barely touched plate, I catch his eye and ask, "Could you wrap this up for me so I can take it home? This is all delicious, but I'm just not hungry." He studies my face briefly, smiles, and nods in agreement.

By Friday, three days later, the pains have become more intense, rolling over and through me in waves, eerily similar to the contractions of labor. I have been unable to eat since Tuesday, and drinking is becoming more difficult. Charles has made daily trips to the pharmacy, returning with Fleets enemas, castor oil, and citrate of magnesia. These serve only to increase the amplitude of the pain.

Charles insists on driving me the thirty miles to work that evening. Soothed by the steady hum of the car, I carefully stretch back and shut my eyes as we loop through the mountain roads.

Charles ventures, "Are you sure you should be doing this?"

"I'll be OK." Offering reassurance that I myself doubt, I am perplexed that this pain has lasted so long, that it is not abating with time. Yet in some way it feels as if a mysterious puzzle were lodged in my belly; I have only to find the key to discover its secrets, and then everything will return to normal. As I walk toward the double doors of the hospital, Charles calls out, "I'll pick you up anytime!" I turn and nod, smiling to reassure him. "Thanks, honey. I'll call you later."

The navy cotton scrubs I slip into have "Eliza Livingston, CNM," embroidered in deep burgundy floss across the pocket. Next, I pull on clean, high, white sneakers and tie my hair back with a silver barrette shaped like a lazy figure eight. Dropping two pens into the pocket of the scrubs, I throw on a white lab coat, push open the double doors marked "STOP: LABOR AND DELIVERY: AUTHORIZED PERSONNEL ONLY," and walk out to the OB floor.

I make rounds on my patients, reviewing their prenatal charts, labs, progress notes, nursing notes, and orders. After seeing one patient, and before seeing the next, I retreat to the call room, take some deep breaths as the pain washes through me, and try to compose myself. Minutes later, poised and smiling, I return to the labor-and-delivery unit to resume periodic patient evaluations.

The laboring women work diligently to prepare their bodies for delivery, responding with sighs, groans, and shrieks to the rise and fall of the contractions grabbing their bellies. They are immersed in the holy agony that heralds the arrival of a tiny infant into waiting hands and arms and hearts. And I, too, labor with intense pain, pain that, like theirs, overwhelms me in rhythmic waves, subsiding only when I feel I can stand it no longer. Comforting them at the same time that their contractions are being mirrored within my own body is surreal.

The staccato *tap-tap-tapping* of the fetal heart makes irregular squiggles on the narrow strip of paper that flows from the squat gray machine at the side of the bed. A laboring mother named Luisa is dozing, released just now from the embrace of the last contraction. Sitting down on the bed, I absentmindedly stroke her legs.

The low grunts that she makes at the peak of her contraction suggest that she will be ready to deliver soon. I check her cervix: eight centimeters and paper thin. "You'll soon have a baby in your arms," I say. Smiling, I sit with her through another contraction. "You are doing such a good job!" During the lull before the next one I explain, "It's not time to push yet. If you really feel you can't help it, try blowing out in little puffs, as if you're blowing out a candle, and keep doing that until the urge passes." She watches me inhale deeply and then exhale in a rhythmic fluttering of shallow pants. She nods, inhales, and slowly lets out the air in light staccato breaths. "Good, Luisa. I'll be back in a few minutes. You're on the home stretch!"

Stepping out to the hall, I walk down to the OR scrub area, take a mask and high paper boots from the shelves, and put them on the delivery table outside Luisa's room.

It is ten-thirty. Since arriving only three hours ago, my patients' labors have progressed, and the pain in my own gut has intensified, rolling over me in waves, before slowly ebbing.

I inform the clerk at the nurses' station that I'll be back in the call room for a few minutes, and I hurry out of the unit. After crawling carefully onto the narrow bed, I curl around my belly. The pain pulls at me, pulls me up to lean against the wall. Finding no relief, I bend over like a jackknife being squeezed closed, grabbing my ankles tightly. Panting, I stifle the groans that form in my throat. Rivulets of sweat run down my neck and face.

Is there a meaning to this pain that leaves me pleading for mercy? I know only that no baby will be my reward for this struggle. I remember my dream, the sense of entrapment, as I lay there spread-eagled on the subterranean altar. Now I am trapped by my body itself, the pain weakening and immobilizing me.

When the pain subsides, I dial the MD call room and try to sound offhand. "I'm having some stomach problems; I'm OK now, but I just want to let you know that I may have to go down to the ER later to get checked out."

"If you feel sick, go to the ER now; there is no reason to wait." There is a pause before the doctor speaks again. "I'll cover the floor."

Returning the receiver to the cradle, I throw my lab coat over my shoulders, walk into labor and delivery, and casually inform the nurse, "I'm going down to the ER to get this cramping checked out—Dr. Jessup will be covering for me." I can feel another pain beginning, and I rush to the elevators. At the lower level, walking down the narrow corridor to the emergency room, I question the actual need for leaving work. Can this be any more than constipation?

**Hints to help you beat the odds. . . .**
**paying attention to your body. . . .**

If you "have a feeling" that something that is going on in your body is deadly serious, pay attention to your hunch. Because most stomachaches are benign and resolve spontaneously, it is easy to convince yourself that everything's fine—that this will pass. When their own health may be compromised, even those in the business of providing healthcare may avoid acknowledging signs and symptoms of serious illness.

The ER is a cluster of small rooms lined with tan plastic chairs. Wheezing, coughing, groaning, grimacing men, women, and children fill those chairs, and more are restlessly milling about. Some have towels pressed to mounds on their heads or arms, and one has a Ziploc bag full of ice resting against his foot. Struggling babies cry with hoarse, weak wails. Overhead lights cast shadows on the tired faces of both staff and patients.

A gray stained carpet is scattered with popcorn kernels and postcard ads that have fallen out of last year's magazines. This feels more like a clinic in the third world than an urban medical center in the United States.

**For your information. . . . emergency room stressors. . . .**

As more and more Americans are without medical insurance, many tend to use emergency room visits for routine and nonemergency care. This overloads the system, forcing personnel to become primary care providers as well as acute care emergency staff.

I take my place against a wall and lean into it for support. Swaying to the ebb and flow of the pain, to the sound of deep coughs from old men, to the croupy cries from babies wrapped in thick layers of cotton flannel, and to the rhythmic *pat-pat-pat* of a mother's hand on her baby's back, wave after wave of pain sweeps over me.

The triage nurse finally calls me into her cubicle.

**For your information. . . . triage nurses. . . .**

Triage nurses evaluate the status of waiting patients and decide in what sequence they will be admitted for examination and treatment. Patients may not be seen in the order in which they enter the ER—they are seen according to the triage nurses' assessment of their status.[1]

From a place of exhaustion and perhaps boredom, she asks a few questions (Where is the pain? How long have you had it?) and takes my temperature and blood pressure.

"What pain medications have you taken?"

"Nothing for pain." I pause and add, "Only some citrate of magnesia."

The nurse's head remains bent over her clipboard. "Well, it will be a while before the doctor can see you; go ahead and take a seat in the waiting room." Grabbing the edge of the desk, I pull myself up to resume my place against the dull gray wall.

**Hints to help you beat the odds . . . help from an ally. . . .**

Try to have an ally with you to keep track of and write down the scenario as it unfolds. An emergency room can be so busy that personnel have difficulty focusing on any one patient; an ally can help by asking questions and advocating for you.

An hour passes—an hour of stabbing pains relieved by brief gaps of quiet. I ask the triage nurse where I am on the list of waiting patients. She responds brusquely that there are many sicker people who need to be seen first. I remind her that I have patients upstairs and need to get back to work. She sighs wearily and suggests that if I need to go back to work, I can go. When it is my turn to be seen, the ER clerk will call me in labor and delivery.

Faced with the prospect of caring for patients as my own focus becomes increasingly blurred by the pain, my reply is terse, "I'll wait."

**Hints to help you beat the odds . . .**
**communicating your distress . . .**

The importance of being clear about the level of pain you are experiencing cannot be stressed enough. Hospitals are frequently understaffed, and amid the demands of many needy patients, the silent sufferer may be left unattended or even ignored.

Returning to my position in the waiting room, I look around, watching the sad little faces of sick babies, hearing the wheezes of old men leaning into uncertain futures, seeing the brusque nurses and tired aides beckoning to this one or that one to step forward, and studying the marks on the walls and the stains on the shabby chairs. People in pain, patiently waiting to be seen, to be medicated, to be admitted, to be reassured, to hear good news, to be sent home.

"Eliza Livingston!" A nurse in worn green scrubs gestures for me to follow and ushers me into a narrow cubicle. Below the striped canvas curtains hanging from metal shower hooks, I can see the feet of people moving about in the adjoining cubicles. There is barely space to walk around the bed. As a nurse, I have passed rows of beds such as these, each one offering an illusion of privacy. The air thickens with the murmur of low voices punctuated by exclamations of pain, the intimate sounds of bodily functions responding to disease, and tired voices reciting the litany of discharge orders. The nurse hands me a wrinkled gown printed with pale tan flowers and snaps at the shoulders.

A harried doctor rushes in and asks a few brief questions: "When did your pain start? What medications have you taken?" Between the pulsations of pain, I tell him that I have been unable to eat since Tuesday and unable to drink since yesterday. I add that I have not had a bowel movement in three days, that I have tried enemas and citrate of magnesia, and that neither has relieved the cramping or constipation.

**Hints to help you beat the odds . . .**
**if you have persistent abdominal pain . . .**

If you have persistent abdominal pain that increases in severity over time, seek the advice of a physician or nurse practioner. Assuming it is simply constipation and treating it as such with laxatives or bowel stimulants can be a risky course. The pain, especially if colicky, may be an indication of serious disease or malfunction, such as a tumor interfering with the passage of bowel contents.[2]

He absently notes my responses as he listens to a message from a disembodied voice behind the curtain, "Patient in 1C allergic to penicillin; what do you want to give her?"

He orders the voice to give ceftriaxone.

"And start an IV on this patient. Give her seventy-five of Demerol."

The scratch of pen on paper pauses, and he nods in my direction. "And we'd better get some abdominals on her, too." And then he is gone.

**For your information . . . abdominal x-rays . . .**

*Abdominals* refers to x-ray films of the abdomen.

Scant minutes pass before the nurse returns with a warm blanket and a loaded syringe. I watch her jam the needle into the port of the IV tubing and slowly push the plunger. Feeling the Demerol sweep over me, releasing the tension in my body and offering respite from the relentless pain, I float into a light sleep.

The doctor returns and repeats some of the same questions. I wince as he presses into my belly.

"Ten years ago I had surgery for a bleeding ulcer; can this pain be from surgical adhesions?"

"Maybe," he pauses. "We'll get some films of your abdomen just to check it out."

**Hints to help you beat the odds . . . telling your story . . .**

Try to give as complete a medical history as possible; medical histories contain important information that will help lead to a correct diagnosis.

I snooze again while waiting for the orderly to take me to x-ray, and I continue to doze as he pushes me through the halls. The radiology technician asks me to get down from the gurney and stand against the film plate. He helps me to the floor, but I am unable to stand straight, and I slide from side to side against the plate. "Stand straight and tall, straight and tall." I know what he wants; I just can't do it. I open my eyes but am unable to focus—the entire room spins like a carousel on uneven ground, and the face of the diligent technician becomes a blurry swirl of features. I slump over the plate, and he agrees, "Well, I guess this is the best you can do . . . it's OK . . . hold still now." I hear the *thunk-chunking* sound signaling that I can move again, and I feel his arms helping me onto the gurney. Back in the curtain-lined cubicle, I sleep.

**For your information . . .**
**narcotic effect augmented by stressors . . .**

The effects of a narcotic analgesic can be intensified by various stressors, such as exhaustion and lack of sleep.

"The x-rays are normal." The doctor's voice startles me. "You can go home now, but come back if the pain persists. I'm sending you home with some pills you can take for the pain." He disappears, and I fall into a dreamless sleep.

I am awakened by a nurse shaking me and speaking to me in loud tones, as if I am deaf or unfamiliar with the language, "Eliza, wake up, wake up, Eliza, you can go home now! Here's your prescription." A plastic packet is shoved into my palm. "We have called your husband to come get you; you can go home now!" I try to see her face, to understand her words. "If you still have the pain tomorrow, come back to the ER. Now sign here." She holds up a clipboard, bracing it with her hand as I feebly sign my name.

**For your information. . . . discharge instructions. . . .**

Patients being discharged are asked to sign a document stating that they have been given discharge instructions, including any medications and directions as to when and under what circumstances to seek further medical attention.

I sleep on the gurney as I am pushed down hallways; I sleep in the wheelchair as I am wheeled out to the car; I sleep in the car as it winds through the mountains; and I sleep at home between the blue-and-white thick flannel sheets.

The cramps start again that evening as the Demerol wears off. My abdomen feels bloated and hard. I am unable to eat or drink. In my pocket, I find the Ziploc bag containing the pills that were given to me last night. The label reads "Hydrocodone bitartrate 5 mg with acetaminophen 500 mg. Take 1–2 tabs every 4–6 hours." Another note, "Take with food," has been scratched out. Fearing that narcotics will serve to mask whatever is going on and very likely exacerbate it, I put the pills aside. When I shuffle to the bathroom, I notice that my urine is meager in volume and the color of ripening apricots.

My son Andrew calls but, too tired to speak or even to think clearly, I pass the phone to Charles. Andrew is an internist and a cardiology fellow at Scripps. I can hear Charles struggling to describe what has happened at the ER and can feel his frustration at trying to answer Andrew's questions.

"Yeah, I will," Charles nods into the phone before handing it back to me.

"Mom, you need to see a surgeon. Go back to the ER, and don't let them send you home until you see a surgeon. OK?"

"OK." I feel embarrassed to be making a fuss about constipation and a bellyache. The medieval dream-figure who sliced through my belly appears in my mind, the mysterious man who cut out the debris and rot inside me.

**Hints to help you beat the odds . . .**
**paying attention to your dreams . . .**

In ancient times, dreams were seen as prophetic. People often looked to their dreams for signs of warning and advice. Dreams provided vital clues for healers and were used to help reach diagnoses. Today, dreams are likely to be prematurely dismissed as meaningless, "coming from nowhere."

Sunday morning, we start back through the mountains, but wanting to avoid my workplace, we go to a different hospital. The ER doctor, after phoning my hospital for the results of the x-rays, determines that I am probably just dehydrated. He orders the nurse to start an IV. I can feel my tissues sucking in the moisture like a dry sponge. Perhaps he is right, perhaps I am just dehydrated. I want to believe him.

**Hints to help you beat the odds . . .**
**know the signs of dehydration . . .**

Pay attention to the warning signs of dehydration,[3] including:

- Dry or sticky mouth
- No or scant urine output; concentrated urine appears dark yellow
- Sunken eyes
- Lethargy or coma (severe dehydration)

Years later, I am appalled to read his notes in my chart: "(Pt.) in NAD [no apparent distress] lying comfortably." The writing is hard to decipher, but it looks like "constipation" is the diagnosis, followed by "doubt appendectomy, gall stones, small bowel obstruction, urinary tract infection."

I ask to see a surgeon, but Dr. Metzger instead pronounces me cured by rehydration and writes my discharge orders.

**For your information. . . . rehydration. . . .**

Rehydration refers to the IV fluids given to correct dehydration. Dehydration commonly results from inadequate fluid intake or from repeated diarrhea and/or vomiting that depletes the body of fluids.

He admonishes me not to take any medication for the pain, declaring that if I *had* had an obstruction, the Demerol I was given Friday night would only have compounded the problem. Am I somehow at fault for having allowed the administration of Demerol?

The nurse starts to disconnect the IV, and I beg her to let me stay, to get a little more fluid. The shift is changing, and the doctor coming on pokes his head through the curtain. "Dr. Metzger has already discharged you, so . . ."

"I don't think I can go home," I appeal to the physician.

"What do you want to do?" He remains poised for flight.

"Can I just finish this IV bottle?" My skin feels painfully dry, and the parched membranes of my mouth make it difficult to speak or swallow.

He frowns. "Well, maybe not the whole bottle, but . . ." He disappears as the curtain he has been holding falls closed.

**For your information . . .**
**diagnostic labs for suspected dehydration . . .**

When a diagnosis of dehydration is being considered, the following labs may be drawn:[4]

- Blood chemistries (to check electrolytes, especially sodium, potassium, and bicarbonate levels)
- Urine specific gravity (a high specific gravity indicates significant dehydration)
- Blood urea nitrogen (BUN)—may be elevated with dehydration)
- Creatinine (may be elevated with dehydration)
- Complete blood count, or CBC (to look for signs of concentrated blood)

Some time after midnight, the nurse returns with discharge instructions, including (1) make an appointment to be seen in the internal medicine clinic in one to two days, and (2) return to the hospital for nausea, vomiting, fever, chills, or increased abdominal pain. Increased abdominal pain? It is hard to imagine this pain increasing.

**Hints to help you beat the odds . . . communicating directly . . .**

Be direct about letting staff know the level of pain you are experiencing. Staff may ask you to rate your pain on a scale of one to ten, ten being the most severe.

The contractions overwhelm me, making it impossible to sleep, or even rest. And with every hour that passes, I feel exhaustion sapping my strength. I wonder if I will reach a point when I simply can no longer cope, when my resources and skills for managing pain wear out, when I will literally go mad from the relentless assault on my body. Winding through the mountains, I can feel the tears sliding down my cheeks and dropping silently onto my shirt.

Weary and discouraged, I lean on Charles as he guides me back into the house. I know that he must be exhausted and frightened as well, but I haven't the strength to help him. As we open the door, the phone is ringing. It is Andrew, asking what transpired at the hospital. When he hears that I am being sent to the internal medicine clinic tomorrow, he is exasperated.

Last night he spoke with Dr. Metzger, who agreed to have me seen by a surgeon. I can hear Andrew's frustration and promise to call him after my appointment with the internist. Passing the phone back to Charles, I curl up on the bed, dozing fitfully between the jabs of pain.

Early Monday morning, sixty hours after my initial ER visit, Charles suggests a shower to soothe me. The drumming of the water on the ceramic tile beats out a comforting rhythm, calming me, distracting me from the pain. I lean against the wall for support and rock my bottom back and forth, swaying in the rhythmic motion of a laboring woman. Waves of nausea roll through me.

Charles helps me dress. Despite the July heat, my teeth chatter and my body trembles. He dials the number of the internal medicine clinic. On hold, he cradles the phone as he helps me slip into my sandals.

"I need to bring my wife in. She was in the ER last night." He pauses. "Abdominal pain." Another pause. "She can't. She's in too much pain."

He covers the mouthpiece with his hand. "The nurse insists she speak to you. I'm not the patient." I nod and listen as Charles holds the phone to my ear.

"What are you coming in for? Who told you to call?"

**For your information. . . . telephone triage. . . .**

In an effort to discourage unnecessary trips to the emergency room, it is possible to make errors in judgment as personnel try to figure out, over the telephone, whether a patient should come in or stay home.

"The ER doc," I explain. "He said to come in." I cannot follow what the voice is saying. "I need to come today," I interrupt. I can feel hot tears rolling down my cheek. Charles grabs the phone and says impatiently, "I'm bringing her in now. She's in terrible pain."

Pressing a soft pillow against my abdomen, I walk out to the car. Back again, weaving through the meandering curves of the mountain road.

When we get to the hospital, I am ushered into the exam room and told to sit on the narrow table. After the medical assistant takes my blood pressure and temperature, the doctor walks in. "I'm Dr. Douglas. So what's happening with you?" he asks. Once again, I begin to tell my story.

He interrupts, chuckling, "You've just been eating too much ice cream lately!" He presses gently on my abdomen; it resists the slightest depression. "Don't be embarrassed. That's one of my weak spots, too." I haven't mentioned ice cream and can't remember when I last ate any. Lying on the exam table, listening to his glib diagnosis of ice cream gluttony, I feel as if I am floating through the looking glass with Alice.

**Hints to help you beat the odds . . . trying to be heard . . .**

If you are in a situation where the healthcare provider is clearly not hearing you, try saying: "You are not hearing me. Please listen to what I am telling you." Or get an ally who is not intimidated by hospitals to come in and advocate for you. Or ask to speak to another doctor or nurse.

He looks down on me, and the image of his face merges with the dream priest looking down on me before slashing crosses in my abdomen. "Well, just to be sure it's nothing else, let's order a flexible sigmoidoscopy."

"When?"

**For your information. . . . flexible sigmoidoscopy. . . .**

A sigmoidoscopy is an exam of the rectum and lower colon using a sigmoidoscope, a flexible tube equipped with a light for viewing the tissues. This test detects about half of all colon cancers.[5]

He replies casually that he will send a referral and that someone will call in the next few weeks to make an appointment. As he walks toward the door, I ask feebly, "In the meantime, what about this pain and constipation?"

"Oh, take some milk of magnesia," he casually replies.

"How much?" Near tears, I can't believe that this visit is ending without resolution. "How often?"

He is in the hallway now and leans against the doorway as he directs, "One tablespoon every six hours until you have a bowel movement." He smiles broadly, playfully shaking his finger at me. "And no more ice cream!" Years later, I read his notes on this visit, which conclude, "NAD, bowel sounds normative, and mild distension."

**For your information . . . NAD . . .**

NAD is medical shorthand for "No Apparent Distress."

Worn out from the relentless pain, I stumble into the waiting room and fall into Charles's arms. Leaning heavily into the ample refuge of his chest, I stagger down the hall and through the courtyard to the parking lot. He drives smoothly and carefully, yet I am carried into every twist and turn of the mountain road and feel every bump and jostle.

Crawling into bed back at home, I curl around my aching belly, but I am unable to find a position that is tolerable. Charles tries to help me settle before calling Andrew, but there is little he can do. Rolling from side to side in a futile attempt to dodge the pain, I can hear him saying into the mouthpiece, "OK. . . . OK."

Unable to smother my groans, I whisper to Charles, "I have to go back—I am in agony. Something is terribly wrong."

"I'm taking her back now," Charles says into the phone. "I'll call you."

Back on the curvy mountain road and back to the ER. Charles helps me into a wheelchair and pushes me to the admitting window. I hold my card up to the hand reaching forward. Like an angry puppet popping up on a stage, a woman with furrowed brows and tight lips leans over the counter and snaps, "What did you come back here for? You should have called an advice nurse. That's what they're for, to take care of things like this over the phone!" I am too astonished to reply.

**For your information . . . gatekeepers of healthcare . . .**

There are many gatekeepers in the US healthcare system. One of their key directives is to determine who is sick enough to need in-hospital care, who can wait for an office visit with a provider, whose case can be resolved over the telephone, and who needs to be seen in the emergency room without delay. The ramifications of error are grave.

Eventually I am wheeled into an exam room, Charles following closely. I see Dr. Metzger walk past the open door and shut my eyes. I hear him take a chart out of the rack, flip through the pages, sigh, and walk in. "Well, you're back. Don't you remember, I said that many times we never know where abdominal pain comes from—we just never know."

"I remember that," I apologize, "but the pain, it's indescribable. Something feels terribly wrong."

He looks at Charles, rolls his eyes, and shrugs. Charles tells him that Andrew wants me to be evaluated by a surgeon. He also notes that Andrew has spoken to one of the staff internists, who wants to be called. Metzger raises his eyebrows in surprise. "If I decide that, in my judgment, she needs to be seen by a surgeon or an internist, I'll call one."

**Suggestions for hospital staff . . .**
**listening with an open mind . . .**

Set assumptions aside, and listen, without judgment, to what a patient is trying to tell you.

Then he looks at me skeptically and suggests that I have been taking pain medicine.

Exasperated, Charles sputters, "She hasn't had any pain medicine! She hasn't had anything to eat or drink for days. Nothing!"

Dr. Metzger appears to doubt our report. He decides to take more abdominal films, and again, he interprets them as normal. "Well, we may never know the cause of this pain," he repeats. "You know, most of the abdominal pain that comes through the ER—we never know what causes it!"

His inability to make a diagnosis is not surprising, given that he has done so little to figure out the etiology of my symptoms.

**For your information . . . etiology . . .**

*Etiology* refers to the reason, the process, causing a syndrome or disease.

I am puzzled that, although I have been seen repeatedly over a period of three days for persistent abdominal pain, no one has done either a pelvic or rectal exam.

**For your information . . . digital rectal and pelvic exam . . .**

Digital rectal exams, simple procedures that take less than a minute, allow the physician to inspect the rectal tissues for abnormalities and can detect rectal cancers that might have otherwise been overlooked. A pelvic exam is done to help rule out a gynecologic basis for persistent abdominal pain.[6]

Even his evaluation of my taut abdomen has been cursory and inattentive. And I suspect that he might be misinterpreting the x-rays. I wonder whether he has consulted with a radiologist. He coaxes me to doubt my memory: Perhaps it hasn't been so long since I have had a bowel movement? And surely, I have tried some pain medications . . . haven't I?

**Hints to help you beat the odds . . .**
**support from your ally . . .**

The potential for miscommunication is intensified by the power imbalance between staff and patients. If at all possible, bring a friend or family member who can advocate for you, asking questions, gathering information, and helping the doctors understand your experience, as well as helping you understand their management.

**For your information . . . causes of dehydration . . .**

Inadequate fluid intake, without question, can cause dehydration. However, the underlying *reason* for the inadequate fluid intake needs to be explored so that it can be addressed.

Again, he decides that dehydration is the problem and orders an IV.

"But . . . there must be something behind the dehydration," Charles stammers. "What's wrong that she can't drink? That she's so dehydrated? That she—"

The doctor interrupts, "She's dehydrated because she's not drinking." His voice lifts in triumph. "It's that simple!"

Toward midnight, at the end of the doctor's shift, he sends a nurse in to disconnect the IV and prepare me for discharge. Discharge teaching includes instructions for the BRAT diet: bananas, rice, applesauce, and toast. I know this diet. It is prescribed for patients with diarrhea. "I do not have diarrhea." The tears are swelling in my throat. "I *wish* I had diarrhea!" Flustered, the nurse flees from the room.

Suddenly, my stomach heaves and, leaning through the metal side rails of the bed, I yell for help. I vomit viscous dark yellow fluid into the murky pink basin that is pushed in front of me. A different nurse is attached to the hand that holds the basin. She touches my hair, offers me a clean towel, and murmurs words of comfort. That tender touch, that voice of compassion from this luminous being kindles in my heart a wavering flame of hope.

Charles asks the doctor who just came in with the new shift about getting a surgical consult. "We only call a second doc if it is, in our opinion, necessary. There is no reason to request a surgical consult for your wife. This is probably just dehydration, and when she gets her flexible sig, that will rule out anything more serious." He ambles out of the cubicle.

**Suggestions for allies . . .**
**identifying people who can understand . . .**

Look for hospital personnel who seem to have the potential to understand the situation, and work with them as best you can in articulating your concerns.

Convinced that this is far more serious than "simple dehydration," I am becoming increasingly frightened. I know that I can no longer think clearly. The days of pain and exhaustion have left me weak and rudderless, a wounded ship adrift on a treacherous sea. "Something is so terribly wrong," I whisper. "I think I am dying." I feel the nurse's calm hands smoothing my hair.

"Yes. I know. You need to stay. I tried to tell him but . . ." She shrugs helplessly. "I'll just take a long time getting you ready to go."

**Suggestions for hospital staff . . . learning to listen . . .**

Listen to what your patients are telling you. Overriding their descriptions of their experiences is denying their reality and ignoring information that may be essential in reaching a diagnosis.

This gracious and discerning woman has looked at me and seen the anguish that no one else seems able to appreciate. My secret ally.

Moaning, I lean between the steel bed rails. More dark yellow bile shoots out of my mouth onto the gray linoleum squares. "I'm sorry. I'm so sorry."

"It's OK. I just didn't get the basin to you in time." The nurse gently draws a cold, wet cloth across my face and props a clean basin by the pillow. Feeling safe for the first time since this siege began, I want her never to leave me.

"Hi." A hesitant voice drifts toward me. "Hi. My name is John. I am a fourth-year medical student. Can I ask you some questions?"

**For your information . . . repeated questioning from staff . . .**

Questions, even repeat questions, elicit important information in assembling an accurate medical history and in figuring out what's going on. In a teaching hospital, the first staff person you might see, after nurses, is often a medical student. He or she collects basic information, frequently repeating questions you have already answered many times. These students are learning, and one of the critical skills they hone is how to take a patient history. Thus the repeat questions. Following the medical student, an intern or resident may examine you and ask more questions, perhaps the same ones. Finally, an attending staff physician may be called into the case by the resident.

A towheaded fellow in green OR scrubs, clutching a clipboard and pen, John stands some distance from the bed as he waits for my response.

"Oh, God, something is terribly wrong."

"I just have to ask you a few questions, and then the surgeons will come in to see you." He hesitates, waiting for encouragement. I am unable to offer any, yet my heart leaps at his mentioning that surgeons are on their way. He draws a deep breath and asks, "When did your pain start?"

"Tuesday."

"Oh, that's seven days!" He hesitates. "Can you describe the pain?"

"Hmmm. It's agony." Hating to let him down, I try to be more precise. "It's rhythmic. Stabbing."

He scribbles onto the clipboard. "And can you tell me what you've done for it?"

"Oh, oh . . . here it comes again." I curl around my belly. "Fleets. Citrate. . . ." The coil of pain wrapping around my bowels leaves me speechless.

He waits quietly until the contraction passes and I uncoil myself.

"When was your last bowel movement?"

"Last Monday."

"Hmm." He taps his pen against the paper pad on the clipboard. "When was your last period?"

"Due tomorrow actually." A deep moan shudders through my body as another pain reaches its zenith.

"That's OK," he pats my shoulder hesitantly. "I'm going to get the surgeon."

"Thank you." Seeing the fear in his eyes, I want to smile, to reassure him, yet my attention and energy are spent. His footsteps fade. A paradox, I think to myself, this young man just beginning his training appears to see a truth that eludes staff physicians with years of experience tucked under their belts.

**For your information . . .**
**accurate determination of illness . . .**

There is a certain skill in being able to look at a patient, swiftly assess the physical condition, and determine whether that patient is critically ill. This medical student appeared to quickly discern that I needed considerable help and rapid intervention.

"Mrs. Livingston!" I hear a clipped British accent. "Mrs. Livingston. Can you open your eyes?" Moaning acknowledgment, I look up. The face is narrow. Dark eyes shine behind steel-rimmed spectacles. "My name is Dr. Narayan. I am the surgical resident."

Relieved as I am to hear that the surgical service is finally getting involved, this information nevertheless troubles me. It is July 2. Two o'clock in the morning, maybe one, maybe three, but in any case, I know that the new residents start every year on July 1. And following that line of reasoning, this nice Dr. Narayan may have been on the surgical service only a few hours. Unless, that is, he is a senior resident. I am surprised and somewhat pleased that I am capable of forming these thoughts and reaching this conclusion.

"But I'm very sick . . . I think . . . an attending . . . it's only July 2—and barely that."

**For your information . . . medical staff training . . .**

Traditionally, rotations for interns and residents end and begin on July 1. Thus, on any July 2, it is *possible* to be cared for by a physician who is only forty-eight hours away from being a medical student. (I learned later that this doctor had already completed three years of surgical residency in England and was beginning his fourth and final year of specialty training.)

"Oh, I assure you, I will be assisting, and Dr. Zang, the attending, will be your surgeon." He smiles kindly. "I know you've told your history far too many times to far too many people already, so I'll just say that we need to open you up to see what's causing all this trouble." He pauses, as if waiting for my response. "I'm afraid we have no alternative," he apologizes. "The x-rays strongly suggest a blockage in the large bowel." *The x-rays that Dr. Metzger insisted were normal,* I think to myself. I am not surprised.

**Hints to help you beat the odds . . .**
**clarifying your situation . . .**

It is possible for medical staff to miss or misjudge an important part of the puzzle in making a diagnosis. If you believe that some information might have been missed or interpreted incorrectly, it might be helpful to ask if something might be reconsidered.

Remembering the hooded dream priests with their knives pulling out the tangles of rot, I wonder whether that dream were a foreshadowing of these capped surgeons with their scalpels. And what would they discover there in the dark confines of my belly? Flooded with relief at the prospect of surgery, I welcome this pending burst of activity.

Dr. Narayan writes some orders on the chart and hands it to the nurse at his side. Asking my permission, he carefully pulls back the bed sheet to expose my abdomen. He gently touches the skin, noticing the heat, the boardlike rigidity, the distension. "Ah, yes, we need waste no time."

A tall man with a gentle concern in his eyes approaches the bedside and looks down into my face. Dr. Narayan speaks again. "This is Dr. Zang. He will be the main surgeon, and as I said, I'll assist."

Dr. Zang looks at me kindly. "We don't know what's causing this blockage: It could be adhesions from your prior surgery. But whatever it is, we need to operate without delay." He touches my shoulder reassuringly. "We'll give you something for the pain and nausea right away and be getting you ready for surgery at the same time."

I close my eyes. What incited these angels of mercy to materialize at my bedside? After days of being dismissed by doctors and staff eager to reduce their ER load, I am being heard. For the first time, I feel that I can begin to relax my vigilance.

A nurse holds a clipboard over me and puts a ballpoint pen in my hand. I reach up to scrawl my name on the consent for surgery.

Dr. Narayan speaks again. "Your son called from Scripps. He is very concerned. Would you like me to call him to tell him what is happening?"

It must be Andrew's repeated calls that account for this sudden revision of care plan that alerted these surgeons to my plight. A piece of the puzzle slips into place.

**Suggestions for allies . . .**
**support from friends with medical backgrounds . . .**

Involve medical friends and family members—they can be helpful in providing a link of understanding between you and medical staff.

"Yes. Yes. Please, tell him everything. Anything at all."

And the nurse, the kindly nurse. If she hadn't delayed my discharge, would I now be back on the mountain road, winding toward home, toward . . . a fate I shudder to contemplate?

"My name is Dr. Kim. I am the anesthesiologist. May I ask you a few questions?" I nod. She asks about allergies, medical history, and family medical history.

**Suggestions for allies and family . . .**
**understanding staff priorities . . .**

If you find yourself in a similar position, try to understand that, in the rush of an emergency procedure, there is a rapid mobilization of personnel working in concert to get the patient to the operating room as quickly as possible. There is little, if any, time for questions or explanations. For someone not familiar with this routine, the sudden buzz of activity can be alarming. Understand that priorities have been set, and allow the staff to proceed without interruption.

More people come into the cubicle: I hear the snap of brakes being released, sense the weight of IV bags being tossed onto my legs, and feel the lurch of the wheels turning, rolling me out of the enclosure. The bed is being pushed through corridors as Dr. Kim continues her questions and descriptions of what to expect. Charles, running to keep up with the speeding gurney, leans over and kisses me as I am propelled through double stainless-steel doors marked "STOP: OPERATING ROOMS: NO ADMITTANCE!"

Someone starts another IV. My gown is removed, circles of foam that I recognize as EKG leads are applied, and my hair is caught up in a paper shower cap.

**For your information . . . surgery protocol . . .**

When a protracted surgery is anticipated, the physician will often want two IV lines in order to be able to quickly and efficiently give medications such as anesthesia, analgesics, and antibiotics. Blood-pressure monitoring and an electrocardiogram (EKG) run throughout the surgery and recovery so that the attendants can monitor vital signs under the stress of surgery and anesthesia.

Dr. Kim leans over me. "Eliza, you should start to feel better now. I've given you some morphine for the pain and some promethazine for the nausea."

The waves of pain soften, and I feel myself floating lazily and peacefully into a sweet haze of opioid relief. My arms are bound to boards extending perpendicular to my body. Spread-eagled. Living the dream.

# *Chapter 2*
# Diagnosis

## *Stage III Colon Cancer*

### DREAMING DEATH

#### *July 1996*

*At the end of a summer day, I am being led through a hardwood forest, a weak wash of sunlight barely warming my skin. My feet are bare, and I wear a white linen gown that falls in billowing folds to just above my ankles. The person leading me is wearing a rough, dark robe akin to a monk's habit. A loose hood conceals his face.*

*Not sure where I am going, I feel a sense of expectancy mixed with apprehension. We are traveling on a well-marked dirt path and come to a clearing on the banks of a river. A boatman stands in the bow of a wooden skiff hauled up into the shallows at the water's edge, and with both hands he clasps a tall, wooden pole. His face is also concealed by a loose hood, and he wears the same plain cloak as the person at my side. He nods when he sees us approaching, and my companion suddenly thrusts me forward toward the mysterious figure poling the craft.*

*Trying to slow my steps propelling me toward the murky stream, it dawns on me that this boatman is Charon, that this river is the River Styx. I panic, looking to either side of me for help, but see only the impassive gazes of oak trees and alders and river willows. Charon nudges his boat further to the shoreline with his pole, and my companion at the same time pushes me forward, closer to the boat. I realize that there is nothing to be gained by protest, that this journey is inescapable.*

"Ms. Livingston—Ms. Livingston, Can you hear me?" My eyelids feel heavy as I strain to open them. Where am I? Huge, cold suns set in shiny metal discs float above me.

**Hints to help you beat the odds . . .**
**relaxing into the experience . . .**

Operating lights in a surgical suite are round, about twenty-four inches in diameter, and very bright. The lights add to the sense of unreality produced by the drugs for pain and anesthesia. If at all possible, relax and give yourself over to this intense experience, without trying to make sense of it. There will be time for that later.

Masked faces look down. Through the foggy mist of anesthesia, I recognize the kind voice of Dr. Zang. "We removed a tumor from your colon." The entire room is turning and rocking. "You have cancer."

**For your information . . . symptoms of colon cancer . . .**

Colon cancer may be preceded by no or few discernible symptoms. Possible signs of colon cancer may include:[1]

- A change in bowel habits
- Blood (either bright red or very dark) in the stool
- Diarrhea, constipation, or feeling that the bowel does not empty completely
- Stool that is narrower than usual
- General abdominal discomfort (frequent gas pains, bloating, fullness, or cramps)
- Weight loss with no known reason
- Constant tiredness
- Vomiting

With those words echoing again and again in my head, the dream I have been living, or the life I have been dreaming, ignites. Is my only escape from this inferno to plunge into the waters of the River Styx?

Thinking of my children, I feel a physical swelling in my chest, an intense love that obliterates any temptation to surrender myself to a dread disease. I will not leave them. I will defy the Fates that consign me to this ferry bound for Hades.

During those painful days preceding surgery, the possibility of cancer never crossed my mind. I always thought I was more likely to drop dead of a heart attack while brushing my hair one morning than to be found peppered with the wayward cells of malignancy. In its stealthy way, cardiovascular disease crept through my father's family. When he was barely seventy, a heart attack killed my grandfather one night as he lay back to edit the revision of *Pain Mechanisms* before going to sleep. At sixty-seven, my robust father was felled by a rogue stroke one Christmas Eve as he settled down to watch his toddler great-grandson carefully setting out cinnamon sugar cookies and Cambric tea for Santa. Among close family members, only my maternal grandmother died of cancer.

**For your information . . .**
**surgical treatment for colon cancer . . .[2]**

Removal of the tumor, along with the removal of a portion of nearby healthy tissue, is the primary treatment for colon cancer. There are three categories of surgical treatments for colon cancer:

- Local excision: If the cancer is found at a very early stage, the surgeon may remove it without cutting through the abdominal wall. Instead, he or she may insert a tube through the rectum into the colon and cut the cancer out. This is called a local excision. If the cancer is found in a polyp (a small bulging piece of tissue), the operation is called a polypectomy.
- Resection: If the cancer is larger, the doctor will remove the cancer and a small amount of healthy tissue around it. An anastomosis then attaches the healthy ends of the colon together. Lymph nodes near the colon will usually be removed and examined under a microscope to see whether they contain cancer cells.
- Resection and colostomy: If the surgeon is not able to sew the two ends of the colon back together, a colostomy is surgically created to facilitate disposal of bodily wastes. The colostomy is needed only until the lower colon has healed; it can eventually be reversed. If the entire lower colon is removed, however, it may be permanent.

I hear another voice, a clipped British accent drifting toward me: "It's in the bucket! Right where it belongs!" The unmistakable voice of the lanky young doctor who came to the emergency room last night as I was once again being prepared for discharge. I strain to focus on that face—it is so like Andrew's: narrow, with a strong jaw and dark eyes. Looking intently at me from behind round, steel-rimmed spectacles, he repeats cheerfully, "It's in the bucket, right where it belongs!" There is not a hint of doubt in his voice or in his sparkling eyes. "We got it all out! You're going to be fine!"

I feel myself folded smoothly into a shadow of light sleep, dreamy images gliding by. Against the backdrop of the River Styx shimmering in the sunlight, and Charon beckoning, images of people I love tug me toward the living world. More bright lights and quiet voices pull me back into the green-tiled room. I know these rooms: operating theaters. I know the shiny tile covering the floors and walls, the stainless steel of the instruments and tables, the silvery glitter of the huge spotlights, the blue paper drapes, the intricate panel of anesthesia controls that looks sufficient to launch a rocket to the moon. Yet I am ordinarily the one wearing scrubs and mask, looking down at the patient on the gurney, comforting and reassuring.

I hear Dr. Zang's voice again. "You have a colostomy."

**For your information . . . a colostomy . . .**

A colostomy is a surgically created opening that diverts the contents of the bowel to the surface of the abdomen, thus bypassing the damaged area of the intestine. A bag attached to the abdomen at the site of the opening, or stoma, collects stool, which the patient empties periodically as needed.

A colostomy may be temporary, allowing the gut time to heal, or permanent, depending upon the circumstances.[3] They are far from routine, yet if you have one or are about to have one, they are entirely manageable and not the nightmare that legend describes. The *idea* of having a colostomy is often more shocking than the reality of having it.

I feel a sharp stab of pain deep in my throat when I begin to move my head in the direction of his voice. Looking up into the shiny silver moons of the operating lights, I find him standing to my right, looking down on me from a great height.

Not, "This tumor looks suspicious." Not, "I think you may need a colostomy." But, "You *have* cancer. You *have* a colostomy." A colostomy? I try to check—but am not quite sure what to look for: a jaunty little Ziploc bag, perhaps, attached to my abdomen? Where? But my hands are fixed in place, immobilized by clusters of tubes that converge at various hubs on my body.

**For your information . . . postsurgical tubes . . .**

During surgery, and perhaps for several days thereafter, you may have the following tubes connected to your body:

- Drip or IV (intravenous infusion), an apparatus inserted into a vein in your arm to give you fluids until you are eating and drinking
- Wound drain, a tube to drain fluids that collect in the surgical site; this facilitates healing
- Catheter, a flexible tube inserted into the bladder to drain urine
- Nasogastric (NG) tube, up your nose and down into your stomach to drain fluids and prevent nausea

*Perhaps,* I muse, *this is an invention of my imagination—I will wake up to find that harmless phantoms have slid into the imagery of a waking dream. I will be whole; I will be well, the colostomy no more than a trick of the mind. The boatman Charon a figment of a dream, nothing more.*

The gurney lurches forward, jolting me awake as the floating metallic suns dim in the distance. Hands beneath me slide my body smoothly from the stretcher to . . . a bed, probably. Even with my eyes closed and my mind clouded, I can imagine the activity. I have rolled countless patients down countless hallways, transferred them from bed to gurney and gurney to bed, assisted at surgeries, and ordered opioids for pain relief. But this time, I am the one being rolled and pushed and pulled and prodded and unwrapped and measured and medicated. As if suddenly the clock speeds back in time, I haven't the strength to take care of my most basic needs or the power to lift my foot to step in the direction of my choice. Self-reliance, initiative, self-responsibility—concepts fundamental to the structure of my life—are no longer possibilities. Yet, perhaps because there is so clearly no alternative, I relax willingly into this alien role of dependent.

From far in the distance, I hear the deep voice of Andrew. Once again, I force my heavy eyelids open to see his tall figure approaching. He comes close to the bed, bends over, and takes my hands. In one smooth motion, still holding my hands in his, he leans over to kiss me. "Hi, Mom." Tears slide down the nasogastric tube, stinging my throat.

**For your information . . . nasogastric (NG) tube . . .**

The "upper end" of the NG tube is taped to the nose for stabilization, and then proceeds to a container in which stomach contents are collected, allowing the stomach to rest and preventing distension.

Andrew lowers the steel rail that keeps me from falling, and he settles into the chair by the bed. His gentle presence breathes peace, rocking me in safety. Floating in and out of sleep, I sense his comfortingly familiar form sitting quietly by the bed, holding my hand in his. Waking up, I am unable to determine whether it has been minutes, hours, or days that have passed since I last opened my eyes. Dozing, I am dimly aware of nurses and aides floating in and out of the room, adjusting pillows and IV flows, emptying Foley bags, cleaning the colostomy pouch, checking IV fluids and antibiotics.

**For your information . . .**
**antibiotic therapy in the postoperative period . . .**

Antibiotics may be administered prophylactically, especially in the case of an emergency surgery, when there has not been time to make the bowel preparations to cleanse and clear the operative site.

Like a camera lens zooming in and out so rapidly that focus blurs, my attempts to reorient myself each time I float back into consciousness fail.

Familiar hospital sounds become the backdrop of a reverie. Floating on a wide river, I am propelled forward by the steady current. Again the dream returns, the River Styx, and Charon waiting for me to step onto his craft. Rings, whirs, and clanks of equipment being moved and adjusted startle me and then blend into the muted sounds of my dream journey.

"We're taking you to get a CT scan, Mom."

**For your information . . . CT scan . . .**

Because colon cancer may spread to other organs, often the liver or the lungs, a CT scan is routinely ordered to rule out further neoplasms. The initials *CT* stand for "computerized tomography." The CT scanner yields images that are like visual slices of the tissue, producing more precise information than a simple x-ray.

Floating on the smooth slumber of chemical sedation, I am pushed down hallways, into elevators, and down more hallways. Now that Andrew has arrived, I can relax my vigilance.

**Hints to help you beat the odds . . .**
**relaxing your vigilance . . .**

You need time and focus to recuperate from surgery and to begin to heal. If you can have a trusted and relaxing family member or friend stay with you to pay attention to what's going on so that you don't have to, you'll be able to focus your energies on your own immediate challenge to heal.

Feeling my body sliding sideways onto another narrow surface, relaxing into the strong and capable hands that move me, I am astonished by my instinctive trust in these strangers.

"Hi, Eliza. Are you comfortable?" Voices begin to give directions, most frequently, "Now hold still." Holding still is not difficult. Tubes and ties bind me to stillness. "I'm going to wrap you tight, OK? You won't be able to move during the test." I can feel my arms being bound against my sides. An adhesive band stretched across my forehead is fastened to steel bars on either side and anchors my head in place. I recall the mummies in the Egyptian section of the Met and Andrew's delight in imagining their lives before being fixed in time and space by the infusions and applications of herbs and by the linen sheets that wrap them in eternal stillness. "It's OK, Mom, I'll be right here . . . this won't take long."

**Hints to help you beat the odds . . . wrapping up for the CT scan . . .**

Because the CT scanner pictures are shot so rapidly, you will be asked to remain still for a prolonged period, unlike the brief, hold-your-breath x-ray stillness. For this reason, you will be wrapped tightly to prevent inadvertent movement as the pictures are being taken. Try to relax and to imagine that sensation of cloth being wrapped around you as holding you securely and safely rather than as an entrapment.

A purring motor sucks my body into the narrow tunnel of a sarcophagus. Opening my eyes, I see the steel walls curving tightly around me. I hear the murmur of voices, then a rapid clicking that reminds me of the snapping whir of locusts targeting an impassive Persian wheat field, shadowing the high desert in darkness. The insects blanket the high plateau, efficiently stripping succulent morsels from the grasses leaning toward the shadow of the sun. Dozing to the monotonous sounds, I sense the light thrumming of locusts against my body. The whirring and clicking of memory alternates with the terse command to hold still.

**Hints to help you beat the odds . . . going with the flow . . .**

You may find that the combination of postsurgical exhaustion and various drugs, including opiates for pain, will affect your thought processes. Again, rather than fighting it and fearing it, try to float on that river of fluid impressions, and go easily where it takes you. Don't try to make sense of it. Just rest peacefully in the present moment.

The staccato clicks slow, aligning with the tempo of the fetal heart, *tap-tap-tapping* against my chest. I am floating through a watery dreamscape.

*I catch the dream baby.*  
*He sits in my palm,*  
*In the waters of my dream,*  
*A tiny baby Buddha*  
*Fallen into a new life.*

When the tapping abruptly stops, I tumble out of my dream, hitting the thin mattress as the tiny Buddha bounces out of my hand and vanishes. Charon, my dream reaper, shimmers and disappears in the distant mist.

Like goods being moved to their destinations along a conveyer belt, I am ejected from the cylinder into the tiled room. My head is released from the band that strapped it in place. My arms are delivered from the tight wrappings. Freed from these shackles, I notice that as they are released, a measure of comfort vanishes. Like the swaddling bands that calm an infant by encircling her in a steady pressure, these immobilizing restraints have also soothed.

I doze amid the buzz of activity and the hum of machines until I am jolted awake by Andrew's whoop across the hall as he runs toward me. He grabs my shoulders, "Your liver's clean, Mom! Your liver's clean! Oh, I'm so happy." I hear the light laughter in his voice, see the clear sparkle in his eyes, and smile. He is jubilant. My chest thickens with unwept tears. I hadn't known enough to be afraid. I hadn't realized that they suspected the scan might reveal a liver spotted like a Dalmatian with dark shadows of spreading tumor. A sleep of trust sweeps over me.

"Hi, Mom." Andrew lightly strokes the back of my hand, skirting the taping that holds the IV catheters in place. "It's morning. Feeling OK?"

"Um-hmm. Fine." I smile at him, surprised that my eyes stay open. How many days have passed?

Looking around, I note that my bed is pushed up against a counter that is jammed with bouquets of flowers, rolls of tape, a pink plastic wash basin, flexible and plastic IV bags, get-well cards propped open, and snapshots of grandchildren. Andy, now fourteen, is about ten years old in the photograph. He holds a bat in his carefully positioned hands and, oblivious to the camera, looks eagerly for the spin of the coming ball. Nico, three-and-a-half and crowned with tight ebony curls, rides a white wooden rocking horse and holds in his hand a cardboard shield on which he has painted a large blue X. Rose, her expectant year-and-a-half-old face encircled with chestnut ringlets, grins out at the camera from the alcove of a window ledge, thin muslin curtains billowing about her.

**Hints to help you beat the odds . . .**
**images of those you love . . .**

Photographs of people you love are reassuring and comforting. If you didn't have time to slip them into your pocket before leaving home, ask a friend or family member to bring them to you.

Turning from the photographs, I can see Charles sitting silently in the far corner of the room, hunched over his laptop computer. My last memory of him is when he ran after the gurney to kiss me good-bye as I was being wheeled through the doors to the OR. Now he seems so inexplicably far away.

By my bed is an armchair where Andrew sits, with papers on his lap and a pen in the hand that doesn't hold mine. He slips around my neck, tucking it underneath the tubes that deliver oxygen and others that drain gastric juices, a pendant of two small figures holding each other. "Rebecca sends you this." Rebecca, home in San Diego with Nico and Rose while Andrew is here with me. I remember this pendant: Friends gave it to her when she was traveling through some darkened landscapes. Now she is passing it from her hands to mine, a talisman to guide me through the coming shadows. The dream returns, my shrouded companion urging me toward the vessel of death, even as I turn to move away from the riverbank.

"Andy's coming to see you tomorrow, Mom. He's on his way back to his dad's after his month at surf camp."

Lifting my wired hand to gesture toward my face and the tubes flowing from it, I protest, "But I don't think he should." My voice is raspy, "He's only fourteen. . . ." Not only is he barely fourteen, but when he was five, his mother, my Zoë, was killed. How will he cope with this frightening news about his grandmother? Hasn't he lost enough?

Andrew takes my hand in his. "He can manage, Mom."

*I know he can*, I think, *but I want him to remember me as strong, tender, and energetic, not confined to a hospital bed, crisscrossed with the paraphernalia of the gravely ill.*

"He'll just be here for the afternoon. It's really important that he see you . . . even like this."

**Hints to help you beat the odds . . .**
**preparing children to visit . . .**

Should you be in similar circumstances, ask a family member to prepare your visiting children for what they will see, and be with them, or quickly available, during your visit. An alternative would be to ask a staff nurse to chat with the child before he or she comes in, describing how you will look and seem.

I study his face. What is he saying? Like a deer caught in the headlights, Charles glances up as Andrew speaks, his expression betraying dismay as well as disbelief. Is it fear that makes him so solitary, so inaccessible?

The following afternoon, Dr. Douglas, the fellow who dismissed my complaints with the admonition that I must have been eating too much ice cream, sidles into the room while my sister-in-law, Vanessa, is with me. Andrew and my brother Luke have gone out for lunch.

"I have bad news for you. The pathology reports that your lymph nodes are positive."

*Why is* this *man telling me this?* I wonder. *Where are my surgeons?*

Vanessa stands up and demands, "Who are you?"

Startled, he shifts his briefcase to the other hand and I answer, "It's Dr. Douglas."

Needing no further explanation, she moves toward him, shepherding him from the room. "We don't want you here delivering this news. We want to hear from her surgeons, not from you."

Closing the door as he backs out of the room, she turns to me, "What is he thinking? He's not your doctor! Now that somebody else has saved you, he suddenly wants to get involved again?"

As if on cue, Dr. Zang and Dr. Narayan come into the room.

Looking up, I volunteer, "I know you have bad news. We've just heard it."

"Heard it from whom?"

"That guy that just left: Dr. Douglas."

"Who's he?"

"He's the internal medicine doc who told me I was eating too much ice cream and sent a referral for a sigmoidoscopy in a few weeks!"

"She doesn't want to see him again," Vanessa broke in. "He's incredibly insensitive."

"She won't have to see him again."

"So he did tell you about the positive lymph nodes," Dr. Narayan confirms.

"Yes, but nothing else—you're the ones I want to talk to about it, not him!"

"Well, it's disappointing news, but not surprising. It means you will definitely need to have chemotherapy."

**For your information . . . stages of colon cancer . . .**

The extent of disease is described by staging, which tells whether the cancer has spread and to what parts of the body. The stages of colon cancer are:

- Stage 0: The cancer is found in the innermost lining of the colon only. Stage 0 cancer is also called carcinoma in situ.
- Stage I (also called Dukes' A colon cancer): The cancer has spread beyond the innermost lining of the colon to the second and third layers and involves the inside wall of the colon, but it has not spread to the outer wall or outside of the colon.
- Stage II (also called Dukes' B colon cancer): The cancer has spread outside the colon to nearby tissue, but it has not gone into the lymph nodes. (Lymph nodes are small, bean-shaped structures that are found throughout the body. They filter substances in a fluid called lymph and help fight infection and disease.)
- Stage III (also called Dukes' C colon cancer): The cancer has spread to nearby lymph nodes but not to other parts of the body.
- Stage IV (also called Dukes' D colon cancer): The cancer has spread to other parts of the body, such as the liver or lungs.[4]

"I figured that." This is a lot of news to take in, yet now that my doctors are here, I feel as if I can cope with it.

**Hints to help you beat the odds . . . an advocate can help . . .**

Try to have an advocate/friend (or several taking turns) be available and present for you during your stay in the hospital. It helps to be able to rely on that person's strength and perceptions at a time when your perceptions might be dulled and your stamina diminished by not only the aftereffects of surgery but also the medications you may be on, such as narcotics for pain; the fatigue; and the emotional turmoil of integrating your diagnosis into your worldview.

"Hi, Nana." I hear Andy's familiar husky voice and feel his hand on my shoulder. Opening my eyes, I see that his dark hair is cropped short and his skin smooth and tanned. The light fuzz of a nascent moustache marches lightly across his upper lip. Parting the way through the forest of tubes with his hand, he leans over to kiss my cheek. His smile is radiant, his eyes clear.

"Hey, Nana, they really got you tied down here. Guess you won't be going anywhere fast!" He looks at the equipment surrounding the bed and the tubes and hoses connecting me to it. "What's all this stuff for?"

I am amazed and touched by his sweet acceptance of grotesque abnormality.

Just thinking about explaining the medical technology surrounding me is overwhelming; speaking at all is difficult with this tube threaded down my throat and requires considerable effort. "Wait 'til Uncle Andrew gets here—he can tell you."

**Hints to help you beat the odds . . . NG tubes are no fun . . .**

The NG tube can be quite irritating. The nurses may offer you an anesthetic spray that may or may not be helpful. Meditation may also be helpful, as research has shown that it can reduce anxiety, stress, and pain.[5]

"He's already here. He brought me from the airport."

Andrew steps forward. "Hey, Nana, isn't this boy buff?" he exclaims admiringly. "Working those waves really piled on the muscle!"

"Yeah." Andy grins and looks modestly at his feet. "It was so cool!"

This child has so much of his mother in him: a certain warmth, an easy laugh, a tender concern. I watch him as he talks with his uncle, noting in the tilt of his head echoes of my Zoë when she was young, vigorous, and exuberant, when she, too, rushed forward to embrace the hopes and promises she knew were waiting for her.

"But tell me—" Andy clears his throat preparatory to changing the subject. "What are all these contraptions for?" With a nod, he gestures toward the pantaloons covering my legs from the upper thighs to my feet. In a distinct and continuous rhythm, they balloon tightly with air, then pause as if holding their breaths, and finally deflate with a sighing wheeze. A moment of silence, and then the cycle begins again: inflate, hold the pressure, deflate, relax the pressure.

"That's just air pressure against Nana's legs—she's not mobile right now, so those things keep her blood moving." Andy looks at Andrew curiously. "As you walk, the pressure of the contracting leg muscles pushes the blood back to the heart. She's not moving around much right now, so the leggings keep the blood moving by artificially increasing and decreasing the pressure. Once we get her up and walking, she won't need them any longer."

**For your information . . . preventing blood clots . . .**

Deep vein thrombosis (DVT), inflammation of a vein accompanied by a blood clot, may occur in patients recovering from surgery or other conditions requiring prolonged bed rest. Intermittent pneumatic pressure leggings are used to help prevent DVT.[6]

As Andrew speaks, I look over at Charles, wondering whether he is listening, whether these explanations might also ease his mind. He seems totally captivated by the computer screen, oblivious to our conversation. This shocking shift to indifference from the loving attentiveness and concern he'd expressed during those long days of driving to and from the hospital is puzzling. Yet it may be something else—exhaustion, perhaps, or fear.

Andy studies the labeling on one of the flaccid plastic bags dangling from stainless steel hooks attached to the poles. Andrew gestures toward the hanging bags with a nod. "She's getting some antibiotics through the IVs—not because she *has* an infection, but to prevent her from *getting* an infection. And lots of fluids." Andrew turns to me in sympathy. "She can't eat yet."

Andy grimaces. "What a bummer, Nana!"

"It doesn't bother me—really. I'm not even hungry, honey."

"Not even for chocolate?" he grins. Andy and I share a passion for both coffee ice cream and bittersweet chocolate.

I laugh. "No. Not even for chocolate!" I am as surprised as he is.

Andy's eyes follow the clear parallel tubes clipped to my nostrils and then parted to cross over my cheeks and wrap behind each ear, to meet again under my chin. "What's all that for?"

"That's oxygen, to give her an extra boost." Andrew gestures to the receptacle in the wall marked "$O_2$" in large green print. "Her body's been through a lot, and the extra oxygen helps keep her tissues in good shape and undoubtedly makes her feel better, too." Andrew pauses, evidently gauging his audience, wondering whether to elaborate.

**Hints to help you beat the odds . . . supporting children . . .**

Having an adult family member present during visits with young children is very helpful, especially in those early days after surgery, when you are exhausted. If you still have an NG tube inserted, it is even more important, as speaking is difficult, and it can be tiring to respond to the many questions that the young often have.

Andy's attention shifts to the thick yellow tube that snakes from my nostril to the clear plastic jar hanging from the wall. I know it *looks* gross and scary, but I don't mention that it *feels* wretched as well. Every time I speak, swallow, or shift my position, I feel a scrape of pain. Perhaps it cut into the soft tissues of my throat when it was hurriedly inserted in that great rush of emergency surgery.

Andrew puts his hand on his nephew's shoulder. "That's definitely her least favorite!" He smiles sympathetically. "It's to empty her stomach—to give it a rest—it'll come out after a few more days."

I fall asleep to the quiet drone of their voices, the doctor patiently explaining to the curious teenager the mechanisms at play in and around my body.

**Suggestions for allies . . . vocal visits and silent ones . . .**

Recognize that there are times when the person with cancer will want to be alone to rest, without environmental stimuli. There will also be times when she has enough energy to actually have a bit of a dialogue. There will be other times when she may be dozing on and off and at the same time comforted and reassured by the sound of your voices in the room. Just because her eyes are closing doesn't always mean she is not enjoying the sounds of people she loves.

Drifting off, the boatman of my dream reappears, and I feel myself pushing away from the riverbank. As Charon grabs the pole with which he urges his skiff forward across the water, I will grab life and pull myself away from the shadows and toward vigor and health. Yet where will I find the strength to hold on?

Charles continues to come to the hospital every day but remains in the background, avoiding engagement both with his surroundings and with the people who move through it. His hearing is gone in his left ear and is substantially impaired in his right. Because of my sore throat and the obstruction of the NG tube, I am unable to speak loudly and clearly enough to be heard. Unless someone else is there to interpret, I try to limit my communication to customary greetings.

At the end of the day, he drops his computer into the case, walks wearily over to the bed, and nervously parts the tubes that crisscross my face. He gives me a peck on the cheek, asks me if I need anything, and adds hoarsely, "See you tomorrow, honey." I smile and say, "Drive carefully," or "Sleep well," or "Yeah, see you tomorrow." Never sure he's heard correctly, he tries to wedge his ear to my mouth, yet the pressure displaces the NG tube in such a way that it burns against the back of my throat, crushing my bruised nostril. Wincing, I gesture with my hands to never mind. His inaccessibility might be terrifying were it not for the ready availability and energetic support of others.

**Hints to help you beat the odds . . .**
**being heard despite the NG tube . . .**

If necessary, ask someone whose hearing is close to perfect to be your "interpreter" so that you won't have to exhaust yourself trying to make yourself understood.

The surgeons visit often, several times a day, and enthusiastically cheer me on the way to recovery. Openly alarmed at the handling of my case by the ER doctors, they report that a meeting was called subsequent to my admission, and existing protocol was altered to require surgical consults on *all* ER patients with diagnoses of abdominal pain of unknown origin. I ask them what might have happened had I actually been sent home that night rather than to the operating room. They shudder and turn away. "Let's not even talk about that!" Accustomed to the tight-lipped medical establishment, I am surprised that these surgeons are not tempted to downplay the gravity of my situation or the shortcomings of the ER management prior to my admission.

Sometimes they have hushed conversations in the hallway with Andrew. More often, they sit on the edge of the bed, chat for a minute or two about kids, theirs or mine, and then are on their way to their next case. Dr. Narayan has a son Nico's age, and we compare notes, share photographs, and plan to get the boys together when I'm well again.

At least once a day during their visits, I point to the NG tube that is threaded up my nose and down into my stomach and gesture yanking it out. And they chuckle sympathetically and say, "No, not yet."

**Hints to help you beat the odds . . .**
**assessing bowel activity . . .**

The NG tube is left in place until the doctors are assured that the patient's bowels have begun to work again. Nurses and physicians will monitor GI activity by listening with a stethoscope for bowel sounds, gurgling that can be heard through the abdominal wall. Bowel motility is also evaluated by asking the patient: "Have you passed gas yet?" Pay attention to what is going on in your body; your report is an important piece of information in assessing your progress.

When the tube becomes particularly painful, the nurses spray a local anesthetic in the back of my throat. Its container comes with a metal wand (reminiscent of the slender, plastic, red tube on the WD-40 canister) for confining the arc of anesthetic. The spray tastes like artificial banana flavoring, and the relief it provides is limited in both duration and effect.

On Sunday morning, Dr. Zang and Dr. Narayan sail in, amazed by my smooth recovery, pleased by my progress. Again, I mime pulling out the NG tube.

Dr. Narayan laughs and says, "Maybe tomorrow."

Cocking his head to one side, Dr. Zang counters, "Well, let's try it now!" He turns to Dr. Narayan, "If worse comes to worse, we'll put it back again."

I raise my fist in triumph and joy. I was not awake when it was inserted nearly a week ago and don't know to dread the prospect of putting it back. Dr. Zang starts peeling back the adhesive that attaches the tube to my nose. Dr. Narayan grabs a paper towel from the stack above the sink.

Feeling the scrape of the tube passing through the raw membranes of my esophagus, throat, and nose, I am swept up in the exhilaration of freedom as it is dumped unceremoniously into the waste bin. Now I can speak without impediment, I can move my head without the constraint of the rubber tube threaded through my neck, and I can move my whole body without the restraining tether joining my nose to the suction bottle attached to the wall above the bed. For the first time in days, I can smile fully, speak freely, and move unencumbered!

During the first several days after surgery, kind nurses bathe me, help me brush my teeth, comb my hair, and care for the colostomy, cleaning it meticulously. When they drain the stool and irrigate the bag, I avoid watching, ignoring their ministrations entirely except to say thank you. As I slowly begin to regain strength, and to awaken to my surroundings, I start participating in my personal care. The nurse brings me a basin of warm water, several washcloths and towels, soap, mouthwash, toothbrush and toothpaste, and a brush and comb. She cranks the bed up into a high-seated position, swings the bed table over my legs, closes the privacy curtains, and leaves.

The only thing I need help with is getting out of one gown and into another one. Once, when I tried doing it myself, the IV apparatus got snagged on the sleeve, and I had to ring for the nurse. Despite the intravenous lines encumbering my range of motion, I love being able to move my hands at will and am reassured by my growing capabilities of caring for myself again. The colostomy, however, might as well be attached to someone else's abdomen. I keep it carefully covered with a folded flannel sheet while I wash myself and otherwise ignore it.

In a strange way, time has lost its meaning: It collapses and expands with fluidity and caprice. When I awaken from a doze, it feels quite possible that I have been sleeping for days or equally possible that I might have shut my eyes only moments ago. Familiar voices and faces, many having come from far away, appear briefly at the side of my bed. Although appearances are somewhat obscured by the mists that cloud my mind, I feel their love and hear their words and am comforted.

And throughout, Charles sits at a distance, intently studying the computer screen. When he arrives in the morning, he kisses my cheek lightly before he settles in the high-backed chair in the corner of the room. He seems unaware of activity and conversations. Perhaps it is his poor hearing that isolates him. Perhaps it is fear.

**Suggestions for allies . . .**
**family and partners need support . . .**

The abrupt diagnosis of catastrophic illness is devastating. Attention is understandably focused on the patient, and it infrequently occurs to those in attendance that the now-silent partner may be scared speechless and unable to voice growing terrors and concerns, nearly immobilized by fear.

I am saddened by his retreat, aware that he must be lonely and probably frightened. Perhaps he feels unnecessary, now that there are doctors and nurses to take care of me. It could be that he feels eclipsed by family members who are fluent in the medical language and culture of the hospital, who encircle me with loving hands and hearts and buoy me with unbridled optimism. Until my admission, he cared for me with a touching tenderness. I wonder whether he feels obsolete, superfluous, now that I am surrounded by professional competence and skill. Is his present indifference a thin mask for feelings of inadequacy? Or is he utterly worn out by days of worry and confusion, of holding me in my pain, of trundling back and forth to and from the hospital?

**Hints to help you beat the odds . . .**
**being sensitive to your partner . . .**

If you become suddenly and gravely ill, your partner may be sidelined by doctors, nurses, and other hospital personnel. Until now an essential and competent caretaker, he or she may feel replaced by those professionally trained to care for you. Being aware of this dynamic will help both of you get through it more easily.

The dream returns, the dream of resisting the wordless invitation of Charon, of turning away from the river that takes us to that place of eternal darkness. Am I compelled to embark on his craft now, or can I choose to delay that journey? Not knowing how my story will end, I do know that it will require strength and fortitude to back away from a release that can sometimes be seductive. Charon's ferry beguiles me into taking refuge in the shadow of its sail. When abandoning this struggle to survive seems so much easier than crossing the river of no return.

# *Chapter 3*
# Settling In

## DREAMING A SANITARIUM

### *July 1996*

*Charles is taking me to a TB sanitarium that is perched high up on a sharp stone peak, a castle guarding itself against marauders. Walking up a narrow footpath, we are each carrying a small suitcase. People there seem to know Charles, and he goes ahead of me, apparently to his room. Alone, I am not sure where to go and start following the curved path around the building. The layout of the place resembles the coil of an enormous snail shell, curving round to resemble a chambered nautilus.*

*Halls to unknown destinations go off to the left in several places. Exterior corridors skirt the wards, in which rows of beds are lined up side by side, all looking out through the windows opening onto the valley hundreds of feet below. People lying in these beds, I realize, can see only sky, as this coiled building is high on the peak of the mountain, well above any vegetation. As I walk, I look to my right, away from the wards, and see a steep precipice. It seems possible that the slightest misstep on this narrow trail will cause me to tumble right down onto the jagged gray rocks lining the embankment.*

*Not sure of my role here, I wonder, am I a patient? Am I a healer?*

A patient? A staff person? The dream speaks to the difficulty I feel in defining this new role.

**Hints to help you beat the odds . . .
being a patient takes patience . . .**

Be prepared for the sense of upheaval as you, now a "patient," are compelled to surrender certain familiar roles, such as breadwinner and nurturer. Moving from roles of independence and perhaps power, you will become dependent, vulnerable, and relatively powerless. Instead of fighting that transition, try to relax into being cared for, and rely on the vigilance and advocacy of your allies to monitor your care.

A patient, yes, that is what I have become in these last days. Am I more than that? Is there a me that extends beyond that label on the end of my bed that reads, "Pt: Eliza Livingston. MD: Zang. Service: Surgery"?

My brother, Luke, appears daily for several days during my hospital stay, to be joined later by his wife, Vanessa. He becomes my energy catalyst, infusing me with exuberance and hope and a commitment to work hard at getting well.

**Suggestions for allies . . . exuberance:
helpful or overwhelming? . . .**

When your patient is flattened by exhaustion and pain, a friend's cheerfulness and liveliness can seem abrasive, yet a few days later, or even later that same day, that same cheer and exuberance may be just what helps her heal. Family and friends will play different roles in helping assist the recovery, each, in their own way, as essential as the next. Various individuals will be more or less helpful at different times, depending on the current situation. You may be able to help the patient articulate her range of needs for company and solitude.

As soon as he arrives in the morning, Luke urges me out of bed, throws my flannel wrapper around my shoulders, unplugs the power cords and tubes that tether me to the wall, shoves my feet into pressed wool clogs, and guides me out into the hallway. Each with a hand resting on the IV pole, we take a few steps, then a few more, until my energy is spent. Every day we increase our pace and our duration, until by the seventh or eighth day we are zipping down the hallway to the pediatric ICU, then back to the last room on the surgical ward, then out the doors to the lanai that wraps around the patient rooms in a long, rectangular loop. As we hurry down the hallways, the doorways to rooms unfold like the sanatorium of my dream, like the chambers of a nautilus. In time we are actually running, the IV pole clattering between us, my wrapper flying out like a nun's habit, both of us laughing, aware of the odd spectacle we are making, and exuberant that rather than weakening, my strength is increasing daily.

**Hints to help you beat the odds . . . it's good to move . . .**

Get moving as soon as possible after surgery! Bed rest, oddly enough, carries its own risks, primarily of developing blood clots and of pneumonia. Even while you are still in bed, your nurses will encourage you to breathe deeply, cough, and move your legs. Walking and moving about improves circulation, helps the bowels to swing into action and clear the chest of fluids, and can relieve gas pains.[1]

The first time Luke sees the shiny staples marching from my belly button to the lip of the sheet drawn across my hips, he exclaims, "Geez, you've got the Ho Chi Minh trail carved north to south on your belly!" His wry humor, even on the bleakest of occasions, once again lifts me out of that place of futility and despair.

Late Monday morning, after taking me on the loop run down the hallways and around the lanai, Luke leans against the wide windowsill reading the *New York Times.* Andrew has gone off to get some lunch. They have persuaded Charles to take a day off, to forego his hospital vigil for today. I am relieved. I haven't the energy to negotiate this startling shift in the dynamics of our relationship. Whether it is fear for my life, fear for his life without me, or irritation at the chaos this disease has thrown into our lives, his remote stance has thrown an enormous chasm between us.

A slight man wearing a lab coat and a solemn face walks into the room. "I am Dr. Liu—the oncologist."

"Oh, yes," I remember. "Dr. Zang said you would be coming."

Luke puts down the paper and turns to Dr. Liu. "I'm Luke, Eliza's brother." Dr. Liu shakes his extended hand politely, and then turns back to me.

"How are you feeling?"

"Better, especially since the NG tube came out."

"Good." He pauses and sits down on the edge of the bed.

**Considerations for hospital staff . . . building rapport . . .**

Sitting down on the edge of the bed, or on a chair pulled up next to the bed, can establish a tone of informality and acceptance that is less likely to be reached when you stand towering above the bed or leaning against the door frame, easing your way out of the room.

"I want to tell you about the chemotherapy you'll be receiving." He is solemn and speaks quietly, without the playful banter shared by the surgeons, who by now seem like old friends.

"You'll be getting 5FU and leukovorin, drugs that have been around a long time and whose side effects are generally pretty tolerable." He hands me a printed sheet on which are listed the possible adverse drug reactions. "You can read that later—it's more for your reference."

**For your information . . . 5FU chemotherapy . . .**

Fluorouracil (5FU) may be included in the chemotherapy regimen for bowel cancer. It is given by injection through a fine tube inserted into a vein in the hand or arm or through a cannula inserted into a vein near the collarbone.

Possible side effects include sore mouth and taste change, gritty eyes and blurred vision, diarrhea, skin changes, tiredness, and general weakness, as well as bone marrow depression, a temporary reduction in the production of blood cells by the bone marrow.

A patient on 5FU chemotherapy may also experience nausea and vomiting, hair loss, nail changes, sensitivity of the skin to sunlight, rashes, soreness and redness of the palms of the hands and soles of the feet, and increased production of tears.

Dr. Liu pauses while I hand the paper to Luke. "You will come here, to the oncology clinic on the third floor, every day for five days and will get the medicine through an IV. Then you wait three weeks and start another cycle. Each cycle consists of four weeks: one week of daily chemo, followed by three weeks of waiting for your body to recover before starting again. There will be six cycles."

I stare at him, trying to remember what I have just been told. Instead of reciting to myself what he said a moment ago, my mind flashes back to the dream of being in the sanatorium, of not being sure whether I might be the patient or the practitioner.

Confirming my role as patient, he continues, "We'll start the chemo next week."

This information puzzles me. Dr. Narayan predicted a six-week interlude between surgery and starting chemotherapy. "I thought—"

"We used to wait five or six weeks, but now we're finding that the wounds of surgery generally heal well even if we start chemo right away. And starting right away gives us an edge on getting the cancer." He pauses and explains, "Dr. Narayan was trained in London, and British protocol tends more toward waiting. It's only recently that we have changed ours to start chemo close on the heels of surgery."

Nodding, *I see*, the barrage of new information is blurring my focus, and I don't really see at all. I do feel, however, that I can trust this man, that I can believe his counsel.

**Hints to help you beat the odds . . .**
**bringing your ally in . . . again . . .**

For conversations like these, you *must* have an ally with you, as the magnitude of the information you are being given will be difficult, if not impossible, for you to remember on your own.

"I'll come by tomorrow or the next day. Perhaps you'll think of some questions." As he starts to leave, Andrew arrives and introduces himself. The two doctors confer quietly in the hall before Dr. Liu goes on his way and Andrew returns to my bedside.

"He seems nice enough, Mom. And his training is hard to beat: Harvard Medical School, Sloan-Kettering Residency and Fellowship . . . I think he did his undergraduate in Shanghai."

He shifts in his chair. "Remember though, the protocol for this cancer hasn't changed appreciably in thirty years." He hesitates. "But there are some clinical trials going on if you're interested, one using monoclonal antibodies."

> **For your information . . . research and clinical trials . . .**
>
> Clinical trials, research studies to evaluate promising new options for the treatment of cancer, offer patients the possibility of receiving drugs that have not yet been approved by the FDA for standard use. Depending upon the study, all the patients in the trial may be given the same new drug being studied, or some may be given the standard treatment and some the new drug, or some may be given the new drug, and others a placebo. For more information, go to the National Cancer Institute (NCI) Web site at www.nci.nih.gov or the National Institutes of Health (NIH) Web site at www.clinicaltrials.gov.[2]

Beyond the windowpane, clouds float carelessly through space, skimming the pine trees outlined against the horizon. An image of the dream sanatorium is outlined against the deep-blue sky, bringing me back to that aerie, echoing my confusion. "What do *you* think?" Wishing for a straightforward and clear solution, I press my son to lead me toward it.

"I really don't know. Nobody knows. The known versus the unknown. The known protocol that will increase your chance of survival by 10 percent. The unknown experimental drugs that may have no effect at all or may wipe out the cancer entirely." I can see the strain in his face, the exhaustion.

"What would you do?" I persist. "What if I were *your* patient?"

"It's still your decision," he says gently, taking my hand in his. "No one can make it for you."

My attention returns to the fluffs of cotton wool drifting across the cobalt dish of sky. I want someone to make this decision for me. I want that security of childhood, when the grown-ups led us toward the choices that would be "good for us."

"Think about it. Take your time."

Thinking requires enormous effort. And pondering options to arrive at a reasonable decision seems a nearly impossible task.

**Hints to help you beat the odds . . .**
**having to make decisions quickly . . .**

In many situations, people have time and energy prior to surgery to explore various options for treatment. However, when the surgery and subsequent diagnosis occur over mere minutes and perhaps hours, the suddenness with which you are called upon to digest that life-changing information can numb you. Making decisions is a monumental challenge; this is a time during which your ally can help you think through your options.

"You really need to be comfortable with your choices. Try to put out of your mind what you think I want you to do . . . or anyone else. It's your body, your decision." He's quiet for a moment. "I know it's hard. There's not a clear answer." Leaning forward with his chin in his hand, he added, "I wish I could help you here, but Mom, this is for you to decide."

On Wednesday, seven days after surgery, a new nurse walks in, introduces herself, and asks, "How's your colostomy care going?"

I stare at her politely as I try to figure out just what she is asking. "Hmmm," I blink and wait.

"You're not doing your colostomy care yet?" She sounds surprised. I am startled at the thought of having anything at all to do with the plastic bag filling with stool.

"No," I stammer. "I don't know how." Suddenly, after days of being cared for and lulled into a serene space of dreams and denial, the practical questioning of this nurse prompts me to confront the obvious. That yes, this colostomy will be going home with me, that yes, I will need to learn to care for it. These are realities that, until now, I have been able to avoid.

**Hints to help you beat the odds . . . denial as a strategy . . .**

Denial is not necessarily a bad thing. When you have to adjust to overwhelming changes in circumstance, denial of one or some of the new realities can be helpful, giving you a temporary break from the work of integrating this new reality. However, denial may be more useful for offering a temporary respite rather than a long-term coping mechanism.

When aides have periodically come in to care for this contraption, I have fallen into the habit of engaging them in brisk conversation while staring at the ceiling or just lying there with my eyes closed, feigning sleep. Now I begin to take note.

The colostomy bag is about the size and shape of a child's hot-water bottle, made of a thin, translucent plastic, rather like a heavy Ziploc bag. There is a hole in the bottom through which the nurses drain the waste into a plastic basin. Then they take enormous syringes and fill them with warm water, which they squirt into the bag, washing the sides clean. Afterward they take a plastic clip, roll the "sleeve" of the bag a few times around it, and then fasten it tightly with a smart snap. And through it all, I feel nothing, neither the warmth of the rushing water nor the jostle of the attachment as they manipulate the pouch.

**For your information . . . describing a colostomy . . .**

A colostomy is a surgically created opening in the abdomen to facilitate the elimination of waste. The healthy end of the colon is brought out through this opening and formed into a stoma, an abdominal opening located at various sites, depending upon which segment of colon has been removed. Stool passes through the stoma and into a small plastic bag attached to the abdominal skin around the stoma with a special paste.[3]

The door to the veranda off the hospital room has a big sign on it: "THIS DOOR TO REMAIN CLOSED AT ALL TIMES!"

*Then why have a veranda?* I wonder.

"I brought a Scrabble board." My cousin Laura stands by the bed hesitantly. "But you may be too tired to play."

I am rarely too tired to play Scrabble, and Laura and I have a long history of playing this game every time we are together and even through the mail we send each other that shuttle up and down the West Coast.

"How about if we play outside?" Laura catches me looking at the ominous sign. "Oh, we can ignore that!" she laughs. "Who's ever going to care? Who here has time to care!"

She drags out a table and two chairs and helps me shuffle from my bed out onto the veranda. We sit in the late afternoon sunlight, seven stories above the car park and the traffic and the boxlike buildings of Santa

Clara Valley, playing a leisurely game of Scrabble against the pastoral backdrop of jack pine etched against the indigo ocean of sky. We pretend we are at a fancy resort.

**Suggestions for allies . . . having fun . . .**

There are so many chores involved in being a patient, some of them painful and many of them unpleasant, that offering some everyday fun activities, such as Scrabble, can provide a wonderful counterpoint. Adjusting the environment to eliminate or hide the "supplies and paraphernalia of sickness" helps as well.

On Thursday morning, a woman dressed in a white lab coat and carrying a basin overflowing with supplies introduces herself as Marcella, the ostomy nurse.

**Hints to help you beat the odds . . . the ostomy nurse . . .**

The ostomy nurse, or the enterostomal therapist, is your ally. He or she will teach you about the care of the colostomy, such as how to keep the area clean to prevent irritation and infection and which specific appliances might be best suited to your situation. *When she gives you a business card, hold on to it and call her when you have questions or need reassurance.*

She cheerily asks me whether I have seen the stoma. *Now how can that have happened?* I wonder. *Surely I would not go investigating on my own.* Just thinking about it makes me feel queasy.

Vanessa, coffee mug in hand, slips off the window seat and comes to stand at the end of the bed. I am relieved that she'll be here to remember what I forget, that I'll have a witness to this visit.

With a businesslike air, Marcella pulls back the covers, "Oh, it's a Hollister!" she exclaims. "Is it working pretty well?" I don't know what "pretty well" is, nor do I know what she means by naming it a "Hollister," so I just nod.

**For your information . . . colostomy bags . . .**

The bags are plastic, either opaque or translucent. They may be closed bags, with no opening other than the communication with the stoma, or they may have a second opening from which to drain the waste without taking the appliance off. If you can imagine a light, plastic, old-fashioned hot-water bottle dangling from just below your waist, with the cork end turned inward to your abdomen, and a hole cut in the lower end, you'll have a rough picture of the layout.

Bags can have other features, such as charcoal filters to diminish the malodorous impact of escaping gas. The filters can be changed as needed, each time allowing built-up gases to escape. The bag may also have plastic snaps on either side, to which can be attached an elastic band. The band goes around the body, and gently stretches the bag so it lays flat against the abdomen. Without that elastic stabilizer, a bag may hang in such a way as to clump, looking as if there's a bird's nest under your clothes!

"Oh, just a minute," Vanessa raises her hand to request a recess. "Charles needs to hear this." She turns to him and asks, her voice louder now to accommodate his poor hearing, "Charles, don't you want to hear this? You know, Eliza might need assistance with her colostomy sometime, and you might be the only one there to help her."

**Hints to help you beat the odds . . .**
**colostomy care support . . .**

Talk to your stoma nurse about the kind of support you might need at home. Before you leave hospital, it may be helpful to have a close relative or friend shown how to look after the colostomy so he or she can help out when you get home.

Charles looks up from his computer screen and says tersely, "No, thank you. When I need to learn about that thing, I'll learn about it." Before the last words were uttered, his head was down, back to the screen. Surprised, Vanessa gasps at his rebuff. Our eyes meet, and I know she understands my fear.

She and Luke will be returning to Portland in two days. Andrew is coming back the day before discharge and will stay only two nights before he has to get back to San Diego. My mother is here now for a few days, but she has to get back to houseguests and the rhythm of her life in the Oregon Cascades. Vanessa shrugs, and we both turn our attention back to Marcella and her plastic basin full of mysterious devices.

She starts to peel away the large hard patch that attaches the bag to the skin. Suddenly, there's the opening, a big, sloppy, bright, red, roselike thing protruding out onto the skin of my abdomen.

**For your information . . . stomas change over time . . .**

The stoma, the abdominal opening, will initially be bright red, swollen, and floppy postsurgery. In time it will calm down, but because it will be shrinking and even changing its shape in the first few weeks, your needs as to appliances will be changing also.

"Oh, very nice," coos Marcella. "This really looks fine."

*Fine?* I wonder. How can "fine" describe this distortion of normal?

Watching me, Vanessa smiles as she cautions Marcella, "I don't think 'fine' is a word she'd use to describe it."

I think it vaguely resembles a very tired, very floppy cervix, one that is utterly worn out from stretching to accommodate the passage of too many big babies.

"It's pretty shocking to look at," Vanessa muses.

**Suggestions for allies (and everyone else involved) . . . responding honestly . . .**

Your honest response can actually be helpful, as it validates the patient's own perceptions of reality. Your acknowledgment of the truth may help the patient to accept the changes.

Looking toward Charles, seeing him still fully fastened to his computer, I am both saddened and relieved that he remains oblivious to the revelations of my abdomen. Saddened because I need him not only to accept this sea change in my body but also to help me to do so myself. Yet relieved that I have not had to witness his revulsion at the sight of this crimson peonylike pom-pom of intestine winking balefully at the overhead light.

Marcella, I notice, is touching the glistening petals of the scarlet rose with her gloved hand, yet I am feeling nothing. It seems so strange that a piece of my body that appears so vulnerable, so unprotected, is inaccessible to perceptions of caress or injury.

**Hints to help you beat the odds . . . protecting your colon . . .**

If you have a colostomy, whether temporary or permanent, remember that the colon does not register pain in response to tissue trauma. Therefore, be careful not to injure it because you won't be able to feel if you have done any damage.

Marcella reassures me that the opening, which she calls the "stoma," will become smaller and smaller and also "neater" in time. She removes the bag, leaving the circular flange attached to my skin. She examines the stoma, pronouncing it healthy and healing well. She also describes an array of bags and flanges, promising that, by trial and error, we will find the one that works best for me.

**For your information . . . a flange . . .**

A flange is a ring of rubbery, pliable material that is attached to the skin around the stoma. The bag is then snapped onto the flange. The bag can be changed as often as needed, and the flange can stay in place for up to a week.[15]

I glance at the wound that stretches from my belly button to below the pubic hairline. The stainless steel staples mark a shiny trail that splits my abdomen and pelvis roughly in half.

I recall wielding the stapler myself at the close of a C-section, challenging myself to make the closure smooth and tight, without puckers or gaps. And now someone else has stapled me back together, except that a deadly tumor was lifted from the cavern of my pelvis instead of a startled baby.

Marcella tugs gently at the fastening device to remove it, measures the inside dimensions of the stoma, and cuts a hole in a new cardboard flange to approximate the shape of the opening. She then applies some "stoma paste" to the side of the flange that will be attached to the skin. While the paste is drying, she wipes around the edges of the stoma with a gauze sponge. I feel the wet warmth against the skin of my abdomen, but when she swipes the gauze over my everted gut, I feel nothing.

Suddenly I am lifted out of the emotional upheaval of getting used to a colostomy and become the curious scientist learning the intricacies of a new gadget. Listening to her talk about the technological variations of ostomy supplies, I wish Charles were part of this conversation.

"There's a long list of devices to choose from and lots of different kinds of bags: throw-aways, closed bags, filtered bags."

She sounds so matter-of-fact. *Of course she does*, I think to myself, *she's not the one with the colostomy.*

"Also the gas emissions diminish in time." Marcella starts to pack up her gear into the pink basin and promises to come back the next day.

For several days following surgery, my nourishment comes from IV fluids dripping into translucent tubes that lead to various punctures in my body.

**For your information . . . IV hydration and nourishment . . .**

Immediately postsurgery, patients are kept NPO, "Nihil per os," Latin for "nothing by mouth." Hydration is maintained through IVs, and some surgeons allow their patients to suck on wet gauze sponges to relieve the dry mouth. When bowel sounds are heard, indicating that the bowel is awakening from its induced sleep, food is slowly introduced, starting with clear fluids.

Not actually hungry, but chronically thirsty and bothered by "cotton mouth," I am grateful for the water-soaked gauze sponges the nurses bring me to suck on. After a few noneventful days pass subsequent to the withdrawal of the NG tube, bowel sounds are detected. I am allowed clear fluids by mouth.

The first breakfast consists of a cup of apple juice and another of green Jell-O. It tastes delicious. At around eleven o'clock, a dietary aide brings in a tray. "Eliza?" she sings out. "Here's your lunch!"

On the tray is a cup of lukewarm water against which leans a small white envelope. I pick it up and strain to read the diminutive green print: "Contains chicken flavored freeze-dried broth granules." There are also plastic cups of reconstituted cranberry and apple juice. In the middle of the tray is a rectangular plastic dish of rainbow-colored cubes of dense Jell-O.

Sometime in the late afternoon, I am roused by the light scrape of a tray being slid onto the bed table. "Dinner's here! Spaghetti and meatballs!" I open my eyes to see a portly man with a fringe of wavy white hair circling his crown. He wears the snappy white jacket of the dietary department, and his name tag says "Phil" in large block letters.

His announcement astonishes me. Spaghetti and meatballs following one breakfast of broth and one lunch of juices and Jell-Os? Following a week of nothing by mouth?

**For your information . . . advancing the diet . . .**

Once a post-op patient has tolerated clear fluids, the diet is routinely advanced to "full fluids," consisting of fluids you can't necessarily see through, such as chicken broth, pureed soups, applesauce, and custard. A "soft diet" generally comes next, introducing foods such as bananas, eggs, and soft pasta.

The friendly man smiles as he lifts the warming dome. A thick white sauce, not the red marinara I would have expected, coats the dull gray of the meatballs and clings to strands of pale pasta. Sensing my disappointment, Phil's smile fades as he replaces the dome and quietly leaves the room.

Just then, Luke's wife, Vanessa, breezes in; sees the tray; and says, "Food at last! How exciting!"

"Umhmm," I smile, "Check it out!"

Whipping off the nickel dome with a theatrical flourish, her smile fades as she gasps, "Spaghetti and meatballs?"

Luke, striding in behind her, leans over the once-steaming plate. "Well, I guess a hospital is one of the last places to give you food that's actually good for you!" Making only a feeble attempt to suppress the derision in his voice, he continues, "It looks like a close second to one of the plates of dusty plastic pastas that the folks at DaVinci's Diner put in the window to advertise the specials."

**Hints to help you beat the odds . . .**
**foods that suit your taste . . .**

Let friends who know your culinary persuasions bring you food from home, as it is likely to be tastier and more nutritious than hospital food. (Although there are exceptions, hospitals are generally not known for their cuisine, either from a nutritional point of view or a gastronomic one.)

Vanessa, herself an ICU nurse, turns to question an RN who walks in on her nightly round of blood pressures and temperatures. "Spaghetti and meatballs! Can this perhaps be someone else's tray?"

"No, this is Eliza's tray." The nurse frowns. "Doesn't she like spaghetti and meatballs?"

"But she's had nothing by mouth for over a week . . . until this morning, when she had Jell-O and juice." Vanessa tries to be calm. "And all the disruption of GI surgery . . . I don't see how she can move from clear fluids right to spaghetti and meatballs."

The nurse shrugs. "That's just what they sent."

"Isn't there something a little lighter that she can start with?" Vanessa persists. "Like plain rice or steamed vegetables?"

The beleaguered nurse glances at the bulbous mound. "Yeah, that does look pretty heavy." Turning back to Vanessa, she explains, "I understand your point, but we don't have a kitchen here."

"Where did this food come from?"

"From Marriott Food Services—on contract."

Baffled, Vanessa sputters, "The hotel chain?"

"Yes. Several years ago the hospital closed the kitchen here, and now all our meals are brought in."

"So . . . there's no way to get something else?" Vanessa's frustration is obscuring her innate courtesy.

"No . . . that's the biggest problem with this shift to meals on contract. . . . There's not a kitchen we can call to make last-minute requests or changes." The nurse shrugs helplessly, her gaze coming back to me. "Is there something that might taste good to you?"

"Maybe a plain baked potato?"

The nurse apologizes. "I'm sorry, but there's no place to get a potato —not now." Turning back to Luke and Vanessa, she suggests, "Not unless you want to go to that deli on the corner—they might have something like that."

"Let's go!" Starting out the door, Luke announces slowly, enunciating each word with equal emphasis, "We are going to get a baked potato," and cheerily concludes, "be back momentarily!"

Less than twenty minutes later, they return to place on the bedside table a small baked potato in a white cardboard bowl. A few bites go down without incident. Unless I run into trouble in the next few hours, there should be no further obstacles to going home.

**Hints to help you beat the odds . . .**
**leaving the hospital, heading home . . .**

When you leave the hospital with a bag of supplies, a hole in your abdomen, and a rerouted GI system, you are likely to feel overwhelmed and be convinced that you have been given an impossible task. Rest assured, however; you will learn to manage this new contraption, and you will be able to continue the activities you have always enjoyed, including tennis, swimming, sailing, and making love.

I entered this hospital a practicing midwife with a bad bellyache; I will be leaving it a cancer patient with a surgical wound, a colostomy, and a timetable for chemotherapy. After spending many years learning about new procedures and policies in obstetrics, I will now be learning about the procedure of caring for a colostomy and the protocols and side effects of chemotherapy. The ambiguity of the dream lingers despite the obvious fact that my current role is plainly defined: No longer signing patient charts with a flourish of Eliza Livingston, CNM, doctors and nurses will be making notes in *my* chart, documenting diagnoses and guessing prognoses. I am now the patient.

# *Chapter 4*
# Coming Home

## SEEKING SHELTER

### *July 1996*

*Carrying two valises, I am on a small island, walking along a seashore trail that is taking me to either a hospital or a school, where I will be staying for some time. The terrain seems familiar yet threatening: a place of exile perhaps, as well as a place of no exit. Suddenly, the trail is under deep water, and, struggling against the current, I realize that I have not accounted for the changing tides.*

*Close to my destination, I must still traverse a long part of the trail that was a jetty yesterday but today is a walkway that sinks deeper and deeper before reaching the dry shore. Panicked at my precarious situation, I realize that there is no going back: The tide is still coming in, and I cannot reverse my steps.*

*Scanning the beach in the distance, I notice several small groups of fishermen silently watching me. Something about them makes me afraid—if I lose my footing entirely, I have no confidence that they will come to my aid, nor do I feel sure that they will leave me alone when I hit the dry land. However, realizing that to dally further would worsen my predicament, I continue.*

*Holding the suitcases high over my head, the thin fabric of my dress swirling in the turbulence of the tide, I slowly make my way down the underwater jetty. The pit of my stomach aches with anxiety and dread, yet I nonetheless feel that I have a chance of making it, and I keep in my mind the image of the school/hospital that might be my sanctuary.*

The night before discharge, Gemma flies out from New York to help with my first week at home. She and I were classmates in nursing school and, despite the thousands of miles that now separate us, we nurture a close connection.

Andrew picks her up at the airport, and by the time they get to the hospital room, they are well into talking about his growing-up days in New York, twenty-five years ago. At that time, Gemma became part of our household, frequently staying for meals, sometimes for the night, and accompanying us on vacations. She was every child's dream of a fairy godmother. The ultimate jokester, she made the most common activity, if not enriching, amusing: While playing her guitar, she sang in a rich, haunting voice folk songs, Broadway hits, and plaintive Irish tunes; she sprang to the children's defense when my rules or expectations became excessive; and she championed their rights when the roller coaster of adolescence swept them out of the dreamy landscape of childhood. Twelve years younger than I and eleven years older than Andrew, she was a bridge that linked the shores of our generations.

As Gemma and Andrew come into the room, they interrupt their reminiscing. Gemma drops her bag on a chair and runs to the bed. "Oh, Eliza, I can't believe this—I can't believe this is happening to you." She leans down and hugs me tightly. Stepping back, she holds my face in her hands and coos, "But you're still beautiful!"

"I don't think so." I have been up, have stood before a mirror. I know what I look like. "I'm going to be OK though—seeing you is making me better already!"

**Hints to help you beat the odds . . .**
**nourishing power of loved ones . . .**

The nourishing power of being with old and dear friends or relatives, people with whom you have shared history and linked hearts, cannot be overstated. If someone in this category wants to be with you, welcome it. On the other hand, if a friend or relative is not particularly nurturing, delay that visit until you are stronger. This is the time to acknowledge the primacy of what helps *you* rather than responding on the basis of what might make someone else feel better.

"Yes, of course!" Standing back, hands on hips, she declares, "You're going to be OK, because we *insist*—we're going to *make* you OK—right, Andrew?" Her dark hair is longer, in a pageboy, and she wears a black dress scattered with white polka dots. Like mine, her narrow waist has thickened since we were in nursing school.

Andrew stands behind her, his hands resting affectionately on her shoulders. "Yeah. Right, Mom?" It is sweet seeing Andrew, who once reached Gemma's knee, now towering over her, tenderly reassuring her.

"Right, . . . Just having you two here next to me is already making me better."

"This is so great seeing Andrew!" Grabbing him at both elbows, Gemma stretches out her arms and stands back, the artist admiring the portrait. "It's been so long. And you're so tall!" Giggling, she moves closer and slides her hand from the top of her head to his chest. "I can barely reach your armpits!"

Gemma turns back to me. "And I'm remembering so much about the old days . . . like when he'd leave those tiny Legos on the floor, and then," she extends her arms to the side like a tightrope walker, "stumbling to the bathroom in the middle of the night, *I'd* step on them . . . and boy, did they hurt!"

"I loved Legos!" Andrew protests. "I still play Legos . . . with Nico."

"I know you love Legos," she teases, "but you could have picked them up!"

Spinning the hands of the clock back a couple of decades, they are amused and comforted in recalling the sweetness and mischief of another time. It is reassuring for me to see them return to the affectionate banter of Andrew's childhood.

"On that note, I think I'm going to take off. . . . I'll stay with Charles tonight, and then in the morning we'll both come in to get you." Andrew has been sleeping on the gurney nearly every night, and I am relieved that he's going to get a break.

**Hints to help you beat the odds . . .**
**reminiscing with friends and family . . .**

Reminiscing, or listening to the reminiscing of those you love, can stimulate endorphins with the attendant pleasure of remembering happy times.

"Good-bye, honey—see you in the morning."

Gemma turns to me. "What a darling, Eliza. But we always knew that. He really hasn't changed at all . . . still plays with Lego even! He's his same, sweet self."

"He really is. And seeing you has to be a real treat for him—you were a big part of his growing up, you know." I think she has no idea how her presence in our household enriched and lightened our lives.

"I haven't seen Andy since he was six years old and building sand castles in the wind at Arch Cape. And the other two, Nico and Rose—I haven't even met them!" Her voice rises in frustration. "There's just too much space between coasts."

"But we have to make more effort to visit." Even as I say that, I know that expectations for me to do any future visiting are low. Any future anything is . . . maybe not impossible, but improbable. I know that I am Stage III, so named because the cancer has extended beyond the colon to the lymph system. And I know that Stage IV is reached when the cancer spreads to other organs beyond the original site. I also know that there is no Stage V. One stage between *being* and *not being*.

**Hints to help you beat the odds . . .**
**imagining the future . . .**

You may experience panic when you begin to make plans for the future, and then realize with a start that that future you are contemplating may occur without you. In time, although your faith in a future may be restored to a greater or lesser extent, it is likely that your intense and intimate experience with catastrophic disease will continue to sharpen your awareness and appreciation of the slender thread that holds us to the life being lived.

I don't want to know any details of my prognosis, and I really don't care to learn much about colon cancer beyond how I can get rid of it. By disposition curious, my inclination to avoid learning more about this disease surprises me.

I must believe that once again we'll wing across the country to see each other. "And," I add, "way more often than we have in the past—like, yearly at least."

**Suggestions for allies . . .**
**letting the patient set the pace of disclosure . . .**

Take cues from the person with cancer regarding how much she knows and wants to know and when. Let her set the timetable for discussions, for sharing fears and anxieties, and allow time for shared silences without pushing for disclosure.

"Yeah, enough of this every couple of years routine! I've missed you so much." She hesitates. "But you know, as the old saying goes, 'Be careful what you wish for!' A few weeks ago, I was just yearning to see you, thinking if only we could have some time together without husbands, without children . . . and now here we are." She shudders. "Just us . . . I guess I got my wish!"

"And I was wanting to lose some weight," I remember, "wishing to be thin again! I guess I'll get that wish now, too!"

"There you go!" She looks out the window at a thin sliver of moon rising against the darkening blue of twilight. "I never dreamed we would be brought together by—by this."

"No. You know, even with all the pain, even while I was being discharged after limping once again to the emergency room, it never occurred to me that this might be cancer!" I am astonished, all over again, at my capacity for denial.

"And that's the first thing I would have thought of!" Gemma's two aunts and an uncle had died of colon cancer. Her mother died of lung cancer. Her father died of leukemia. And Gemma herself worked on the oncology ward after graduation. Every twinge and bump, she was sure, must signify a stealth tumor poised for ambush.

"I know, but it's almost as if you did all the cancer worrying for both of us!"

"Yeah, I do enough for ten of us!" Her hands fly up to her breasts, shielding them. "I *know* I'll get it next . . . if not breast, colon." Her hands move down to cradle her abdomen. "And if not colon, lung." She keeps one hand curving around her abdomen and raises the other to fan her fingers out over her chest. "It makes me sick just to think of the possibilities!"

"Don't count on it. Maybe you don't have to get cancer at all . . . maybe I'm having it for both of us!"

Rolling her eyes, she exclaims, "I should be so lucky!"

"Maybe you will be."

The nurses' aide comes in to take my blood pressure and temperature. Gemma sits on the wide windowsill and peruses a magazine.

"Oh, your blood pressure is really low," the nurse says. I glance over at the readout: 80/37.

"But it's always low, and I promise you I'm OK."

"Do you feel faint when you get up?"

"No, I promise. I feel fine." Eager to go home, I reassure her. "I'm not faint, not light-headed, not dizzy."

**Hints to help you beat the odds . . .**
**knowing your own normal blood pressure . . .**

If you know your baseline blood pressure, you can help identify a deviation. What is very low for one person may be normal for another. Symptoms of low blood pressure include light-headedness and dizziness, especially when moving from supine to sitting position or from sitting to standing.

"OK." She hesitates. "But let me know if you start to feel weak or anything."

"I will." She packs up her equipment and starts for the next room.

Looking up, Gemma speaks slowly, emphasizing each *low*. "Your blood pressure has *always* been *low*: Your blood pressure's *low*, your temperature's *low*, your respirations are *slow*—don't they know that yet?" She sounds baffled. "They've been taking care of you nearly two weeks already!"

"They know in a way, but it still makes some of them nervous. I tell them I feel fine, don't worry, this is my normal baseline, but sometimes they call the resident down here (sometimes even in the middle of the night, poor thing), to 'assess' my condition!"

"Well, I wish I were your nurse!"

"There's nobody better!" I mean it. She is all I want in a nurse: knowledgeable, skilled, kind, and sensitive. "You're a natural."

"That's because I *love* bedside nursing!" she insists. "And despite all those efforts by our professors to derail us toward research and teaching! They just couldn't believe that we *like* taking care of people." Her voice rises in frustration. "That's why we went into nursing!"

We both laugh at the irony that has followed us since we first enrolled in nursing school: We wanted to be RNs so that we could be nurses, while our nursing professors were researchers who really didn't seem to like doing the things that nurses traditionally do. "Some of them didn't even know how to care for patients! We'd get on a ward and have to ask the 'real nurses,' the staff nurses, how to do things." We both laugh at the memory.

Gemma concludes, "And some of these RNs and LPNs here probably learned from nurses who didn't really know *how* to be nurses."

"Right. So we should be patient." I continue, "And besides, most of them have been superb. They have been amazingly kind. Actually, other than that struggle to get admitted in the first place, I have had wonderful care. This one is just nervous about making a mistake—and we both know that feeling!"

Suddenly Gemma sits up on the gurney and turns toward me. "Eliza, do you remember that guy with the colostomy?" She laughs and covers her face. "We were so *dumb*!"

I remember. We were in our third year of a baccalaureate program that emphasized theory and research over actual nursing skills. We knew theories and principles but felt woefully unprepared to actually care for a living patient. We were terrified of hurting somebody.

On this particular morning, we walked up the two flights of stairs to the surgical floor, eager to take this one more small step toward becoming full-fledged nurses.

Finding our patients' charts on the rack at the nursing station, we read through the medical histories, admitting notes, progress notes, lab reports, and orders for labs, medications, and care parameters.

Holding our heads high to suggest the professional confidence we were trying to cultivate, we tucked the charts under our arms and walked down the hall toward our patients' six-bed ward. Stepping through the doorway, trying not to betray our discomfort, we glanced quickly about the room, scanning the faces and surroundings for information.

Before we could identify our assigned patients, a man standing by the side of a bed gestured toward us, plaintively calling, "Nurse! Nurse! I need help! My colostomy . . . help!" He wore a wrinkled cotton hospital gown and gestured with a skinny arm.

Momentarily struck dumb, we froze in space and time. We knew nothing about colostomies to begin with, and since this man was not our assigned patient, neither of us read anything about them in preparation for our clinical day. Moreover, resounding in our heads was the admonition to give no patient care without prior approval from the instructor.

And lastly, we were immobilized by the deep fear of dealing with a part of the body that, under normal circumstances, is entirely hidden.

Like statues suddenly released by a touch in the child's game, we bolted for the door. Mortified by our ineptitude and desperate to escape, we turned and ran down the corridor, calling, "Nurse! Nurse! Somebody needs a nurse!"

"Oh, I can't believe we did that!" she grimaces at the memory. "We must have looked so goofy."

"What'd we think *we* looked like? Librarians?" Remembering our starched white pinafores over blue uniforms, our white stockings and polished white shoes, I recall our pride in wearing these clothes that identified us as nursing students.

Joining her laughter, I wince at the sharp pain in my belly, and Gemma rushes to splint my abdomen with a firm pillow. "Thanks, nurse!" Encircling the pillow with my arms and pressing hard, I can giggle without pulling at the edges of my wound. "Oh, this laughing feels good to me!" Turning to my side, I look at Gemma. "That's part of what's so great having you here: You *always* make me laugh!"

We are both quiet a moment before Gemma muses, "We never saw that guy again." Surprised at the sudden somber turn in her voice, I agree, "No, we didn't. I wonder what happened to him? I wonder if anyone helped him?"

"Of course someone helped him!" She becomes pensive again. "But . . . it wasn't us." Pausing again, she continues, "I still can't believe we didn't even try to comfort him."

"No . . . but we were young . . . and so very green," I stop myself, unable to justify our behavior. The shame returns once again to snake up my back and wrap around my throat. How could we have turned our backs on this man who was living with who could know what sadness? It was fear that suspended us in that space of inaction. Bald fear. And ignorance. Acutely aware of our inexperience in skills and techniques, we failed to recognize that simple kindness and compassion were also essential to patient care. A kind word, a gesture, a reassurance that we would get help for him. Memories of his humble appeal remind me of being in the ER only days ago, pleading for help from people who seemed to neither see nor hear me. Are those people the men of my dreams? Present, yet chillingly disconnected?

"This *is* kind of a karmic payback." I hope my smile reassures her that I am joking.

"No, this is just bum luck."

**Hints to help you beat the odds . . . avoiding self-blame . . .**

There is a growing trend in the United States to assign blame to the victim of a devastating disease, and the question may be bluntly asked, "Why did you need this disease?" or "What do you suppose this disease is trying to tell you?" Although there are lots of lessons to be learned from experiences with serious illness, I make a distinction between needing the illness to learn something and learning something because one has a certain illness.

"Yeah, I guess . . . the random arrow of chance."

In the pause of conversation, we can hear the echo of televisions in neighboring rooms, the murmur of staff members conferring in hallways, the soft squeak of rubber-soled shoes walking down the hall to answer a call light, the muffled slam of a refrigerator door closing, the purr of traffic seven stories below.

"So here we are together. Just like the old times." Sliding from her perch on the window ledge, Gemma corrects herself. "Well, not exactly."

"No," I admit. "Those old times now seem so innocent, so full of hope. Anything and everything seemed possible."

"And we had so much fun then." Gemma stretches out on the narrow gurney at the end of the bed. "Oh, this feels so good just to lie down." She props herself up on one elbow and adds, "But tonight my bedtime reading will be these booklets on colostomies!"

**Hints to help you beat the odds . . .**
**getting written information about your care . . .**

Written information about colostomies is available from hospitals, physicians, and nurses. If you have not been given booklets or informational sheets before your discharge, ask for them. Once away from staff support, you may need the reminder of the written word as you try to remember your instructions regarding colostomy care.

"That might really put you to sleep fast!"

She starts pouring through the pile of handouts and brochures, making notes and asking questions, such as "How does the gas escape from this thing anyway?" or "Where do we get all this stuff they say we need?"

**For your information . . .**
**heading home with ostomy supplies . . .**

Your ostomy nurse will send you home with enough equipment for the next couple of days and instruct you and your support person as to how to order and obtain ongoing supplies.

At the conclusion of my midnight blood pressure and temperature monitoring, we turn off the lights and settle down. Drifting off to sleep, reassured by the smooth rhythm of Gemma's breathing, I imagine home. I am aching to be held in the warmth of Charles's arms, yet I'm also kept at bay by his new cool distance. Hungering for the garden, for the feathery rustle of wind in the trees, for the soft thud of ripe fruit hitting the ground, for the glory of full-blown ivory and yellow dahlias on sturdy stems, and, most of all, for the splashing rhythm of the creek burbling down the hillside on its way to the sea.

**Hints to help you beat the odds . . .**
**an ally keeping watch . . .**

You may sleep better if an ally can sleep on a cot in your room. It can allow you to let go of your watchfulness and really relax.

Morning comes, and Charles and Andrew drive separately to the hospital. To carry the flowers and plants as well as Gemma and me, two cars will be needed for the trip back through the mountain roads. Charles stands in the hall while Andrew and Gemma listen to the nurses giving me instructions for going home.

Nurses have been coming in since early morning, saying good-bye, bringing small tokens of affection, and offering words of encouragement. While Gemma packs up flowers and clothing, Angie, my assigned nurse, helps me dress. The clothes she drops over my head seem familiar yet strange, and I recall how foreign even my own nightdresses seemed after days of wearing only the rough cotton hospital gowns. In this in-between place of being discharged but not yet home, I realize that the steady and

**Hints to help you beat the odds . . .**
**bringing an ally to hear discharge instructions . . .**

Hospital personnel will insist on some friend or family member taking you home from the hospital. You cannot go home alone. Make sure that that person comes up to your room and is a second pair of ears to hear the instructions you are given prior to discharge. Although some of it will be written down as well as spoken, it is recommended that another person be there not only to listen to your discharge orders but also to ask questions that you may be too overwhelmed to even think about.

predictable rhythm of these hospital days has offered a safety and security that is now hard to leave. Trying to reach home and shelter, am I heading for the flooding jetty of my dream? Were it not for Gemma's and Andrew's presence during this transition, I would be flooded with anxiety.

I ride with Andrew, and Charles takes Gemma. Although leaving the hospital room itself is difficult and even scary, once we are in the car headed for home, I feel excited. And going through the mountain curves, I am riding these roads without the spasms of pain that marked each mile of so many futile trips to the ER.

It feels odd traveling these same roads that we retraced so many times in the days leading up to my admission. Sensing a fundamental shift in the way I experience the world, I notice that the sky looks bluer, a marine backdrop to trails of cottony clouds stealing over the horizon. The leaves of olive trees flicker yellow in the sun and dusky gray in the shadow, the coastal air feels fresher and blows sweeter across my face.

My mother, Tashie, who has flown down from her home in the Oregon Cascades, greets me when I walk into the house after an absence of eleven days and well into the beginning steps of a precarious journey. "Oh, sweetheart, there you are!" She hurries to my side, hugging me carefully and kissing the top of my head. "Where do you want to sit?" she asks anxiously. "Or do you want to go right to bed?" Stooped over my belly, I smile, so glad to be home, glad to find her waiting. Ever the mother, she fusses to make me comfortable, pulling a chair next to me and dashing over with fluffy pillows, but I am hungry to go outside, to wander through the garden.

"I'm not ready to do either right now."

"Here, take this." She presses a pillow to my abdomen, and I hold it with both hands, like a baby in a low-slung front pack.

**Hints to help you beat the odds . . .
stabilizing your abdominal wound . . .**

When you move, cough, laugh, or sneeze, press a firm pillow to your abdomen, and hold it tight by grasping it with both hands and forearms. Splinting it in this way protects the healing wound from the jostling and tugging created by motion.

Shuffling through the dining room and out to the garden, I watch the stream tumbling through the watercress and over the weir toward the ocean. The burgundy leaves of the Japanese maple flutter in the light breeze, the deep yellow quinces glow in the sunlight, the sun-splashed patio beckons. A blue dragonfly with glints of silver on its wings darts under the green canvas umbrella. Doves, wavering on the power line, coo softly.

On home turf at last, I sense a familiarity, a safety, and a security at the same time that I feel myself to be a tenuous traveler happening onto a strange land. Everything looks different somehow. Even objects seem alive, laced with an energy that is palpable. The furniture inside, furniture I have lived with for decades, now seems changed: It watches me expectantly, inquisitive. This is my familiar and well-loved home, yet a curiously altered one as well.

"You shouldn't be out here! You're just home from the hospital!" Charles reaches for my hand. "I'll help you into bed."

*But I don't want to go to bed. I have been in bed for nearly two weeks. I want to be here.* I can feel a contest beginning. Where is Gemma? I need her to reassure him. She speaks with a confidence he can hear and with an affec-

**Hints to help you beat the odds . . . finding the balance . . .**

Finding the balance between taking care of your plundered body, and beginning to move away from the sick role, is always difficult, as your needs are in flux depending upon the relative strength and stamina of your body. It is sometimes only after overdoing it that we realize that we have done too much. In time, you will begin to get cues from your physical body and learn to anticipate how it will respond in certain situations. With that information, you will be better able to know, and communicate to your support people, what measure of independence versus dependence is appropriate.

tion that inspires hope. As objects seem altered, he does as well; I feel so far from him, so deeply disconnected. When all these people go home to their lives, leaving us alone, who will take care of me? Charles? But he is drifting so far away. Perhaps I can take care of myself. Perhaps not.

"I feel OK being up, truly." I begin walking toward the arched cedar bridge that spans the narrow creek. "Just give me a few minutes here . . . I've really really missed home . . . more than I knew." Leaning on the bridge rail, I can smell the red ginger blossoms on the stream bank.

"But you're weak, you've been so sick." Looking toward Charles, I hold my post on the bridge. Generally compliant, eager to acquiesce to avoid conflict, I astonish him with my intransigence. Frustrated, he sighs audibly, "Well, whatever you want to do." He shoves his hands into his pockets and walks toward the house. My guilt at upsetting him casts a dark shadow across the sun.

**Hints to help you beat the odds . . .**
**communicating clearly . . .**

Exchanges like this leave both people upset and create conflict that can stay unresolved. Make every attempt to be clear and direct about what specifically would be helpful to you.

Is he one of the dream men on the shore? One of the men whose inclinations were not clear? Will he help me, or on the other hand, will he harm me? No, there was something vaguely sinister about these men of my dreams. They could not echo Charles, who, despite his present fear and distance, I know to be gentle and kind. I think back through the decades, remembering when Gemma and I were in nursing school, and the oncology patient implored us to help with his colostomy. And I shudder at the memory of that primeval fear that hastened our flight from his pathetic supplications. Is it that same fear that keeps Charles so far away now?

Continuing to hold my belly, I carefully walk down the pebble pathway, passing lilac bushes, the persimmon tree laden with hard green knobs of fruit, and the pomegranate weighted with small, green spheres streaked with crimson. Crossing the stone bridge to the other side, I wind around past the limes and clementines, the dahlias and larkspur, and back to the dark brick patio. My thoughts return to the dream. Perhaps that cluster of fishermen symbolizes the chemo agents, the agents that can hurt as well as heal, kill as well as cure. And my struggle to reach the sanctuary—the struggle for life itself.

**For your information . . . a chemotherapy challenge . . .**

Chemotherapy travels via the vascular system, reaching and affecting cells throughout the entire body. A systemic drug, it attacks not only cancer cells that are threatening your life but also healthy cells that help you live. This makes the weighing of risks and balances difficult as well as essential: Will the potential benefit of this drug outweigh the potential harm?[1]

Stepping out of my dream, out of the quiet of the garden and into the house, I find myself amid a hub of activity. Gemma takes my elbow and starts guiding me to the bedroom. "I want to check out the colostomy and supplies before we actually need them . . . 'cause God forbid we should need them and not have them later when the world's asleep and the pharmacies are closed!" Direct and practical, her forthright approach to all that has to be dealt with makes me feel safe. Safe and loved without condition. Warmth creeps through me. She laughs and adds, "And I also want to go to the video store and get *My Cousin Vinnie* for you—it's really, really funny!"

"I'm ready for funny!" I agree. "Funny books, funny movies, funny stories. Humor heals. It has to! Funny feels so good!"

"OK, after this, I'll go to the video store. Right now, let's just change the bag while we don't need to, and we can practice, and then be ready and organized when we *really* need to!" She speaks enthusiastically, as if she were talking about something interesting, the details of glassblowing

**Hints to help you beat the odds . . .**
**the healing power of humor . . .**

The healing power of humor and laughter has been discussed by many scientists and philosophers, most notably Norman Cousins, editor of *Saturday Review* and author of *The Anatomy of an Illness as Perceived by the Patient*[2] and *The Healing Heart*.[3] He commented, "Laughter is a form of internal jogging. It moves your internal organs around. It enhances respirations. It is an igniter of great expectations."

perhaps. I dread dealing with this device in any way, yet know that there is nobody better to have here with me than Gemma. Smart, calm, practical, and kind, she will help me through this with a minimum loss of dignity and a maximum gain of acceptance. And throughout, her humor will ease me over the humiliation and awkwardness of adapting to catching my shit in a plastic bag hanging from my abdomen.

"So!" She pats the bulge over the left side of my abdomen. "How do we get this stuff off?"

"I don't remember." I try to recall the instructions I was given. "An ostomy nurse visited me in the hospital room a couple of times to explain how it all works, but I think I have information overload . . . too many new details to take in and remember."

"That's why you need someone with you to take notes," Gemma cautions.

"That's part of it," I try to explain, "but the other part is that everyone seems to think I know more than I know, just because I'm a nurse, 'in the business,' so to speak. But I'm not in *this* business. I know little more than the next person about cancer and colostomies!" With both hands, I clasp the warm bulge on my abdomen as I speak.

"That's always a problem. . . . It's like when we have patients in labor who are doctors or nurses, we assume they know what's going on, when maybe they don't." Gemma brings us back to the moment with her admonition, "You need to ask them to tell you whatever they would tell a librarian or an architect or a kindergarten teacher or anyone else not professionally connected to healthcare."

"I know. I began to once I realized it was happening, but. . . ." I am becoming frustrated not knowing what to do with this device but also trusting Gemma's skill and creativity. "Oh, it's so hard remembering what they *did* tell me!"

**Hints to help you beat the odds . . .**
**recording information and instructions . . .**

For hospital stays as well as clinic visits, take a pencil and paper or a tape recorder with you, as well as an ally who can be recording, either through tape or the written word, allowing you to focus on listening. If you have many and perhaps complex questions to discuss with your doctor, let the office know ahead of time so that they can plan accordingly.[4]

"Well, we can figure this out even so." She picks up the bag of colostomy supplies and pulls out a brochure. "Why don't you lie down on your nice, clean bed while I read the instructions." Supporting me carefully as I lean back on a pile of pillows, she then turns her attention to the brochure until I ask, "What do you think is happening with Charles? He's so . . . so not here. Not with me. Not with any of us."

"No, he sure isn't!" She laughs. "He's always with that wretched computer!" Her face grows pensive. "I think he's scared. And he doesn't know what to do."

"I'm scared! I'm scared about when everyone is gone and he and I are here alone, and I need him but he won't be here . . ." I correct myself. "I mean, he'll be here but he won't." *It would almost be easier not to have him here at all*, I think to myself, *to dispel the illusion that I have help and support.*

"You know, I'm sure he'll step up to the plate when he has to."

"What do you mean 'when he has to'?" I know she doesn't mean when I die, but I wonder.

"I mean, when you two are here alone—maybe all these people make him retreat, especially a doctor, a nurse, a mother. Poor guy. He's probably intimidated, and figures he doesn't know anything helpful."

"Maybe." I am not convinced.

"Well, think about it," she pursues, "here he is, a contractor, and here you are, a nurse, a midwife. And not only that, here is Andrew, a cardiologist; here am I, an oncology nurse; and then your mom, who's lived around medicine practically all her life. In that mix, Charles is undoubtedly convinced he has nothing to offer except to cooperate by staying out of the way!"

"You're right, that all makes sense," I realize, "and he's always been afraid to interject himself into a situation where he feels he can't, in his

**Suggestions for allies . . .**
**each person can help in unique ways . . .**

The person you love who has cancer is going to need support in a range of areas. Medical expertise may be crucial at one point, playing Scrabble may be the perfect support another time, bringing a platter of peeled fruit may be exactly what is needed yet another time. Each of you brings your own special gifts and talents that can catalyze healing.

words, 'add something.'" I wonder: *Is he feeling excluded? Is he glad to be on the periphery of these mysteries? Does he feel the distance between us? Does that distance make him feel safe? Or sad?*

**Hints to help you beat the odds . . .**
**empathy for a partner . . .**

Difficult as it is, try to imagine what your partner's experience may be during this time and leave openings for discussions. So much of the misunderstandings happen due to what *is not* said rather than what *is* said. Communicating clearly can help derail misunderstandings.

Beginning to appreciate his experience, so vastly different from mine yet at the same time so intimately entwined with my own, I return to the immediate concern. "But I wish I could feel more confident that he'll reconnect with me when we're alone together."

"Tashie tells me that there are lots of people who want to help—let them! Let them come stay with you."

Suddenly I was tired of fretting about it. "It'll work out, I guess. Mostly I just want my husband back."

"I know. He'll come back—he's just scared shitless right now!" Clasping her hand to her mouth, she laughs, "I really didn't intend that play on words . . . but, I guess in a way that's what this is all about: shit."

Gemma, my Gemma: never one to avoid the obvious.

"So speaking of shit, let's get back to it." She picks up the handouts from the Ostomy Association. I watch her read against the backdrop of sounds of supper being prepared and the low murmur of voices in other rooms.

Lulled into a daze by the safety of being cared for, by Gemma's ample warmth sitting next to me on the bed, sheltering me, my dream returns, the sense of no exit, of there being danger in every direction. I must summon from within the deepest parts of me the courage and strength to stay on that precarious trail, to go ahead even when injury and annihilation threaten. Preparing me for what is to come, the dream perhaps warns of the temptation to succumb rather than face the seemingly overwhelming odds staring me in the face. I must remember this later, when the devastation of the chemo might seduce me into abandoning the struggle to survive.

# *Chapter 5*
# Stella the Stoma

## DREAMING MIRACLES

### *September 1996*

*Miniature St. Nicholases are tumbling from the open end of my colostomy bag. Wearing on their heads high bishop's miters trimmed with gold piping, they are robed in long, crimson gowns with finely pleated edges. The thick, gold threads that embellish the pleats and folds shimmer in the sunlight. In their right hands, they carry high staffs that curl at the top like shepherd's crooks.*

*Their cheeks are rosy like polished Macoun apples. When they smile, the deep lapis of their eyes sparkle with mirth, and their tawny skin crinkles into a web of tiny laugh lines. Feeling an intense joy, I smile back. Their lightheartedness, their cheerful glow, is palpable, their presence a miracle. There is no shit at all, just these jolly St. Nicks. Following the brilliant torrent of St. Nicks, a flutter of delicate white creatures floats down from the bag. Tiny, snowy angels with soft feathery wings, generous folds of white diaphanous gowns swirl about them as they fall. As the saint's faces are fully extroverted, ebullient and friendly, these angels are quiet, turned into themselves, and contemplative.*

In the languid days of late summer, toward the end of my second cycle of chemotherapy, I have my first major colostomy accident. Nudged out of the wondrous yet perplexing dream of Saint Nicholases and snowy white angels tumbling from the pouch, I am dismayed by a strong odor that at first seems to be part of another dream but that quickly declares itself a physical reality. Still half asleep, I reach to touch my abdomen where the flange seals in the waste. In the habit of frequently checking this attachment, I am jolted further out of my dreamy state by the warm, muddy sensation that meets my groping fingertips. I get a sudden flash of memory: the bubbling squishy silt of the Calistoga mud baths. I remember the giddy promise that floating in a sea of volcanic ash and hot spring water will cleanse impurities and detoxify and soothe the system. What irony, that the mud of purification and the muck of human waste feels, and even looks, the same!

"Charles! Charles!" I whisper loudly, astonished that he is not also awakened by the stench that fills the room.

"What is it? Are you OK?" He reaches over to turn on the lamp by the bed.

"I'm OK, but look at this! Don't you smell it?" I lift up the sheet covering us to reveal the plastic bag that has slid to the side, exposing the naked stoma, the deep-red, peonylike opening, spilling out rivulets of feces. Mortified, I close my eyes.

"It's only poop! All it takes is some soap and water and an open window."

"But it's so disgusting! And it's all over the sheets, too!"

"They'll wash!" he cheerfully reminds me. "As I said, all it takes is some soap and water."

By this time he has gotten up and is gingerly removing the soiled top sheet. He cleans off my abdomen with a towel, then helps me into the shower. I never imagined that running water could ever feel so extraordinarily soothing, cleansing, and purifying. Ignoring the drought, I linger under the low-flow showerhead, basking in the warmth and comfort of feeling clean again.

Charles brings a fresh towel and helps pat me dry. Walking over to the bed, I find that the sheets are clean, the room is aired, and all the supplies are laid out for a new flange and bag. I feel so lucky: Here while I was relaxing in the shower, Charles was cleaning up Stella's mess.

He sits next to me as I lay on the bed, reassuring me that we have survived this crisis just fine and chuckling affectionately at my humiliation

**Hints to help you beat the odds . . . being prepared . . .**

Keep everything you need to change your colostomy together in a bag or in one place. That way, you won't be halfway through and realize that something vital is missing.

and alarm. "After all," he repeats, "it's just a little shit—and let's thank the gods for detergent!"

"Amen!" I agree.

During the weeks following my return home, once we are managing on our own, we learn to deal with the colostomy, developing a routine that we now fold smoothly into our days.

As detached as Charles had become during my hospitalization and the first few days at home, he is now devoted and attentive. Immensely relieved that he is once again engaged, I am feeling safe now in his care. Somehow, that transition has been occurring without my noticing it: The distance between us has quietly closed.

I remember the first night at home, when we lay side by side on our queen-sized bed, not touching. He lay staring at the ceiling, arms rigid at his sides, a tin soldier toppled over on its back, lying humbly on the nursery floor. I was afraid to make the first move, afraid he was repelled by my disease and my changed body. It seemed like hours later that I asked timidly, "Will you hold me?"

He turned carefully toward me from his position of staring at the ceiling and asked wonderingly, "I won't hurt you?"

"No, you won't hurt me." I tried to reassure him. "I need you."

He wrapped his hands gently around me, and amid a stifled sob I heard, "Thank you. I need you, too."

**Suggestions for allies . . .**
**a range of responses to changes in body image . . .**

A dramatic change to one's body image can be alarming, as well as a difficult adjustment. One concern is that the change, such as a colostomy, will repel the very people most needed. Try to be sensitive to what your friend or family member is saying, what the body language might be trying to convey, and let her or him know that you are open to listening, to talking, or just to physically holding, all of which convey messages of acceptance.

Grateful that I took the risk of asking that night, I am astonished all over again that I had so misread his distance and reserve. Now I sleep in the safety and comfort of his arms every night, and an intimate tenderness has replaced the reticence and withdrawal that so unnerved me.

Aware of the hazards, real and imagined, of the colostomy, I worry that the little plastic bag might leak, that the seal over the stoma might slip, that escaping gas will invite unwelcome attention. Like dreams of being naked in public, I even worry that one day, forgetting to attach a new bag after removing the old one, I might remember my vulnerability only after an accident occurs, when sitting in the doctor's waiting room, or on the highway snaking through the mountains. Should I have an accident while away from home, I keep in the car a navy nylon zipper bag containing all the apparatus needed for an entire replacement: plastic pouch, adhesive disk, clamp, gas filter, adhesive removal swabs, stoma adhesive powder, and aloe-soaked diaper wipes.

**Hints to help you beat the odds . . . emptying the bag . . .**

Emptying the bag is done on an as-needed basis. If your bag has an opening at the bottom, find a camp stool or something similar, and place it in front of the toilet, just touching the edge of the bowl. Sit down facing the toilet, lean slightly forward, and allow the bag to drop into the bowl. Reach down and unclip the fastener at the bottom of the bag, allowing the contents to flow into the toilet. First with toilet paper, and finally with a moist soft cloth, wipe clean the edges of the opening, and refasten securely.[1]

I am not sure who first starts using the name Stella: "Stella the Stoma." This appellation provides welcome comic relief and a linguistic conceit for the exchange of intimate information. In mixed company, I can ask for help with Stella, Charles can suggest that Stella might need some attention, and Luke can inquire after Stella's well-being. And we can all express frustration with the gaseous eruptions that punctuate conversations with sputters and sighs, recalling to mind the low whistle of air escaping a collapsing balloon.

Speaking of Stella as a character to be respected, cared for, and cajoled when necessary allows me to accept the entire ordeal as a mere inconvenience. When Luke visits, he always inquires after Stella's welfare

> **Hints to help you beat the odds . . .**
> **coping with a colostomy . . .**
>
> If you are one of those persons who will do *anything* to avoid a colostomy, even *die*, please reconsider. With humor, determination, and the support of family and friends, one can adjust to the most outrageous of changes.

and jokes about her unpredictable temperament. When rumbles and wheezes jet out the release valve, he turns toward me, exclaiming, "Good job, Stella!" or "Right on, baby!" with a raised fist of triumph saluting our faithful friend.

Other times he imitates Tennessee Williams's Stanley Kowalski in *A Streetcar Named Desire* and calls through the house in a booming voice: "Stella!" and then repeats, extending both syllables as did the character in the Broadway play, "Stella!" And when he leaves, whether headed for the farmers' market or the airport, he hugs and kisses me, and then pats my belly with a "Ciao, Stella!" lingering on each syllable.

When Luke is not around, friends take responsibility for Stella's occasional outbursts. When she rumbles from beneath the folds of my linen jumper, someone invariably steps forward pleading, "Oh, excuse me, excuse me!" at the same time looking around at whomever might be within earshot, and then muttering, "I am so sorry," while bowing his or her head in apology.

In the spirit of the necromancers in Bertolucci's *Little Buddha*, Luke considers Stella an honored presence and an important prophet of what's to come.

"And how is Stella today?" he asks as I walk into the kitchen one morning.

"She's OK, I guess," I reply guardedly.

"OK?!" Six-foot-three, he stretches taller and repeats in disbelief, "*OK?* Is OK enough for our Stella?" Leaning against the tile counter, he points his finger into the air, striking the pose of Inquisitor. Adopting an Indo-British accent, he continues, "You must remember the seers who analyzed the contents of the little emperor's potty every morning. Stella deserves no less!"

He pantomimes removing the lid from an imaginary potty on the floor and leans down to inhale deeply. Exhaling "Ah," he stands up, still holding the illusory lid. Giggling, I wince at the pain rippling through my still-tender belly. Charles helps me press a firm pillow tightly against my abdomen. "As they foretold the destiny of the small king, Stella will decree your fortunes!" Bowing low, he asks, "Yes?" and immediately answers himself, "Yes."

He stands up in front of me, inclines his head to one side, and inquires, "So, what were the characteristics of Stella's morning's stool, if I may ask?"

"Oh, you don't want to know!" Pushing affectionately against his shoulder, I wave my hand to dismiss his query.

"But I do! This is very important." Taking imaginary pen and paper in hand, the investigator persists. "Now: consistency, size . . ."

"Enough, enough!" Still laughing, I interrupt his list of questions. "Stella's fine, her poop was fine, the kingdom is at peace, and she's tired now." And after the facetious disclosure of zany information regarding Stella's output, the day begins in earnest.

Luke, who has spent hours in the medical school library researching the best diets for people with cancer, specifically colon cancer, starts out with Charles at the farmers' market, collecting heirloom tomatoes, broccoli buds, small Chinese cabbages, melons, kale, red onions, spring leeks (yes, even in autumn), and heads of garlic.

**For your information . . . research into diet and cancer . . .**

A study by the American Institute of Cancer Research reports that "over time, the implementation of one recommendation—consumption of 400 grams/day or more of a variety of vegetables and fruits—could, by itself, decrease overall cancer incidence by at least 20 percent. The evidence is convincing or probable that diets high in vegetables and/or fruits protect against cancers of the mouth and pharynx, esophagus, lung, stomach, colon and rectum, larynx, pancreas, breast, and bladder."[2]

Returning with bags and baskets bulging with the autumn harvest, they pour out their loot onto the kitchen counters, and Luke begins directing the food preparations. Charles is an eager apprentice, perhaps relieved to have a specific physical role in helping maintain my nutrition during the siege of chemo.

Occasionally I help, but more often I stay away, comforted by the low sounds of their conversation and camaraderie as they work. "Charles," I hear Luke explaining, "mince the garlic with *this* knife—don't use that newfangled contraption!" With the two of them in command, I can let go of wondering and doze peacefully on the wooden chaise under the maple tree, their voices drifting through the open kitchen window.

**Suggestions for an allies . . . how friends can help . . .**

Organize a circle of friends to take turns preparing small amounts of various healthy foods that can be available throughout the day, requiring little or no preparation.

In the mail comes a long letter from Vanessa's father, George, who has triumphed over both lung cancer and colon cancer. He also has a colostomy, and his gently reassuring letter is comforting as well as informative. He describes various strategies for making colostomy care more efficient and less traumatic. He sends small flannel squares, which, in his experience, work better than the disposable "wipes" usually recommended by the ostomy information booklets. He writes, "Instead of sitting on the toilet for colostomy care, I use a canvas sling camp stool set in front of it, allowing much more room in which to work." He continues, "I have been able to go anywhere I want. When I travel, I just pack my supplies and my foldable camp stool in my bag, and take off." Always impressed by George's dignity and grace, until now I didn't know that he had had a colostomy for over a decade.

Among the many cards and letters arriving daily, one is a form letter directing me to report to the GI service at 10:40 AM on August 7 for a flexible sigmoidoscopy. This is a full five weeks after the emergency

**For your information . . .**
**disclosing the secret of colon cancer . . .**

You may find that once you are diagnosed with colon cancer, friends may come forward to disclose their similar diagnoses. They can be sources of support for you, and they can also benefit from being able to help someone (you) in similar circumstances. Many cancer survivors report getting immense satisfaction from helping others with similar diagnoses.

surgery for a bowel obstruction. An impersonal command, it stands in stark contrast to the warmth and compassion of the doctors who are now shepherding me through this disease and its treatments. Dumbstruck, I set it aside, shuddering to contemplate my fate had Andrew not intervened that desperate night.

Day after day, our mornings start with a cleansing ritual that takes nearly an hour.

**Hints to help you beat the odds . . . changing the bag . . .**

Before you start to change the bag, assemble all the supplies and equipment you might need, such as the new bag, the new flange, the stoma paste, the pink tape, a charcoal filter, a plastic bag in which to dispose of the discarded materials, warm and moist cloths, a towel, and a washcloth.

Unfolding the turquoise-and-blue-striped camp stool, once a cradle that supported one end of the white Kevlar kayak, Charles places it in front of the toilet. I pull my yellow flannel nightdress off over my head and, facing the toilet, sit down on the faded canvas sling, straddling the bowl and leaning forward to allow the bag to hang freely from my abdomen. Charles fills a plastic liter bottle with warm water and stands behind me, waiting. Slipping the white plastic "barrette" off the end of the bag, and after allowing gravity to drain the first bits of stool into the toilet, I press the ends of the translucent bag between my fingers, working more stool down until it drops into the porcelain bowl. Lifting up the open end of the pouch and holding the edges between my thumbs and forefingers, I signal Charles to begin pouring water into the bag. "Stop now," I say as the bag fills. Holding the ends tightly together, I swish the water about to loosen the stool clinging to the sides of the pouch. Then flipping the opening to point down into the toilet, I release the edges. With gurgles and splashes, the bag empties.

We repeat that routine of filling the bag, swishing it about, and emptying it into the toilet two more times before Charles gives the bottle a final rinse and places it under the sink until next time. Carefully holding the edges of the bag, I wipe them with one of George's moistened flannel squares, dry them carefully, and swab them with witch hazel–soaked gauze sponges. Charles washes the white plastic barrette and hands it to me. Rolling the open edges around the single plastic rod, I clasp the companion rod to it, tightly clamping the edges together. Reaching for a small towel to wipe the entire bag dry, at the same time I check the seal of the adhesive disk for signs of leakage.

**Hints to help you beat the odds . . .**
**cleaning the colostomy bag . . .**

To wash the inside of the bag after emptying it, use a plastic bottle filled with warm water, pour into the bag, swish it around while you hold the opening closed with your fingertips, and then release. Be aware that frequent rinsing can loosen the bond of the flange to the abdominal skin. If it seems that the application is not sticking as it should, it may be that you need to reduce the frequency with which you rinse the bag.

Charles helps me up, and I stand in front of the sink to give myself a sponge bath. Tomorrow I will be changing the bag, the flange, the entire contraption, and I look forward to the long, warm shower I will take between removing the old equipment and attaching the new disk and bag. Too frequent showers risk breaking the seal of the disk that secures the pouch to the skin of my abdomen. Early on, that attachment had broken repeatedly until Anne, my nurse practitioner friend, suggested reinforcing the edges with *pink tape*. When I asked later her why it's called pink tape, she replied simply, "Because it's pink!" That humble product prevented many an embarrassing leak.

In the mirror, I study a face transformed by the pillaging of chemotherapy. The woman staring back at me has sallow skin pulled tightly over angular bones; light-gray shadows sweep small arcs under pale-blue

**Hints to help you beat the odds . . .**
**developing a routine . . .**

Figuring out a routine, not just in caring for the colostomy, but also for scheduling and remembering things such as taking medications, applying sunblock, taking a daily walk, drinking plenty of water, and eating even when you may not be hungry, can help you manage your needs efficiently and smoothly.

eyes. Sparse clumps of dull hair jut out in short spikes. A few stubby eyelashes and just three or four odd hairs mark the eyebrows. It occurs to me that I resemble the mannequins that languish in the display windows at Macy's. I wash my hands thoroughly but carefully: The skin is thin and friable and feels tender to the touch. Filling the sink with warm water, I toss in a sea sponge the size of a mature cabbage. The rough surface softens miraculously in the warm water; so long ago, I used just such a sponge to wash my babies' bottoms.

Squirting on some pale-green body wash, I carefully drag the dripping sponge across my skin. Charles washes my back in slow, smooth strokes. Dunking the sponge in clean water and pressing it between my palms, I wipe off traces of soap. Watching the soapy water spiral down the drain, I marvel at the tiny hairs sticking to the sides of the sink. Reminders of my tenuous hold to this physical life, these wispy hairs are also scattered about the shower drain, the pillowcases, the towels, and the sundry hats and scarves.

My head is getting that moth-eaten look so common to women going through chemo. The few thin strands of hair lie flat, scattered about in meager clumps like islands dotting my pale scalp. I look forward to assuming the quiet elegance of the absolutely bald.

As I wipe a damp cloth over my head, the few little hairs bend over briefly, then abruptly flip back up, powered by cowlicks that even the ravages of chemo cannot subdue. I pat hydrating cream on my face, my arms, my neck—wherever I can reach. It vanishes. I slather a coat of sunblock 30 SPF onto my face and arms. It also disappears. I taste the thirst in my body as a living beast longing for the next drink. Finally, I twist the top off a small plastic tube and smooth moisturizing cream onto my face.

**For your information . . .**
**some common side effects of chemotherapy . . .**

The skin and associated tissues are commonly affected by chemotherapy, as these cells divide rapidly, and become collateral damage—unintended targets of the drug. Side effects include hair loss or thinning, sensitivity to sunlight, skin discoloration, and nail changes.

Hair can become brittle and break off, or it can fall out of the follicle itself. Hair loss generally starts about two weeks after the initiation of chemotherapy and grows back, sometimes with a different color and texture, three to five months after the completion of chemotherapy.[3]

I remember the mouth sores of the last cycle, when brushing my teeth was impossibly painful. The nurse suggested wiping the insides of my cheeks, tongue, and gums with wet gauze sponges, but I wasn't able to get my mouth open far enough. Now, during this lull signaled by the partial recovery of tender tissues, I relish the feeling of the soft bristles sweeping over my gums. As chemo progresses, my pleasures become simpler and simpler, until finally reduced to the elementary.

I turn to the clothes laid out on the blue-tile counter. Leaning against the wall for balance, I step into cotton underpants and carefully bring the elastic band to rest below the disk that holds the colostomy pouch. Next comes the bra, gaping pitifully around wasted breasts that no longer fill the cups. Charles drops the blue-and-white cotton jumper over the white

**Hints to help you beat the odds . . .
mouth care guidelines . . .**

Because the ramifications of mouth sores are serious, and because once established they are troublesome to address, it is important to monitor the state of your mouth and try to prevent their occurrence.

First, maintain meticulous hygiene, keeping the tissues clean and moist. Search out a very soft toothbrush, or if a soft enough one is not to be found, use a sponge swab. Brush or swab very gently, taking care not to damage the tissues. Flossing at this time is probably to be avoided, especially if it hurts or causes bleeding of the gums.

Avoid using commercial mouthwashes, and instead use a salt solution, which can in itself be preventive.

If you start to feel tender spots in your mouth, even if there are not yet any visible ulcers or more subtle changes such as red patches or pimples, take the following precautions: Maintain your fluid intake throughout the day. Because swallowing can become uncomfortable, hydration can be neglected or avoided. Avoid alcohol, as it can be an irritant to the tissues. Hopefully, you're not smoking cigarettes at all, but if you are, stop! Avoid acidic foods such as citrus fruits and tomatoes, as they will further aggravate your condition. Bland foods with minimal spices will be least likely to irritate.[4]

**Hints to help you beat the odds . . . feeling cold . . .**

Feeling cold is not a side effect that I have noticed mentioned in the cancer literature, although it is not an uncommon response to stress. If you also are experiencing cold and chills, dress accordingly, and keep your head under wraps to conserve heat.

turtleneck. It is late September in California and warm, in the high seventies, yet I am chilled.

Fortunately, the styles this summer include rather shapeless dresses that hang loosely from the shoulders. I order a cotton shift the color of buttercups from a catalogue, and Sophie and Vanessa send loose, elastic-waist pants and tent-shaped dresses that provide good camouflage for the contraption that hangs from my belly.

**Suggestions for allies . . . making colostomy bag covers . . .**

A beautiful or whimsical washable cover for the colostomy bag can be a fun present and useful for transforming a mechanical appliance into a lingerie fashion item. Measure the dimensions of the colostomy bag, and then buy appropriate yardage to cover both sides. Sew in snaps for easy application and removal.

Through Stella, I have direct access to the mysteries within: through that scarlet rose nestled on my abdomen, I am privy to the secretive workings of the gut. On the one hand, I perceive the colostomy as a grotesque violation of the most basic laws of nature, yet on the other, Stella becomes my friend and comrade. We develop a rhythm of coexistence that neutralizes the horror that the word *colostomy* might otherwise elicit.

I try to feel pleased when doctors speak to me about the plan to reverse the colostomy and reattach the bowels, but secretly I am scared: scared of more surgery, scared my bowels might forget how to work on their own, scared of losing Stella. Dr. Narayan, one of my surgeons, brings it up when I see him for follow-up care. Sitting on the edge of the exam table, my legs swinging in space, I listen as he explains the plan.

"A month or so after the chemo is finished, we'll take you to surgery again and take down the colostomy . . . reattach the ends of the bowel, and you'll be right back to normal."

**For your information . . .**
**colostomy "take-down"(reanastamosis) . . .**

A "colostomy take-down" describes the surgery to remove a temporary colostomy and reattach the healthy ends of the bowel so that elimination can return to normal. The stoma is sewn shut and in time becomes a pale-pink scar.

He smiles, waiting for questions, and I venture, "You know, I've gotten used to this thing . . . I call her Stella, Stella the Stoma."

**Hints to help you beat the odds . . .**
**getting help with your colostomy . . .**

Recognize that a colostomy can save your life, not wreck it!

Call on your local ostomy association for help. It can be wonderfully supportive and informative, helping you over hurdles that, in the dark of confusion, may seem impossible to overcome.

Try different appliances until you find the one that works best for you.

Gradually make ever-widening forays out into your pre-colostomy world, resuming the activities you love.

"But I can't imagine you've gotten so used to her that you want to keep her!" His laughter suggests that he appreciates the humor of my approach to what might be a dreadful and isolating experience.

**Hints to help you beat the odds . . .**
**unthinkable adjustments are possible!**

If you are in the position of having a permanent colostomy, recognize that in time you will make the necessary adjustments, and life will assume a normal rhythm despite this major change to your anatomy and physiology.

"No," I reassure him. "I guess I'm lucky that this isn't forever for me . . . but still . . . I never thought I would feel this way." I hesitate, looking for the right words. "But if my situation were to change, and for some reason I couldn't have the reversal, I could be OK with that, too."

I am embarrassed to describe my fears about the surgery, losing Stella and trying to find normalcy again. Seeming to read my mind, he surprises me by saying, "You know, all that plumbing's going to work just fine, just the way it did before you got sick. There may be a little adjustment period, but you'll do well . . . I know you will."

I love the way he trusts my body, the way he has faith that I will be OK. I know I may not be, and he certainly knows, but he never reminds me of possibilities I don't care to contemplate. Whatever the precarious nature of my situation, I *don't* necessarily want to hear the truth. I want to hold on to hope, and this gentle man helps me maintain a firm grasp.

**Suggestions for hospital staff . . .**
**being honest without taking away hope . . .**

Take your cues from the patient. In this age of increased disclosure, it is sometimes thought that the naked truth is always the best route. It is possible to tell the truth, or at least part of it, and still convey a message of hope and even optimism.

Pondering my fear of losing Stella, I remember the dream, the dream in which angels and saints are falling from the colostomy bag. That dream must be telling me that nuggets of gold are falling from that bag, as well as chunks of waste.

**For your information . . . dangerous opportunity . . .**

The Chinese ideogram for "crisis" is "dangerous opportunity." It may be hard to see opportunities arising from the crisis of catastrophic disease, but they can and often do: opportunities for growth, for reshuffling priorities, and for a deeper understanding of yourself and your values. Given these new insights, you may begin to look at your life and your world through clearer lenses and choose to make changes you might otherwise not have even contemplated.

The gold? I know that this device is a life-saving measure. Had there been an alternative, other than death, my surgeons would surely have opted for a procedure less radical. Given that Stella is contributing to the preservation of my life, isn't that enough?

Perhaps, but Stella affects me positively in other, more subtle ways. After years of living a few feet from my body, uninterested and unconcerned with its welfare, my mental and emotional life disconnected from my physical body, I suddenly have to confront a colossal failure of its immune system and a massive breakdown in its functioning. The disease and all its sequelae, including Stella, impose on me a startling awareness of this body that contains my physical life, forcing me to befriend its most intimate mechanisms. It is Stella's presence that is becoming a major catalyst in my struggle to heal this split between body and mind.

# *Chapter 6*

# Fires of Transformation

## DREAMING INFERNO

### *September 1996*

*My aching wrists are chained to metal rings high on the wall of a shadowy stone dungeon. Suspended well above the damp clay floor, I can neither sit nor lie down. A soiled, shapeless dress hangs from my shoulders. My punishment seems to be related to a basket full of herbs that I had been carrying.*

*I am suddenly transported from the dungeon to stand on an enormous pile of twigs and boughs, my calves and thighs bound to a thick, wooden pole at my back. Flames are leaping into the air, singeing the ragged hem of my dress and gliding over the skin of my legs, arms, and face, scorching the soles of my feet. After the torture in the cold, bleak dungeon, this blaze seems a peculiar relief. As the underground crypt thrust darkness into me, now I am filled with sky.*

*A small child, perhaps three or four years old, approaches and reaches up to place a basket of herbs in my hands. I feel strengthened by this tender gesture and also by the sight and aroma of the herbs. Taking the basket in both hands, I hold it above my head, an offering to the gods. The fire is consuming me, burnishing my flesh, transmuting my body. I am exhausted but cannot leave. In the stillness of the dying embers, my ashes float to the ground.*

Struggling for release from my dream, I pull myself off the pile of sizzling wood, opening my eyes to secure an anchor that will hold me to the coming day. I feel the flames sweeping over me: My eyes are on fire, my face blazing. The intense heat reminds me of Dante walking through the fire at the top of the Mountain of Purgatory; he recounts that, had there been a vat of molten glass at hand, he would have jumped into it to cool himself. Reaching up, I feel the heat radiating from my cheeks through my palm. With the ghost of my ancestor, Mary Clement, standing beside me, I feel the scorching heat of the flaming pyre and remember my grandfather's sonorous voice as he read aloud an account of the trial.

"Abigail Scattergood," he announced, "reports seeing Mary Clement flying over the town on a broomstick." Another villager reported seeing the hapless Mary in the forest behind the village, signing her name in blood in Lucifer's book.

For these sins and others, she is sentenced to burn at the stake. She might have been a healer. A midwife perhaps? A gentleman farmer from the Plymouth Plantation, undoubtedly a relative, stepped forward to appeal her case. A successful appeal would cleanse the besmirched family name. In an unusual deviation from the expected denial, the judge ruled in her favor. She was released from her prison cell, the sentence of death by burning commuted. *Will my sentence be likewise commuted?* I wonder.

I can feel the silence of the house leaning into the background babble of the creek outside the window. Next to me, Charles sleeps, the familiar deep sighs of his breaths reassuring. It is Sunday. I have completed my second cycle of chemotherapy. My legs are propped up on the wedge that my aunt Pat has made from a trapezoid-shaped chunk of foam covered with pink-striped flannel, a remnant of Christmas nightdresses she made years ago for her girls. The angle of the wedge reduces the pressure on the surgical wound that splices my abdomen and pelvis.

**Suggestions for allies . . .**
**relieving pressure on the surgical wound . . .**

If you don't have a wedge cushion, find someone in the circle of support who can make a similar firm pillow. It can be used to elevate the legs and also the head for activities such as reading, playing Scrabble, and eating. Either position will relieve pressure on the surgical wound.

I hear the hushed voices of three-and-a-half-year-old Nico and twenty-month-old Rose playing with the Brio train set in the next room.

"Put it here!" Rose insists.

"But I want to put a bridge there," Nico explains.

"OK!" Rose agrees cheerfully.

Kitchen sounds, of dishes being put away and cupboards being opened and shut, tell me that Rebecca, Andrew's wife, is already up and tending to breakfast. Early risers, the children may already have eaten.

**Hints to help you beat the odds . . .**
**stating clearly what helps and what doesn't . . .**

The household sounds of activity that I found comforting and nourishing you may find irritating and intrusive. Decide what helps and what hinders your healing, and tell those around you so that they can respond accordingly. Remember, they can't read your mind!

Charles loops his arm across me. "Good morning." He raises himself up on an elbow and studies my face. "Jeez, what's happened overnight? You look so sunburned!"

"I feel sunburned!"

"It must be from the chemo . . . you've barely been in the sun at all. Does it hurt?"

**Hints to help you beat the odds . . . protecting your skin . . .**

When outside, even if briefly, apply sunblock of at least 30 SPF, wear sunglasses, and wear long sleeves and a wide-brimmed hat. A fleeting exposure to sunlight can initiate a significant burn when one is on certain chemotherapeutic drugs, and eyes may become highly sensitive to sunlight.

"A lot . . . as if I'm on fire." My speech is muddled, as if I am talking with a mouth full of marbles. Patches of skin have sloughed off from the insides of my cheeks and palate, which are blistered and raw.

"It really bothers me to see what this chemo is doing to your body."

Charles peers at me. "Hopefully it is as hard on those cancer cells as it is on the rest of you."

"It has to be hammering them, too!"

"God, I hope so." He shakes his head wearily. "I can't imagine what my life would be like without you."

Looking at his forlorn face, I am tempted to reassure him, despite the grim prognosis we have both heard. There is something so childlike about him now, a vulnerability I can't protect. My white count is worrisomely low from the chemo depressing the functioning of my bone marrow. Last week when the nurse told us that I couldn't get chemo until the bone marrow recovered to a safe zone, I couldn't help crying. Charles patted me and cooed reassurances, yet he seemed himself to be stricken with fear.

**Suggestions for allies . . . getting support for you . . .**

When one is stricken with a devastating disease, attention is focused on that person, with little left over for those intimately connected, who will invariably be suffering as well. You also need support and a place in which to discuss your own fears and anxieties. Many cancer centers have support groups for friends and family of those with cancer.

It is hard to picture Charles suddenly alone and figuring out life as a widower. The plans for holidays, the nurturing of relationships with family and friends, the travel, the theater, the music—the day-to-day details that determine the shape of our lives, enriching and broadening our perspectives, are my responsibilities. And despite his ready participation, I cannot imagine him taking the initiative to make these things happen in my absence. Reaching for his hand, I can't think of anything helpful to say except, "I love you."

He takes my hand gently in both of his and continues, "You know, it's you that makes my life interesting and fun. The trips you plan, the stuff that you make happen in our lives."

"I'm doing everything I can to beat this thing, but . . . if this disease *does* overtake me, lots of people who love you and love me will be here to help you through it." I can see the glistening of tears on his cheeks. As has occurred to me many times these last weeks, I think that *watching* me live through this disease is harder than *being* me experiencing it. "I'm going to do everything I can to get well—I am *dying* to live!" We both laugh at the absurdity of the linguistic play.

Recalling my ancestor ghost, I remind him, "And remember Mary Clement—she was scheduled to die by burning, and she *didn't*—she was exonerated!" I can hear a certain triumph in the lift of my scratchy voice. "And I'll be exonerated, just as she was!"

"That's right." Charles turns to me, wiping his eyes with the back of his hand. "Against all odds, she survived. Well, her DNA continues to live in you, so . . ."

"So, I'll be OK."

"Um-hmm. You will." He raises my hand to his lips and kisses it lightly.

As he rolls out of bed and starts for the shower, I am already pondering the fire that consigns me to ashes in the dream and my ghost ancestor who escapes her sentence to burn at the stake. Remembering the heat of the dream pyre, I imagine freeing myself from the ties that bind me to the post. Thick ropes. But now . . . are there other kinds of ties that bind? What are they? I must figure out the requirements for exoneration.

**Hints to help you beat the odds . . .**
**taking the inward journey . . .**

The diagnosis of cancer, or a similarly devastating disease, can lead you on an inward journey: to examine the life you are living, the priorities you have set, and the changes you might consider. Exploring these areas may be part of your work toward healing.

Rebecca passes by the open door. "Good morning, Nana! How was your night?" She steps into the room, a tall glass of iced tea in her hand. "Oh! Does your face feel hot?"

"Really hot! On fire!" I nod, wincing at the burn, remembering the dream blaze. "And my mouth . . . inside . . ."

"It sounds as if the mouth sores are worse today. And this burn on top of that!" Her hand feels cool on my face. "Ooh, your cheeks are burning!" She reaches for the thermometer on the bedside table and carefully slides it under my tongue. "Let's make sure you don't have a temp."

**Hints to help you beat the odds . . .**
**getting help with mouth sores . . .**

Sores and inflammation can occur in the mouth and esophagus and usually appear within a week or two of receiving chemotherapy. Mouth sores can cause pain and tenderness, which can make it difficult to eat, drink, and even swallow, which, in turn, can lead to dehydration. Keep your doctor and nurse informed of your condition, as they may prescribe pain medication, such as a topical anesthetic, as well as antifungal or antiviral agents.[1]

The quiet competence with which she cooks, cleans, and cares for me is reassuring. Grateful for these days that she and the children are here, I avoid thinking of their departure, when the echo of childish voices will grow faint before vanishing into memory.

Waiting for the three minutes to get an accurate temperature, Rebecca busies herself watering flowers and tossing the dead blossoms into the wicker wastebasket.

**Suggestions for allies . . . keeping the environment alive . . .**

Dispose of wilted flowers as soon as you notice them. It can be particularly depressing for a cancer patient to be faced with dying or dead flowers.

There is a tall, green vase filled with lilies, delphiniums, stephanotis, curly willows, and irises on the makeshift altar where she has arranged the talismans, tokens, amulets, prayer wheels, angels, stones, beads, and medicine wheels that have been arriving daily, along with flower arrangements, books, drawings, and cards.

"Well, you don't have a fever! Your temperature isn't even ninety-seven!"

I nod and shrug.

"That's normal for you, isn't it?" Rebecca studies my face, looking for signs of illness, but the burn seems an isolated event, a direct response to the intensity of the chemo. "How about if I get a cool cloth for your face? Would that feel good, do you think?"

The children hear our voices and pad excitedly into the room. "Nana's awake! Nana's awake! Hi, Nana!" Their small hands reach eagerly for mine, Rose plunging her tousled silky curls into my chest. She has wrapped herself in a swathe of silk scarves, one an emerald green rectangle imprinted with golden stars and silver crescent moons. The other was given to me many years ago by the wife of a tribal khan, a fiercely determined woman who rode her silver stallion with a man's confidence, her flaming red hair billowing behind her in the wind, the silky black scarf with burgundy and ochre designs snapping in the gusts sweeping down from the mountains. Rose uses these scarves and others to wrap herself in new personas and experiences, changing characters with each toss of color. Admiring the drape of the scarves on her intent little body, I remember that Mary Clement, according to the records, was cited twice for "lewd behaviors," one described as "wearing around her neck a scarf of immodestly bright color."

"Hello, Princess."

"Um-hmm." She nods. "And today I'm a princess!"

"And I'm Peter Pan!" Over dark green tights, Nico is wearing a green felt tunic with carefully cut points trimming the edges. The matching felt hat sits on his head at an angle, a feather jauntily nodding with each turn of his profile.

"Hey, Peter Pan!" I salute.

Nico grins. "And I'm also a bat, Nana . . . I've been hanging by my feet all night long!"

"But now you're Peter Pan?"

"I'm Peter Pan Bat!" he declares solemnly as he nestles into the bed next to me. "And I'm very tired now from hanging by my feet for the *whole* night!"

"Gentle! Gentle with Nana," reminds their mother as they jostle into position. *This is gentle*, I think to myself, *this cuddling is giving me exactly what I need.* My chest feels tight with the swell of crimson warmth flooding it. Somehow I can override the pain in my throat to speak with them, and however husky or raspy my voice may sound, they seem unperturbed by the change.

**Hints to help you beat the odds . . .**
**loving and connecting . . .**

Being with these little children is nourishing and life-giving. Figure out who in your life can fill a similarly essential and gratifying role, and surround yourself with that love and connection.

Rebecca leaves the room, returning shortly with a cool, moist towel. Carefully laying it over my face, she exclaims, "You're generating your own tropical heat wave!" The coolness feels good. Seconds later, she lifts the steamy cloth. "I think we need some ice for this!"

Rose squirms out of bed and stands by the night table, contemplating the telephone. She lifts the receiver, pushes random buttons on the pad, and starts talking into the mouthpiece, ignoring the dial tone. Suddenly I hear the blare of a strident mechanical voice, "Intruder! Intruder!" Lifting the damp linen from my face, I see Nico startle and sit up in bed, hands clasped over his ears. Rose is looking curiously at the receiver in her hands. Their eyes open wide like saucers, scanning for the source of the disembodied voice, unaware that it has been triggered by Rose's curiosity.

"It's OK," I reassure them. "It's really OK." I cannot help chuckling at the disparity between their innocent alarm and that insistent voice admonishing us. Taking the receiver from Rose, I punch in the code to cancel the alarm that has been sounded by her restless little fingers punching *star-star-star* in quick succession. "Alarm canceled! Alarm canceled! Alarm canceled!" the mechanical voice blares. Words are overlaid with new meanings, words like *intruder*, and *alarm*. If only the intruder in my body could be so easily canceled.

Charles strides out of the bathroom dressed and ready for the day. "Well," he laughs, "I guess we know that panic thing works!" He turns to the children. "Did that noise give you a scare?" he asks. They nod and race toward his open arms.

"Papa, where were you?" Nico asks.

Rose points her finger toward the phone. "Funny lady talking, Papa!"

"I've been in the shower, kids, but I'm ready for the day now." He nods toward the telephone. "I'll bet that noise scared you two, but don't worry, Nana fixed it." Charles sets the children down. "I'm going to get some breakfast. Have you guys had breakfast already?"

"Yup," Nico responds, "Mommy made us pancakes."

"Lucky you!"

"With raspberries and powdered sugar!" he continues.

"That sounds great! But maybe I'll just have the raspberries."

The children turn to me as Charles leaves the room. "See, kids? It's OK." I reach for the children and begin to tell them a favorite story. ". . . And the old woman said to the fire: "Fire fire, burn stick, stick won't beat dog, dog won't bite pig, pig won't jump over the stile, and I'll never get home tonight!"

Rebecca returns and lays an icy towel across my face. "What was that all about?"

I whisper through the cool layers of cloth and ice chips, "Oh, just a false alarm." I smile to myself. "It surprised all of us!"

I can hear the tinkle of ice cubes in Rebecca's glass. "I just don't understand this burn," she puzzles. "It looks as if you've been in a fire."

*I have been in a fire*, I think, *a dream fire*.

She takes a long drink of iced tea. "It just has to be from the chemo. Do you want me to get a hand mirror so you can see it?"

"You needn't—I'll get up in a few minutes and look."

Realizing their Nana has been distracted from storytelling, the children scamper off the bed and head for the next room. "Granny Tashie," they cajole their great-grandmother excitedly, "Can you tell us the pig story? About the old woman and her pig?"

Lying under the melting ice, I listen to my mother recite the rhymes the children love to hear: *The Old Woman and Her Pig*, *The House That Jack Built*, *Little Babaji*. Eighty years old now, her keen mind and sharp memory intact, Tashie tells a wonderful story, full of dramatic pauses, suspense, and surprise. Is that something I will ever do? Tell stories to my great-grandchildren? Tears creep toward the corners of my eyes to suddenly slide off my temples onto the pillow. *Time. I want time. Time with these children, with the people I love*. Thoughts of separation make hollows in my stomach and drain the warmth from my chest. It's not dying that's going to be so hard. It's leaving these cherished ones.

**Hints to help you beat the odds . . .**
**appreciating the now . . .**

Although cancer can take you into a territory of lost innocence, where you can no longer fool yourself that life stretches on without end, it can also shock you into living each day with a fresh intensity and a new appreciation for life.

I see myself swept up in flames that consign my flesh back to nothingness, at the same time lifting from the ashes a spirit freed for the last flight. But perhaps I won't die. Perhaps the ghost of Mary Clement will echo in my own story. Perhaps I, too, will be pardoned.

Rebecca suggests calling the advice nurse to confirm our suspicion that this mysterious burn is actually a side effect of the chemo. Since walking the short distance from the front door to the car, and then from the car park to the hospital, are the only times that the sun hits my skin, I agree and hear Rebecca describing the dramatic burn that appeared in the night.

"A chemical burn?" Pause. "But from what?" There is another pause before Rebecca says thank you and hangs up the telephone. Turning to me, she reports, "It *is* a chemical burn from the chemo. Like a bad sunburn, except you don't need any sun to get it."

*Perhaps this burning is atonement for past transgressions*, I muse. *Is this disease my redemption? Redemption from what?*

Rebecca walks into the kitchen and comes back with another linen towel filled with ice. "Charles is out cutting some aloe strips to lay over the burn." She exchanges the icy towel with the one she had placed on my fiery skin minutes ago. "At least it's not an infection. The advice nurse didn't sound alarmed anyway."

The information handout states that a full 85 percent of the patients getting this chemo tolerate it well, with few and minor side effects. The mouth sores, the chemical burn, and the general attack on my body make me wonder whether I fall into that small group that doesn't.

Mouth sores, otherwise known as oral mucositis, offer one of the biggest challenges to patients receiving chemotherapy for colon cancer. The soft tissues lining the GI tract become inflamed, causing a thinning of the mucosa. That thinning can encourage sloughing off of tissue and painful ulcerations in the mouth and esophagus.

Pressing a pillow to my abdomen for stability, I get up and limp to the bathroom. Grasping the counter for support, I lean into my reflection. My skin is the glistening red of a just-boiled lobster, yet with a purplish cast, and smooth like glass. There is no line at the neck where my shirt stops, no owlish disc of white under my eyes where sunglasses block the sun. Blisters are scattered over my lips, and I can feel them on the insides of my cheeks and the back of my throat. My thoughts flash to the blisters and ulcers that I cannot see, the ones that travel down my esophagus to my stomach and to the bowel.

These painful sores make oral hygiene a particular challenge. Charles searched for a soft-bristle toothbrush, buying several and analyzing the most pliable. But today, the slight opening I can manage is too narrow to allow the passage of the toothbrush: I rinse off the toothpaste in a splash of water and replace the brush. Taking a lemon glycerin swab stick, labeled "toothette," from the drawer, I slide it between my lips and gingerly swab the teeth and the edge of the gums. I start to pour the weak salt-water wash into my mouth but, remembering the burning and stinging of last night, decide against it. Yesterday I was able to drink through a straw and take tiny bites of custard from Zoë's silver baby spoon. Today, though, I can feel pieces of skin peel off my throat when I swallow.

**Hints to help you beat the odds . . .**
**helping mouth sores heal . . .**

Before your chemotherapy begins, schedule a visit with your dentist.

Maintain meticulous oral hygiene, using a soft toothbrush or swab to clean your mouth and gums after each meal and before retiring.

If you develop significant stomatitis, increase the frequency of your mouth care to every two hours.

Suspend flossing until stomatitis clears.

Avoid mouthwashes containing alcohol.

Rinse with warm saline or a bicarbonate solution.

Drink three liters of fluid a day unless advised otherwise.

Avoid spicy foods, alcohol, and tobacco.

Notify your healthcare providers if pain or bleeding in your mouth is hindering you from eating and drinking adequately.[2]

I see in the mirror a visible nakedness that is beginning to reflect the hidden nakedness of my interior world, both open, both unprotected. My cheekbones rise close to the translucent skin, giving me a look of having just been born, of raw newness and vulnerability.

I hear Charles come in from the garden, walk into the kitchen, and wash his hands. He pauses as he passes the door to our room, and then continues down the hall. I imagine him settling onto the pale-green zafu to meditate, and with a deep sigh resting his eyes on the Green Tara Buddha that gazes kindly from the cloth painting.

When we married, he was pulled into our huge and close-knit extended family, leaving behind a familiar pattern of comfortable predictability and surrounded instead by an unaccustomed vigor and spontaneity. Should I die, does he worry that that vigor will be lost? Will his life lose that quality of surprise?

This disease, and the treatments that assail my body, compel me to live very much in the present. Just moving from one moment to the next requires all my focus and attention. There is truly neither time nor inclination to ponder the past or to fret about the future. It is only now, today, that I can commit all my resources to strengthening my body, calming my mind, and committing to life. My concerns range from the comfort measures that will make me more relaxed this minute, this hour, to pondering the complex meanings of this journey. This is not a trip to which I would ever have agreed, yet now that unseen hands have hurled me this far into space, I am awed and curious about the landscape through which I am passing. I feel myself in a state of flux, in a place of becoming.

The burn fades over the following days, and the glistening surface of my skin begins to quiet, the blaze of scarlet cooling and dimming under the aloe leaves and the melting ice. These changes help me to remain conscious, to remain connected to these monumental revisions happening in my body. I am certain that this chaotic transformation deserves my attention and respect.

Yet, even as I wonder about the meaning of life and the cosmic implications of a disease that literally consumes one's body, there are the mundane practical details that absorb my time day to day. Plagued with persistent mouth sores, I eat doll-sized meals composed of "smooth foods." The doctors and nurses urge me to drink water and give me a special mouthwash to discourage infection of the ulcers.

Since starting chemotherapy, Charles and I are following a modified macrobiotic diet, and the chopping and the steaming have become meditations in themselves.

Because I move so slowly and rest so frequently, tasks that take a well person a short time can consume a major portion of my days. All these adjustments and requirements impose a structure on my time that is calming in its essential qualities: The simple, concrete goals are aimed toward sustaining life.

In September, we are given a brochure titled "Cancer as a Turning Point," which describes a free two-day conference for women with cancer. Families are also welcome to attend.

"Do you want to go?" asks Charles.

"I don't know," I answer, unable to decide. "You tell me!"

"Well, let's go. It may be boring and not worthwhile, in which case we can leave, or it may be really helpful, and we'll be glad we're there." He pauses, waiting for my response, before continuing. "Only by going can we find out."

**For your information . . . choosing what to eat . . .**

Diet affects every system in our bodies to one degree or another. Which diet is most beneficial under which circumstances differs with each person and his or her individual constitution. Foods to *reduce* or *avoid* entirely include red meat,[3] processed foods, cakes and pastries, and anything with added sugar, as well as alcohol. Foods to *choose* include whole grain cereals and breads, high-fiber fruits and vegetables, low-fat dairy, lean protein such as fish and poultry, and healthy fats such as olive oil and trans-fat-free margarines. A recent Harvard study correlates higher rates of colon cancer in women with a higher intake of carbohydrates,[4] another reason to choose the veggie platter over the pastry tray!

He's so very sensible, and as he speaks, I realize that this decision is not so hard after all. It's not that I don't know *how* to make choices these days—it's just that I don't have the *energy* to make them.

Up early on the day of the conference, Charles helps me empty and clean the colostomy, and he packs spare supplies in a canvas bag. Approaching the campus building, we are greeted by welcoming signs and balloons. As we walk into the building, I am struck by radiant smiles set in gaunt faces, by colorful scarves, loose hats, and shiny scalps.

After introductions are made, the moderator asks, "Will everyone who has cancer, please stand." With the vast majority of people in the room, and with Charles' steadying hand, I rise. She asks for those who have cared for people with cancer to stand, and Charles joins the many who are here supporting partners and friends, children and parents. After a lingering round of enthusiastic clapping, those who have been standing sit, and we settle back in our chairs, ready for the next segment of the program.

But yet another request surprises me. "And now," the speaker says, "will everyone who has outlived her or his prognosis, please stand." Chairs creak again with shifting weight, and I am astonished to see tens and even hundreds of women rising to a thunderous roar of applause. Electrified by the enormous power generated in these links that bind us one to another, I feel as if I have entered a hallowed sisterhood of shared experience.

The speeches that follow underscore that exuberance of hope without minimizing the terrors of our journeys. Although famous authors speak eloquently about their experiences with cancer, and health

**For your information . . . Cancer as a Turning Point . . .**

Jan Adrian of *Healing Journeys* produces these free conferences, "Cancer as a Turning Point," two to three times a year. Information may be found at the Web site www.healingjourneys.com.

providers describe promising new theories, my favorite speakers are the everyday women who tell their stories of living with cancer.

I am exhilarated by one woman's story of climbing a twelve-thousand-foot peak in the Andes during what would have been her final week of chemotherapy. She and a handful of other women with breast cancer challenged their bodies to complete the arduous ascent. Reaching the summit became less important than having the courage and fortitude to begin the journey at all. These women summoned physical, spiritual, and emotional strengths to defy the odds against such achievement amid the devastation of cancer and chemotherapy. Listening to the speaker describe the triumph of making that climb, I am elated, floating on the exhilaration of boundless possibility.

I am further inspired by a woman who whittles larger-than-life figures of animals, taking up a nearly forgotten family tradition of woodcarving. She describes the participation of these various creatures in her healing, in working through the vicissitudes of her disease. One is a towering rabbit, "Harvey," which she wheels onto stage. A graceful giraffe follows, gliding into the limelight on small wheels.

Cancer has pushed these women to shift their directions, to approach challenges head on, and to discover new ways of being in their bodies and in the world. They have walked through their illnesses and emerged not only intact but also enriched and deepened into themselves. Wondering whether I will reach that point one day, I am unable to imagine having the strength even to accomplish the most ordinary tasks of living. Imagining my own wellness requires a physical energy and a trust that I cannot conjure in my present depleted state. What will have to happen to bring me to that place of belief in myself, in my power to heal? My capacities for projecting myself into a better future seem to have shut down.

Listening to those women and others, I begin to understand the potential for cancer opening doors to rooms hitherto closed or perhaps not previously known. "I'm glad we came to this," Charles says as we walk out to the car at the end of the day.

"Me, too. Thank you for bringing me." I am too tired to say more, but I think he senses the fullness of my heart and mind.

**Hints to help you beat the odds . . . coping with fatigue . . .**

Fatigue is one of the most frustrating and stressful side effects of chemotherapy, and it has an enormous impact on your quality of life. Manifestations of this fatigue include difficulty concentrating, forgetfulness, weakness, lack of energy, and a diminished ability to accomplish mental and physical tasks. Unrelated to physical activity, it is not resolved with sleep and rest.

Ironically, pushing yourself to participate in some form of mild exercise, such as walking, can help alleviate the fatigue. Start with short walks on level surfaces, and increase the distance gradually. Also, remember that inadequate water intake can cause or exacerbate symptoms of fatigue.[5]

"Thank you for bringing me!" he counters. "I had no idea what this would be like, but I'm really grateful to have heard all those people full of hope."

Although I actually found a place to lie down during the lunch break, I am exhausted and doze on the way home. That openness to possibility, that sense that anything can happen, buzzes excitedly in my head. Tired as my body is, my mind has been fired by the stories of hope and healing.

Through family, I meet Julie, a woman who was diagnosed with Stage III colon cancer just weeks after I was. Our chemotherapy protocol is the same, and our schedules roughly parallel each other: one week of chemo daily for five days, followed by three weeks for our bodies to recover before beginning again. We are "chemo buddies," supporting each other through our travels in this hostile land.

Fat continues to be very difficult to digest, so my diet remains restricted. Once a week, Julie and I meet for lunch at a sushi bar, where I can get food without the high levels of fat characteristic of most other cuisines. Miyako, the owner, has a face like the moon, smooth, round, and serene. Her eyes miss nothing, scanning the room for tea cups needing refills, dropped chopsticks, and plates ready for removal. She also seems to realize how we are feeling.

"Hijiki good today," she begins, and we nod, knowing that we are in competent hands.

"Very good, very good." She nods. "You looking good today." She smiles proudly, satisfied that things are going well.

She directs Nari, the petite and lovely sushi chef, to prepare a fortifying and immune-building combination of vegetable and seaweed sushi.

Under the tutelage of this healer in disguise, we learn about the medicinal powers of food, such as burdock root and shitake mushrooms.

Over time, Miyako becomes my "sushi doctor," always curious to know my progress, adjusting my food to my current condition.

"How you feel today?' she calls as we walk through the door. She stands in the back of the small restaurant, short blue-and-white kimono wrapped around her, a rolled circle of bandana crowning her head.

"My mouth is hurting," I tell her.

"You need shiitake mushroom . . . build up your immune system." Looking at me for a response, she inclines her head and revises her prescription. "Your mouth hurting, I think maybe no sushi today. Maybe just green tea, miso soup."

**For your information . . . mushrooms for healing . . .**

Traditional Asian medicine describes various mushrooms as potent healing foods. Shitake, as well as astragalus and cordyceps, is believed to boost the immune system. Research investigating the relevance of complementary and alternative medicines such as mushrooms is currently being conducted at the National Institute of Health's National Center for Complementary and Alternative Medicine.

When she looks at both of us for affirmation, Julie states firmly, "That's fine for Eliza, but my mouth feels fine and I want sushi!"

Miyako laughs heartily and agrees, "Yes, I make sushi for you. You want . . ."

"Whatever we usually get . . . you know." Turning to me she says, "I never can remember what we order that tastes so good."

Miyako leans toward us, pen in hand. "How about edamame? Can you eat edamame today? That very healthy!"

"Yes! Edamame sounds good."

Her concern for our nutritional needs is touching. She turns to Nari to discuss our order, and Julie and I are left to talk while we wait for the plate of steaming edamame garnished with thin slices of lemon and coarse salt.

"So, how are you doing?" Looking at me, Julie rests her chin on her hand, and we settle in for our time of checking in.

**For your information . . . edamame . . .**

*Edamame* is the Japanese word for soybean, in this case steamed and sprinkled with salt and juice from a fresh lemon.

"I'm just putting one foot in front of the other," I say. "I feel as if I don't have the strength to do anything else!"

When Julie begins to feel sorry for me, I stop her. "But if this is what the chemo is doing to me, imagine what it's doing to the cancer cells!"

"But then I should worry that I don't feel worse!" she exclaims.

"No, I don't think so . . . who knows anyway? For me, thinking that way has become a device for getting through the worst times."

"Who does know?" she agrees.

We compare nausea, hair loss, mouth sores, joint pain, running eyes, fatigue, and doctor visits. We also talk about our families—the impact this is having on them. This is our time to say whatever we want without having to be brave or light-hearted or strong.

Some months later, Julie brings a friend who has been diagnosed with breast cancer to join us for lunch. Our duo quickly becomes a trio, and in time, as more friends and friends of friends are diagnosed, we evolve into a large group of ten to twelve women. For reasons of space and time, we move from the sushi bar to meeting in different houses for sandwiches and salads. Cancer is one of many topics, which include children and grandchildren, jobs and travel, and the chitchat of friends.

For the first time in my life, I am required by my physical circumstances to take in what I am given, to consider what I am offered, and yet to know that I can give nothing in return. For a woman, especially for a professional nurse, this is a nearly overwhelming challenge. My mind has been so tuned in to what *others* need and want and expect from me that I literally have not known what I need and want for myself. Now my body has been felled by a disease that forces me to consider only myself—there is neither time nor energy to address any but my own most essential needs.

I think about being a woman, being a nurse, and the dream flashes back to me, and my ghost ancestor with it. It seems that accused witches were often either flirts or healers, and since she was fifty-five at the time of her trial, it is more likely she applied herself to the healing arts rather than those of seduction. I surmise that her greatest offenses involved healing and perhaps midwifery. Was my becoming a midwife an unconscious retracing of the steps of this ghost ancestor?

**Hints to help you beat the odds . . .**
**joining a support group . . .**

Whether you join a formal support group or simply gather with others on your own, being with peers who are diagnosed with a similar disease and who are enduring similar treatments provides a setting in which there is a common understanding of shared experiences. The value of this kind of support, where you need not explain yourself, is immeasurable. Dr. David Spiegel, chief investigator of a Stanford University study looking at the effects of support-group attendance on women with advanced breast cancer, is finding evidence that, not only is their quality of life improved, but their lives may actually be prolonged.[6]

My days become a kaleidoscope of shifting patterns. At times I return to the burning dream and others, looking for meaning in that florid and often terrifying landscape. At times I ponder my death and grieve not at the thought of dying but at the thought of separating from those I love. And throughout these times of reverie, there is interwoven in my days the details and minutiae of living with cancer and chemotherapy amid the intense love and concern of family and friends.

A flood of gifts, letters, and flowers arrives daily. I contemplate how to respond in kind. I receive a letter from work, notifying me that midwives, nurses, and doctors are giving me many hours of their hard-earned vacation time. I panic, wondering how I can ever repay them. Andrew puts his hand on my knee. "Mom, for so many years, you have been here for all of us. You have helped so many people—now it's your turn. If one of your friends were sick, would you give whatever you could to help them?"

"Of course."

"So why can't you let them do the same for you?"

The habits of a lifetime are not easily shifted to integrate a new awareness. In taking in the love and generosity that is coming to me, I am hoping for the grace to be able to accept so much without simultaneously worrying about what I can do or give in response.

A more subtle shift in my inner world has been to listen to my heart and mind and body to detect what I need. Am I tired? Am I hungry? Am I needing time alone? Is this conversation getting too depressing? Do I

**Hints to help you beat the odds . . . learning to receive . . .**

Try to relax into being cared for, and suspend worries about "owing" or "paying back." In the past, you may have helped out those who are helping you now, or you may be able to do so in the future. Sometimes, we may never have the chance to give back to someone who has been essential support for us. Yet in some ways, allowing people who love us to help us and care for us at this time may actually be, in and of itself, a gift to them.

need help with something? Do I need somebody to be with me right now? Do I need a different person to be with me? Does this hurt?

Responding honestly and clearly to my inner cues has historically been a challenge. From some Spartan construct deeply imbedded in my cells, I have been so ready to override pain and discomfort that I have difficulty even recognizing them. Now it is essential that I quickly identify and acknowledge them: My life may literally depend upon it. The denial of physicality and the shame of bodily weakness are a paralyzing inheritance, an unbidden legacy from my austere Puritan ancestors. My task now is to face my physical body head on and care for it respectfully. For every time I override pains and ignore disabilities, I am pushing this body beyond its natural capacity.

The many doctors whom I have seen since this diagnosis have all asked about ominous symptoms that might have signaled the disease taking hold. I was not aware of any red flags, but as I wasn't actually observing the state of my body at all, it is hard to say now whether there were symptoms.

**For your information . . .**
**more about the symptoms of colon cancer . . .**

Although some people, at the time of diagnosis, report noticing no precursor symptoms whatsoever, symptoms of colorectal cancer include rectal bleeding, blood in the stool, abdominal pain and bloating, and a change in bowel habits (notably constipation or diarrhea, a narrowing of the stool, or a sensation of incomplete emptying of the bowel). For some, the only noticeable symptom may be a general weakness and lassitude due to anemia.[7]

The experience of this disease has propelled me into another time and space: I seem to live in a sort of bubble that separates me from the world I have known. It is a place of lost innocence, a place suspended between the familiar world of the living and the world of the dead into which I have peered but not yet entered. Gazing into the dark face of death has given me access to this space between the worlds, the space where I now live.

The chemotherapy itself represents a quality of energy, of everything being reamed out, a discarding of the old and a making way for the new. It seems a chance to discard the nonessentials, to strip life down to the bare bones of necessity. I thrill to the power of these liquids coursing through my body and am encouraged by the extreme side effects that surely reflect the severity of damage to the proliferating cells.

**Hints to help you beat the odds . . .**
**magical thinking can be helpful . . .**

If you have few side effects, you can convince yourself that this must signify that the cancer cells are being overwhelmed. You can develop your own mythology to cope with the side effects, and it doesn't need to be concordant with findings of medical research. Rather, it needs to be a story that helps you through this experience.

On the other hand, I do not envision a war taking place. I think of these cells less as alien enemies and more as my own body's darkest shadows. They are due a certain respect: They are powerful, they are persistent, and they are stealthy. My hope is that they will dissolve in the blaze of chemotherapy or at least be transmuted into light.

Perhaps it was not I that burned to ashes in the dream—perhaps it was the cancer cells that were transformed into the ashes that floated to the ground. But where was I then? My ghost ancestor reminds me that she, condemned to die, surprised herself and her entire village when the magistrates commuted her sentence. I feel her strength and courage seeping into my bones. She triumphed over extremely poor odds. I solemnly swear that this Mary Clement, this grandmother of many generations ago, will live in me and steady my hand and heart as I reach for absolution.

# *Chapter* 7
# Ebbing Power

## DREAMING THE BABUSHKA

### *October 1996*

*The left side of my chest feels metallic, heavy, encapsulated, and disconnected from the rest of my body. A rainbow composed of shades of gray arcs from the left side of my chest up and over to the right. I understand that the dull particles that make up the rainbow are composed of the toxins being jettisoned from my body and out into space.*

*A stooped old woman appears, entirely bowed inward, well toward closing the circle of her life. She wears a simple black frock and pushes a broom. In the manner of a babushka, she wears a white headscarf fastened under her chin. She studies the ground in front of her, piling up debris, and with great difficulty scoops it onto the broom fronds and drops it into a dustbin that's nearly as tall as she. I understand that this debris is composed of the toxic substances radiating from my body and that the babushka is helping to cleanse and purify me.*

It is a Wednesday in October, the third day of my third cycle of chemotherapy. Already I am feeling very tired and vaguely nauseated.

**Hints to help you beat the odds . . .
pacing your periods of rest and activity . . .**

Set realistic and workable goals for your patterns of rest and activity. Naps and quiet times during the day can be interspersed with activities, which need to be paced according to your energy level. If you have an unusually active day, the following day might be primarily one of rest and recuperation. Try to plan twenty to thirty minutes daily of mild exercise, such as walking.

Dropping a floppy linen hat on my head, I remember the dream and the old woman with the white scarf concealing her face, the dull black cloth covering her body. The white of transformation, of entering into mysteries of death and rebirth. And the black of mourning, of melancholy, of the dark earth from which new life emerges. Will I be freshly born after this chemo takes me to the brink of death? Or will the chemo be unable to thwart the cancer? Are the gods of my dreams preparing me to die?

Putting on a pair of dark wraparound sunglasses, I step out onto the covered porch and sit down on the bench next to a lopsided angel I have been shaping from clay.

Last month, I started going to weekly pottery sessions with a group of women who meet at a studio overlooking Monterey Bay. Against the backdrop of the surf's mighty roar below, we can watch it pound the shore as we find our stories deep within the earth. The teacher, Fiona, is a celebrated sculptor, yet her expectations for us are not that we create great works of art but that we discover and explore our inner lives through the process of working with the clay. I am soothed by the smooth coils in my hands, by the women around me working quietly on their pieces, and by the rhythmic crash of the surf on the sand below.

**For your information . . . art as a tool for healing . . .**

Various art therapies are gaining more and more credibility as research is finding that art is indeed a powerful vehicle for healing. It is believed that the act of creating art can help people to express hidden emotions and to reduce stress, fear, and anxiety. Art therapists also believe the act of creating influences brain wave patterns and the chemicals released by the brain.[1]

When Fiona suggests I shape the clay into my impression of the disease in my body, the creature that reveals herself is small, hunched over, and dark gunmetal gray. The next week, Fiona asks me to fashion the being that I will need to heal, and a tall robust woman with gold and green lightninglike spikes snaking up her spine emerges. The figure sitting on the bench is an attempt at a more traditional angel, with raised wings and gown billowing behind. Except that as I mentioned, she is lopsided, and the gown falls in heavy clumps rather than billowing folds.

I brought her home under a swathe of damp muslin so that I could work on her between classes, lift her wings higher, and smooth her chunky gown. Lifting her shroud, I peek at her bent halo and dull eyes. "She looks as if her body is breaking down the way mine is . . ."

"She's strong though . . ." Charles counters. "Look at the determined tilt of her head!"

"And she'll get stronger," I agree, dropping the moist cloth over her.

Charles helps me slip into the faded Birkenstocks he takes from the shoe rack. Walking to the car, he carries under his arm a pillow that he took from the carved rosewood bed.

Settling into the passenger seat, a pillow under my head, I close my eyes, reassured by the steady hum of the car as it rounds the curves through the mountains. As the miles collapse into themselves, I can feel the anxiety start to push against my chest. It is almost a physical takeover: I feel swallowed by a heightened alertness, a watchful waiting. Trying to meditate, I visualize the chemo rushing though my veins, sweeping the wayward cells into the dustbin.

**Hints to help you beat the odds . . .**
**the power of your imagination . . .**

This may be when telling yourself a story comes in to play, a story that calms you as you approach the time and place where you will be receiving chemotherapeutic drugs. (Physical reactions to the anticipation of chemotherapy can even include vomiting.) Imagery, meditation, and storytelling can all help you through this scary place. If you have ever cried at a movie, you know the power of imagination. Although you know that what is taking place on the screen is not real, your imagination can stimulate a real physical response. So imagine yourself somewhere peaceful and secure, far away from the fear and anxiety.[2]

Charles parks under a twisted Monterey cypress, and we walk through the courtyard between the parking lot and the building. Doctors and nurses sit in the sun drinking coffee or tea and talking quietly. They wear scrubs; some wear white lab coats embroidered in blue thread with their names and departments. Some have masks dangling around their necks, and others have stethoscopes trailing from their pockets. I was once in groups such as these. I wore my loose green scrubs, the lab coat with "Eliza Livingston, CNM" embroidered in dark-blue script over the pocket, and below my name, "Department of Obstetrics and Gynecology." Sitting in the sun, drinking tea, I have watched people pass by as they walk through their diseases, on their way to dates with doctors. Now, I myself am the patient walking by, the ill woman leaning on the arm of her husband.

Tucked into the small elevator, we float to the fourth floor. There are two fellow travelers: a short, blonde woman with a round face and long spirals of coiled hair flying out like a nun's wimple and an even shorter man, dark, with thick shiny coarse hair that falls over his brow. They seem reluctant sojourners. I wonder if they have anything contagious. I hold my breath, but quietly, so that no one will be offended. The possibility of inhaling air that might be laced with exhaled germs frightens me. Knowing my bone marrow functioning has been suppressed by the chemo, I am fearful of the innocent cough, the breath exhaled. The woman gets off on three, the gynecology clinic, and the man gets off with us on four, the internal medicine floor.

**For your information . . . preventing infections . . .**

Most anticancer drugs affect rapidly dividing cells, including blood cells, which fight infection, help the blood to clot, and carry oxygen to all parts of the body. Patients whose blood cells are compromised are more likely to develop infections, bruise, or bleed easily and have less energy. To prevent infections, patients on chemotherapy should wash their hands frequently, avoid sick people and crowds, immediately clean cuts and scrapes, avoid contact with animal waste, and notify their doctor if they develop chills, sweats, or fever of 101 degrees or greater.[3]

I hand my card to the clerk, who slides it into a port in her computer. Jolted into action, the printer spews out an appointment confirmation slip, which the clerk clips to the card before handing it back to me. Smiling, she directs us down the hall. I am surprised that she does not recognize that I am a regular, that she has checked me in countless times. Each day she greets me cordially and coolly, as if I am a total stranger. Yet during the many minutes I have stood in front of this desk, I have memorized the photographs pressed under the glass top: the little girl wearing the white cotton gown festooned with scarlet ribbons and crowned with Santa Lucia's wreath; the toddler in the sandbox, squinting up at the photographer standing in front of the sun; the family picture, mom and dad carefully smiling, the little girl's grin showing the gap of fallen baby teeth, the little boy solemnly staring into the camera. I feel that I know this woman's family, that I care about them, yet each day the clerk greets me as if I were here for the first time.

We walk to the oncology waiting room, and I drop the card and appointment slip into the wire basket at the nurses' station. Sitting next to Charles on the blue upholstered armchair, I catch my breath. Already I am tired. A woman to my right sits forward with her chin in her hand, and I can see that her wig has slipped, coming down to cover her brow and at the same time exposing the back of her bald head. Several friends assumed I would want a wig and sent telephone numbers, pamphlets, articles, and sketches to suggest styles.

**Hints to help you beat the odds . . . coping with hair loss . . .**

- Remember that hair loss is almost always temporary!
- Consider the possibilities (wig, hats, scarves), and explore options in anticipation of losing your hair.
- Use a mild shampoo.
- Avoid chemical treatments such as coloring and permanent waves.
- *Avoid using heated rollers.*[4]

I face the prospect of baldness not with despair but with curiosity. My growing hat collection includes a red angora toque that hugs me to sleep at night; a deep-purple-and-maroon beret with an exaggerated crown, similar to hats worn by Dante; tall, Elizabethan-type hats woven from hemp and linen, and a Patagonia polar fleece hat that's periwinkle on one side and red on the other. Hats for varying weather, for fluctuations in my body warmth, for fluctuations in my mood. The same friends that offered wig information now send hats and scarves. Curving his hands over my smooth pate, Luke calls me Sinead.

Charles picks up an old *New Yorker*, but I look at the worn pages and imagine the germs tucked secretly into the stories, the cartoons, and the elegant ads for Baccarat glass sculptures and Ferragamo shoes. I push my hands into the deep square pockets of my jumper, lean on Charles's shoulder, and close my eyes.

"Orange or cherry?" Angela stands in front of us, holding the Ziploc bag containing syringes filled with 5FU and leukovorin. I don't want a popsicle; the sweetness makes me sick to my stomach. "Could I have some crushed ice instead, please?"

**Hints to help you beat the odds . . . ice for prevention . . .**

Sucking on ice chips or popsicles prior to the administration of 5FU can reduce the chances of developing stomatitis, mouth sores. If you have difficulty tolerating the sweetness of the popsicles, try holding ice chips in your mouth.[5]

Angela is terse in her reply. "Well, you know you can get that for yourself down in the cafeteria." I am startled and look to Charles for help. This is the same Angela who, just weeks ago, was so kind. She looks down on us, her lips pressed tightly together in disapproval, her loose, dark curls pushed against her head. She is actually only a bit over five feet tall, yet she towers over us now as we look up at her from the waiting room chairs.

Charles gathers himself, "Is a cupful enough?" At Angela's nod, he heads down to the cafeteria.

I am puzzled by Angela's hostility. She was my nurse for the first cycle of chemo. For five consecutive days, she pumped my body full of the chemicals consigned to wage war against the wayward cells. She was kind and even cheerful at times. I felt very safe in her care. Yet today she is without sympathy, concern, or even kindness. And she, like the clerk who checked me in, seems to have no recollection of having met me before. *Am I a figment of my own imagination?* Even if she doesn't remember me, she would see her signature in my chart, her testament to having cared for me.

I dutifully follow her across the hall, through another waiting room, and down a corridor into the familiar cramped chemo room. A gray computer smudged with fingerprints and the soot of time sits on a small desk wedged up against a wall. Next to it is a high stack of hospital charts—worn manila folders that hold the secrets of patients' lives, sicknesses, and treatments. Not two feet from the desk is an overstuffed armchair covered with maroon Naugahyde that is punched at the seams with bright-yellow brass tacks. Next to the chair is a metal stool on wheels. An IV pole, also on wheels, stands discreetly behind the chair. Against the wall is a cupboard that holds Band-Aids, nausea medicine, adhesive tape, IV supplies, needles, syringes, and alcohol pads. In the corner next to the door is a matte-blue, molded plastic chair. If there are two visitors, one has to stand.

I settle into the soft cushions of the dark-red chair, relaxing into the support of generously wide armrests. I am hoping that Angela might wait for Charles and the ice. I am also hoping that she might remember that we have met before.

**Considerations for hospital staff . . .**
**understanding your power . . .**

Although you are seeing patients at a dizzying pace throughout the day, for each patient you see, you are, with few exceptions, the only one administering chemotherapy. Try to remember that your importance in their eyes is huge: You are the one with the power and the authority. Your gestures, your words, all that you communicate by silence and implication as well as directly, assume an enormous importance to the patient who not only depends upon your skill but also can be strengthened and exhilarated, or diminished and disempowered, by the way in which you communicate compassion and empathy versus indifference and even hostility.

Impatiently, she pulls the rolling metal stool next to the chair, and arranges the iodine, the butterfly needle, the tape, and the gauze squares on her lap.

She takes my hand in hers. Searching for veins, she studies the back of the scrawny hand, the narrow wrists, the spindly forearms. She sighs heavily, and I feel as if I am letting her down. She picks up an alcohol swab and rubs concentric circles on my wrist, starting from the center and moving out. She leans down and blows close to the skin. The intimacy of that gesture makes me hope that she will see me and remember

**For your information . . . the butterfly needle . . .**

The butterfly needle, also referred to as a winged infusion set or blood collection set, is the most commonly used intravenous device. It is a stainless-steel beveled needle and tube with attached plastic wings on one end. It is used in the collection of blood from patients who are difficult to stick by conventional methods. These would include geriatric patients, cancer patients, and children.[6]

and, in the wash of memory, will soften her stance. Watching her, I recall blowing on steaming spoonfuls of soup to cool them before tipping them into my babies' mouths.

She quickly picks up the butterfly from her lap and jabs the needle into the skin at the inner aspect of my wrist but is unable to find a vein. She moves the needle around under the skin, and I hold my breath and look away.

When she finally takes it out, the skin fills quickly, forming a small balloon. She slaps a square of gauze down on it. "Press hard here," she directs grimly, pointing to the swelling. I meekly obey, hoping that my eager compliance will remind her what an easy patient I am.

She wads two gauze pads into a small square and presses them hard onto the swelling wrist before smoothing tape tightly around it. She reaches up into the cupboard for another butterfly and again places it on her lap. Taking the other hand, she finds a tiny blue tracing on the outer edge of the palm. She pushes the needle through the skin, threading the catheter through the vein. This time I can see the fine line of blood passing through the narrow translucent tube, confirming that the stick has been successful.

Expecting to see IV tubing plugged into the butterfly, I watch horrified as Angela connects the syringe full of 5FU directly to the butterfly port. Alarmed by the prospect of chemicals being injected directly into my veins, I remind her that, because of the chemical phlebitis, I am to get the chemo diluted through an IV solution.

Visibly irritated, she mumbles that no one told *her* this and that she hasn't sufficient time in her schedule. She tears a piece of paper tape from the turquoise plastic dispenser, presses it onto the butterfly to hold it in place, and leaves the room. Leaning back, I close my eyes, relieved to have spoken, to have held my ground and not hastily apologized in the dark shadow of the nurse's anger. Yet I also feel troubled to have so thor-

**For your information . . . chemical phlebitis . . .**

Providing that the veins maintain their integrity, administering chemotherapeutic drugs directly is faster and easier than diluting them. However, when chemical phlebitis occurs, diluting the drugs with an IV solution is an option that will be less irritating to the already inflamed vessels. Another option is starting a central line, which has a lower infection rate.[7]

oughly annoyed Angela, whose shift from cold indifference to muted rage is palpable.

When it became apparent two weeks ago that my veins were severely inflamed by the chemotherapy, another oncology nurse had offered me a semipermanent port that would be inserted into a central vein and stay there for the duration of chemotherapy. There would be no more needles and no more sticks, but there would be the threat of infection around the port and the general anxiety in having tubing threaded through veins lying deeply in my body.

**For your information. . . . A semipermanent port. . . .**

If you have veins that are hard to find, or if you need to receive multiple drugs, a semipermanent type of IV called a vascular access device (VAD) may be recommended by your doctor or nurse.[8] It may also be an option if your veins become inflamed from the frequent administration of irritating drugs.

The oncologist, understanding my reluctance to have a permanent port inserted, ordered that the chemo be diluted with generous amounts of fluid. This method would diminish the severity of chemical phlebitis, allowing the vein walls to heal.

*Is Angela's rage due to my having declined the offer of a main line?*

During Angela's absence, Charles returns and hands me a little paper Dixie cup filled with crushed ice and printed on the outside with blue forget-me-nots with tiny yellow centers. He sits down in the visitor chair and looks at me, glancing at the green plastic butterfly taped to my hand. Too tired to explain Angela's absence, I follow his glance and notice a purple bruise radiating out from the pressure bandage and moving toward my elbow. Feeling for the hematoma under the gauze pad, I hold it between my thumb and index finger like a large chestnut.

Angela returns, carrying a 250-cubic-centimeter flexible plastic IV bag filled with normal saline. After hanging the bag from the metal IV pole behind the chair, she returns to her stool. When she connects the IV tubing to the butterfly resting on the edge of my hand, I look up to watch the steady drip of fluid filling the tubing.

Angela takes out the bigger syringe: It is fat and holds twenty cubic centimeters of 5FU injection. Inserting it into the IV port, she pushes the plunger forward with her thumb. I watch and see that with her other hand, she is kinking the IV tubing so that undiluted chemo is entering my body. It burns under the skin, and when I ask her to open the line to the normal saline, she doesn't move. Just when I open my mouth to speak again, her hand falls away and the fluid is free to flow again. She looks at her watch. I wish she would look at me. Notice me. Only a few CCs of the chemo have gone in, so she repeats the process: closes off the IV tubing, pushes the barrel of the syringe to empty it of another few CCs of chemo, opens the IV tubing, and begins again. Watching carefully, I am hypnotized by the fear that she might push in the undiluted chemo all at once.

Remembering the dream rainbow, I imagine it sucking away all the debris of cancer. Still wincing from Angela's rough words, I try to imagine her dark energy wafting away on the gray-hued rainbow.

**Hints to help you beat the odds . . . .**
**meditating your way out of stress . . .**

If you are feeling captive in a situation such as this, without an advocate to help you, try to remember that the nurse's reaction probably has little to do with you and may more accurately reflect difficult challenges in her personal life. This is not to excuse it but to free you of responsibility for provoking her anger or indifference. That said, you can lift yourself up out of the immediacy of the situation and concentrate on meditating or imaging being in a peaceful place with positive changes taking place in your body.[9]

Looking up to watch the drip of the IV fluid, I notice that it has stopped, even though the line is not kinked. I wait for Angela to notice the blockage, but she continues to push chemo through directly, without the IV fluid running. I groan with the burning under my skin and point out that the dripping has stopped. Angela looks at her watch and sighs audibly as she stands up. When she extends the IV pole to raise the bag up higher toward the ceiling, the drips resume.

"Thank you," I murmur apologetically.

Saying nothing, she sits down wearily on the stool. I try to catch her eye, to smile in sympathy for her busy schedule, for her heavy patient load, for whatever burdens are weighing on her so heavily.

I try to visualize the chemo healing my body as it washes through the tunnels of my veins, but I cannot concentrate. I am distracted by fear—not fear of the chemo or even of the cancer, but fear of Angela.

**Considerations for hospital staff . . .
recognizing the power imbalance . . .**

The power imbalance in hospitals can transform capable private citizens into timid and even cowering patients. Remember how huge you become in your role as medical care provider and how your tact, compassion, and understanding are essential to healing.

The big syringe is finally empty, and next she attaches the smaller one containing leukovorin. I look casually at the label and am reassured: "Eliza Livingston" is neatly printed in bold, black letters on the glossy white rectangle wrapped around the barrel of the syringe.

Finally it is over—the syringes are tossed into the plastic biohazards sharps barrel, and Angela starts to remove the IV. I appeal to her to leave it in for a few minutes so that the fluid can wash through the veins, which still burn. Still silent, she leaves the IV intact and walks out of the room.

A few minutes later, she returns: "Had enough now?" She looks in my direction but does not meet my eyes. "I guess so . . . thanks." I would have preferred to finish the bag but don't want to further irritate her. She pulls the fine catheter out of the vein. Over the hole that made a tiny O in the dry skin, she presses a shiny blue Band-Aid printed with the image of a black-and-white Orca. I thank her as she turns away and, without speaking, walks out of the room.

Charles helps me up out of the chair and carries the Dixie cup with the remaining chunks of ice as we walk slowly to the car. I try to hold a cube in my mouth but am feeling sick to my stomach. I lie back on the blue flannel-covered pillow and doze. Driving through the mountains, my hand aches and also the wrist with the chestnut hematoma.

*When I get home*, I muse, *I will soak both hands in warm water. I will cut a leaf from the aloe plant in the garden and make strips to tape to the knot on my wrist.* Even as I plan, I know that I will have to ask Charles to get the aloe: I cannot risk touching the dirt that might be on the plant.

**For your information . . . guarding against infection . . .**

As mentioned earlier, if your white count falls low enough, indicating bone marrow depression, you may be forewarned against exposing yourself unnecessarily to garden dirt, as well as unpeeled and uncooked vegetables and fruits harvested from the garden.[10]

Charles will cut the leaf, scrub it with the vegetable brush, cut it into strips, and wrap these living bandages around my hands. Yawning, I tuck my head to the side, out of the glare of the noonday sun.

# *Chapter 8*
# Perilous Waters

## DREAMING DANGER

### *October 1996*

*I am walking on a narrow sea wall that rises twenty or thirty feet above the surf, perpendicular to the shore. The sky is metallic gray, the air is chilly, the wind blows, yet the water is a turquoise Caribbean blue, a marked contrast to the mighty storm raging in the air.*

*I hold by the hand a small child, three or four years old. Waves far below us break over the wall, washing over our feet. Upon reaching the end of the bulwark, we plan to dive into the water and swim to shore.*

*We finally reach the end of the rampart, yet now it seems to be parallel to the beach, rather like a reef, except man-made, apparently of cement, narrow and dizzyingly high. When I see blood in the water that is swirling around our legs, I realize that this will attract the sharks, and I decide against swimming.*

*The wind blows harder and the air grows increasingly chilly as I grip the child's hand tighter, and we carefully reverse our steps. Nearing the shore, we see a Greek woman, a nanny who apparently lives with us, waiting. She is large, zaftig, the mother of all mothers, and welcomes us into her warmth.*

*The raging of the storm quiets; I am flooded with relief. In her hand, the Greek woman holds a pair of scissors and prepares to cut the child's hair. The child seems to understand that this is necessary and patiently watches the clumps of hair fall to the sand.*

Stirring from sleep, I open my eyes to see the yellow sun splashing lacy patterns on the peach wall. Feeling the warm sand of the dream, at the same time I shudder, remembering the chill of the wind and sky. The dissonance is reflected now in the warmth of a late-summer midmorning as backdrop to the wintry chill in my chemo-ravaged body. Charles hums in the shower, the steady thrumming of the water intersecting with the pulsing rhythm of the surf of my dream. Fearing a fall from the high rampart, I am having difficulty leaving the dream behind and walking into the light of a new morning: Walking toward safety, navigating stormy seas and maneuvering through precarious paths. Isn't that my present challenge—to recognize the danger confronting me, and then maintain my balance as I back away into safety? Does the height of the dream wall suggest that my healing depends upon forces beyond the ordinary? Does its solidity suggest a firm foundation under my feet, a structure that will support me?

Charles wraps a towel around his waist and sits down beside me on the bed. "You're halfway through, honey." He rubs my back gently. "Three behind us—three to go!" It is October. Yesterday I finished my third cycle of chemotherapy.

"Yeah. It feels like forever in a way. And it also feels like a quick flash in time." The dream tugs at me once more. "I just had this dream, of walking with a small child on a narrow sea wall in the midst of a terrible storm—I felt surrounded by danger: by the storm, by the possibility of falling from the wall, by the difficulty of holding onto the child amid the wind and waves, and then by the sudden appearance of blood in the water, and the fear that it would attract sharks." Remembering the balance required to back out if this precarious place, I continue, "But in the end, we were safely walking toward the shore, where, remarkably, the sand was warm and the storm forgotten." I smile at the memory.

"Well, you have been in a dangerous place." He pauses. "Who do you think the child is?"

"I imagine it's me, a part of me. The new-life part, the fresh-start part, perhaps." Images of the dream replay themselves in my head. "And since I am protecting the little child, doesn't that mean I want to live, to find that place of safety?"

**Hints to help you beat the odds . . .**
**recording your dreams . . .**

Listen to and watch your dreams, and think about their messages. You might want to keep a dream journal by your bed, to track the themes and patterns as they emerge during this journey of the body, mind, and heart. If you decide to record your dreams, start as soon as you awaken, as they tend to vanish very quickly after waking up.[1]

"It sounds like a possibility." He turns to me and grins playfully. "I hope you want to live because I sure want you to keep living!"

"I do. I really do. It's not that I'm afraid to die exactly—but I just don't want to leave the people I love."

Charles helps me swing my legs over the bed. Walking into the bathroom, I see that he has already laid out the supplies for cleaning the colostomy. "I can't believe you're not totally grossed out by this stuff. You're truly a patient man." I am grateful for his help and even more thankful for the grace with which it is given.

"Well, it's just part of what we have to do now. It's a mechanical intervention! . . . which, by the way, allows you to live . . . and for that reason, I appreciate it and can overlook any offensive aspects."

After tending to the colostomy, he leaves me to wash and dress. I see in the mirror that the downy scattering of hair no longer covers the imperfections of my scalp. I notice scars from long-forgotten tumbles from tree branches and bikes and collisions with cupboard corners.

My eyebrows and eyelashes are so sparse as to give the impression of complete nakedness. Again, I am reminded of the smiling ceramic mannequins in Macy's windows waiting to be dressed and groomed.

With the shearing of the long locks, which in June had reached nearly to my waist, I feel as if I am stepping into another dimension, as if I am being initiated into secret rites. There is an intentionality in shaving my head that confers a certain power, the power of making choices. Waiting patiently for my hair to thin and fall out in random clumps seems, for me, a poor alternative. My mother smiles. "You look like a

Buddhist nun who has just taken her vows." This naked crown marks my initiation into another dimension, another time and place.

The Greek woman of my dream, the woman who cuts the child's hair, reappears to me. The warm mother, instinctive, fiercely connected to life. Like her, I have cut the things that need to be cut. Now I must toss aside the nonessentials that obscure the light and pay close attention to the choices that are shaping my life.

I recall the Jungian notion that cutting the hair or shaving the head in a dream may herald an initiation or transformation.

**For your information . . . hair as defining one's femininity . . .**

Hair can be the very definition of one's life as a female. A girl or woman with long, flowing hair is usually considered more feminine. The shearing of a girl's hair can be not only a physical event but also a symbolic one; removing her hair can mean that you are removing her femininity. In the Greek mythology, Medusa's hair was transformed into actual serpents when she dared to compare her beauty to that of the gods.[2]

The hair needs to be shed prior to engaging in a battle for dominance, a skirmish in which the prevailing participant will triumph. I have heard descriptions of the cropped heads of Catholic nuns, the nakedness concealed by flamboyant black-and-white, starched headdresses. I remember Orthodox Jewish patients, their shorn heads covered by stiff acrylic wigs that frame their faces in somber taupe.

I have read of maidens whose long, flowing tresses, upon marriage, are gathered up into tight buns and fastened with pins at the napes of their necks. I watched the Samurai warriors in *Rashomon*, their hair cut and bound tightly for going into battle. I remember photographs of the shorn heads of Buddhist nuns, shining in the dusky candlelight as they bend in prayer.

The ring of the telephone interrupts my reverie. The voice on the other end is offering me an 800 number I can call to get a wig, free for cancer patients. "I really appreciate the information, but I don't think I'll be needing a wig."

The light-hearted voice continues, "We find that cancer patients feel so much better about themselves if they can look normal—and we can help you do that."

**Hints to help you beat the odd . . .**
**deciding on a wig . . . or not . . .**

Wearing a wig is a very personal choice. Make your decisions based upon what feels right to you, with no apology. If you choose to wear a wig, many healthcare plans cover some measure of the cost. Local cancer support groups also may provide them, as well as the Look Good, Feel Better program administered by the American Cancer Society.[3]

There is a peculiar irony in the suggestion that there can be anything normal about this experience. How can I begin to understand the mysteries occurring in my inner world if I suppress the physical changes reflected in the mirror? How can I understand the extraordinary events happening in my life if I pretend they are not happening?

"That's very kind of you," I begin, "and I'll keep your telephone number and call you if I need your help at some later time."

There was a time in my life that I would have accepted her help so as to not reject her, when I would have made the changes recommended so as to not offend her. But today I am holding onto what I want long enough to examine it, identify it, and name it before it gets diluted in the stream of advice and opinions that swirl in the bubbling cauldron of choices, options, and decisions.

"Oh!" she says in a surprised voice.

In the brief pause that follows, before she can continue, I quickly add, "I really appreciate your call. Thank you."

Not interested in continuing the conversation, I draw it to a close. Before cancer, I might well have allowed her to keep me on the phone far longer than I wished just because I feel sympathetic to her need to talk, for her need to be needed. Concerns such as these are now crowded out by the elementary needs of survival. Knowing that my resources are finite, I must choose carefully where and with whom I spend my time and energies.

I could have told her that keeping a wig looking natural and tidy would be frustrating for me, and she would undoubtedly have explained strategies for making it easier. I could have told her that keeping track of my own hair, when I had it, was hard enough, and she might have given me enthusiastic beauty tips.

Running my hands over the smooth contours of my skull, I consider the uncovering of my life as well as my scalp. This awesome disease is pushing me toward an intimate examination of my existence, to an uncovering of the devices and deceits with which I have habitually covered pain, difficulty, and sorrow.

Despite my reassurances to the contrary, friends worry that I must be depressed by my baldness, so they continue to send hats and suggestions for wigs and telephone numbers where I can get hints, such as tips for looking your best while on chemo. Welcoming the hats, I decline the recommendations for wigs. In the oncology waiting room, I notice them slipping and sliding from bald shiny heads, slowly migrating to end up just above their brows, tilting to one side, or crawling down the neck until the hairline appears to start at the crown of the head.

**Hints to help you beat the odds . . .**
**wigs? . . . hats? . . . scarves? . . .**

A whole range of responses to this loss is possible, from not really caring that much to baldness being one of the most dreaded experiences unfolding. Some people prefer to keep every remaining strand left, and others choose to clip or shave off the meager patches scattered over the scalp. Some choose glamorous wigs, others elegant hats and scarves. Whatever your emotional response, honor it.

But there is a deeper meaning to my resisting camouflage, to my not wanting to hide or deny my naked scalp. Inclined to study and explore this disease and its enormous power, I remember my father enduring the ravages of malaria in Iran. Even as the cyclic fevers shook his body without mercy, he watched the tempest taking place within him and noticed the course of symptoms. As soon as the shaking ceased and his teeth stopped chattering, he smiled and commented on the manifestations of the disease and the life cycles of the larvae in his body that were reflected in the waxing and waning of the dreaded fevers. Always curious, even as he himself was assailed with disease, he continued to observe and analyze it from the stance of medical investigator.

Now deep in the experience of my disease, I can understand his approach in a new way. It is truly fascinating, albeit terrifying, to contemplate tiny microbes wielding such awesome power, ripping through ones vigorous and robust body and leaving trails of devastation in their wake. Leaning back and away from my intense experience, looking at it from the distance of scientist, helps me to endure unthinkable pain and humiliation.

**Hints to help you beat the odds . . .**
**5FU and palmar-plantar syndrome . . .**

Soreness and redness of the palms of the hands and soles of the feet (sometimes known as palmar-plantar syndrome, or hand-and-foot syndrome) can be a side effect of 5FU and is more likely to happen when the drug is given continuously or over a long period of time. Your doctor or nurse practitioner may prescribe vitamin B6 (pyridoxine), which can help to alleviate this side effect. It is temporary and improves when the treatment is finished.[4]

My eyes are chronically weeping, and even my nose runs clear fluid with no warning. The chemo seems to have opened all the sluices, recalling to mind the flooded rice paddies lining the highways of the Sacramento Valley. The drugs also seem to override the normal warnings that signal that the nose is about to drip or that tears are beginning to overflow. I have grown accustomed to finding myself in midsentence, horrified to discover a bead of translucent fluid gathering at the end of my nose or to feel the wash of tears sliding down my cheeks without the preamble sensation of feeling them build up behind my eyeballs. This peculiarity illustrates the futility of anticipation, reinforcing the focus on the present: This moment is the only moment I can address; this moment is the moment I am living now.

My gums ache and recede, and my teeth loosen. Despite the sores lining the insides of my cheeks, I try to keep my mouth meticulously clean. The irony is that meticulous oral hygiene will diminish the chances of ulcers, yet that very hygiene is painful if not impossible to execute due to those same mouth sores. Dr. Liu gives me a special mouthwash packed with antibiotics and analgesics and some topical Xylocaine gel. It allows me to clean with less pain and dulls my perception of skin sloughing off my throat each time I swallow.

**For your information . . .**
**chemotherapy affecting the GI system . . .**

The gastrointestinal system, another area of rapid cell production, is also vulnerable to the damaging effects of chemotherapy. Common GI-related side effects include loss of appetite, nausea and vomiting, diarrhea, constipation, and stomatitis (sores in the mouth and esophagus).

My burning eyelids feel gritty and are so tender they feel as if they have been turned inside out.

**Hints to help you beat the odds . . .**
**5FU's effects on the eyes . . .**

Gritty eyes and even blurred vision can be side effects of 5FU. If this happens to you, eye drops may be prescribed to soothe the tissues.

My joints ache: my knees, my wrists, my hips. I move like an old woman, slowly and with the precision born of the fear of injury. Compounding the skeletal compromises, the chemo itself weakens me, accentuating my tenuous shuffle. It surprises me that lingering traces of vanity have vanished: My singular focus is on getting where I need to go without stumbling. Even my craving for dignity is diluted by the overwhelming requirements for day-to-day survival.

Following the first cycle of chemotherapy, looking down at my fingernails, I noticed one slender white ridge radiating in a crescent that followed the outline of the moon. More fine white parallel arcs are accumulating with the completion of each cycle of chemotherapy. They curve around the half-moons, resembling the marks left by receding waves on wet beach sand. I feel along each arc a tiny ridge and smile at their resemblance to diminutive pink washboards.

From the spot where the chemo is injected through IVs, angry red-and-purple streaks shoot up my arms clear to my shoulders. Chemical phlebitis. Chemical inflammation of the veins. When I was in graduate school, I was the favorite for fellow students to practice IV starts, my veins being "pipes" that were easy to find and easy to thread. Now I imagine those clear pipes being cluttered with debris, peppered with holes, and burned by the chemicals that I hope are saving my life. The dull ache persists. Charles wrings hot water from towels and wraps them, steaming, around my injured arms.

**Hints to help you beat the odds . . .**
**comfort measures for chemical phlebitis . . .**

If you develop chemical phlebitis, warm, moist packs wrapped around the site can help ease the discomfort and reduce the swelling.

Friends are eager to prescribe medications and potions to eliminate the side effects of chemotherapy, claiming that if I take this tablet or that tonic, I will feel "almost normal." *But what is there that is normal about this experience?* I think of my laboring mothers and the choices they make. Some want to be awake and aware of their bodies' struggles and triumphs as the babies strain to descend through the narrow circuitous portal and into the world beyond the womb. Others choose to read magazines, *People*, *Elle*, *Cosmopolitan*, and *Martha Stewart*, or to watch football games, cartoons, soaps, and game shows while an epidural removes them from the extraordinary experience taking place in their bodies.

"You should really let them give you some Decadron," a friend suggests.

Remembering that unpleasant feeling of being jittery and unable to relax, I reply, "They gave it to me once, and I felt . . . well, my mother's description would be 'like a flea on a hot griddle!' I didn't like it at all."

"Oh, you didn't?" she wonders. "Well, we're all different, I guess."

Unwilling to separate myself from the experience happening inside my body, I am reluctant to take medications to alleviate the side effects unless they become intolerable. It seems foolhardy to disregard the signs that may herald evolving injuries and assaults by either the disease or the treatments. In making the choice to be alert to the transformation happening to my ravaged body, I also choose to listen to the changes in my interior world. I am awed by the power of both the disease and also the drugs being infused to obliterate it.

The profound depletion of my body has weakened my tolerance for the ordinary stimulus of day-to-day events and compromised my ability to make simple decisions. People are repeatedly asking, How can I help?

**Hints to help you beat the odds . . .**
**dealing with loss of appetite . . .**

(Cancer itself, as well as the treatment, can alter the way food tastes. You may experience a complete or partial loss of appetite. You may perceive a metallic taste on your tongue, and foods you once liked may no longer taste the same.)

- Report weight loss to your doctor or nurse practitioner.
- Eat high-protein, high-carbohydrate foods.
- Eat small frequent meals.
- Consider taking an appetite stimulant if prescribed by your doctor.

and I am stymied for a response. The attention and energy required to figure out what I need is more than I can muster. Not wanting to sink into the mire of self-pity and despair, I know that I want to stay close to laughter amid all this and ferret out the humor in a world that risks becoming eclipsed by sorrow.

Humorous books and tapes start arriving, and I laugh through *My Cousin Vinnie* and *Mr. Hulot's Holiday* and chuckle reading *Karma-Cola* and *The Queen and I.* I avoid reading the survival statistics for Stage III colon cancer, fearful that the grim prognosis, should it become imbedded in my belief system, will become a self-fulfilling prophecy.

Diagnosed with Stage III colon cancer within weeks of my surgery, my friend Julie comes with me to a drop-in support group at Women-CARE, a local agency that offers free support and education for women with cancer. The space is crowded and hot, and the women's stories are heartbreaking. Consumed by the sorrow in the room, we both realize that, despite friends' insistence that support groups are essential to those living with cancer, we will not be returning. Overwhelmed by listening to so many sad stories, we instinctively recognize that we have no energy to take them in without further depleting ourselves.

When Vanessa and Luke return in November, as always, seeing them is energizing. We go to the Saturday Farmers' Market, and Luke eats oysters on the half shell while negotiating the purchase of a Bodega Bay salmon. Laden with fresh organic vegetables and fruit, we come home, where I lie down on the sofa, dozing contentedly to the background buzz of groceries being unpacked and dinner being planned.

**Hints to help you beat the odds . . .**
**making every morsel count . . .**

Eat locally grown organic food, processed as little as possible, and reduce fats and refined sugars. When you are able to eat so little, it becomes more important that whatever goes into your mouth is beneficial.

Later Luke brings me a small bowl of miso soup with buckwheat spouts, shitake mushrooms, and scallions, and then takes me on a slow walk around the garden. Passing by the kitchen, I can see Charles chopping green papaya for salsa and Vanessa preparing a mound of garlic cloves.

**Hints to help you beat the odds . . .**
**including garlic and onions . . .**

There is some evidence that daily consumption of allium vegetables such as garlic and onions may inhibit cancer. You might want to include them in your daily intake to reduce your risk of recurrence.[5]

Luke guides me back into the bedroom, and I sleep until dinner.

On the patio by the stream, I find that Luke has arranged miniature portions for me on Rose's doll china. Max and Pat join us for a supper of grilled salmon stuffed with fresh anise, tarragon, and parsley, boiled yellow Finn potatoes with chives and olive oil, and roasted chestnuts. There is salad and fruit also, persimmons and Asian pears, but I am able only to enjoy the sight of them. Uncooked foods, camouflage for bacterial assailants, remain forbidden.

After supper, Luke instructs Charles in the art of filling the brass marijuana pipe. Taking a pungent bud from the white plastic yogurt container, Luke explains, "You take about this much." Demonstrating with a pinch of dried leaves on the tip of his finger, he continues, "and tamp it down with this guy." He picks up the brass instrument that looks like tiny ice tongs and taps at the cluster of herb. "Don't push it down too hard or the air won't be able to get through." He hands the oval pipe to Charles, and their contented voices lull me to sleep.

**Hints to help you beat the odds . . .**
**reducing your risk of infection . . .**

- Report any signs of infection, including fever, chills, sore throat, cough, burning while urinating, or redness or swelling at the site of an injury.
- Maintain a safe and clean environment.
- Avoid people who have colds, flu, or other infections.
- Avoid eating raw fruits and vegetables.
- Avoid gardening, handling plants and flowers.
- Avoid handling pet waste, such as kitty litter.
- Maintain meticulous hygiene:
  —Bathe daily.
  —Brush or swab teeth at least twice daily.
  —Wash hands carefully and thoroughly.
  —Empty bladder at least every three to four hours.
- Drink at least eight glasses of fluid daily.
- Eat a diet rich in proteins, carbohydrates, and beta-carotene.[6]

"Hey, Eliza!" I am roused by Luke's voice.

"Eliza! Don't you want to try some of this gold? Charles has it dialed in—he's a champ!" They stand beside the bed, grinning down at me like two schoolboys eager to demonstrate their latest magic trick. Charles holds the brass pipe in his hand, and in the casual camaraderie of brothers, Luke wraps his arm loosely around Charles's shoulder.

"But I'm OK now," I begin. Right now, the nausea is bothersome but tolerable. "I don't want to use it unless I really can't stand it."

"But why wait until you're miserable?" Luke cajoles.

"Yeah," Charles joins in, "take a puff now before it ploughs you under."

I relent, not because I change my mind about the degree of nausea I'm feeling, but because their preparations have made them so pleased with themselves, and so eager to demonstrate their prowess, that I myself want to see and feel their excitement when the drug makes me feel better.

Charles leans down and kneels by the bed while I turn to my side, supporting my head on my arm. Luke strikes a match and instructs Charles, "Now take some puffs yourself to get it started, and then hold it to Eliza's lips."

"Oh, no, please," I plead. "These sores have made my lips are so tender—let me hold it!"

**Hints to help you beat the odds . . .**
**saying what's on your mind . . .**

Be clear in your communications with people trying to help you. If whatever they are doing is not helpful, tell them! They can't read your mind.

Just one puff helps the nausea. Curling up on the bed and watching the room tip and sway, I am given a peaceful respite from the churning within my gut. At the same time, the smoke burns my throat, mouth, and lungs, so I make note to use it only when desperate.

Each time thereafter, Charles is careful to prepare the pipe exactly as Luke instructs, meticulously attending to every detail, resisting my urging to shortcut the routine he's learned. When he notices my step faltering or hears my moans, he kneels by the side of the bed and whispers, "Just try it . . . it always helps." And I sometimes accept his offer, and more often decline when I sense that the smoke will hurt the tender gaping sores lining my mouth and esophagus.

**Suggestions for allies . . . recognizing changing needs . . .**

Be aware that some of the comfort measures and advice you offer will be turned down, so try not to take it personally. What helps one day may be irritating on another.

Returning a few weeks later, Luke puzzles over the problem of nausea, determined to find a formula that will allow me the relief of marijuana without the irritation to my mouth and throat. With great care, he makes chocolate brownies laced with ghee in which he has soaked crushed marijuana buds for a day and a night.

We sample them while watching Danny Kaye in *The Court Jester*. The roughness of the crumbs hurts my mouth, so I take only a tiny sliver. The nausea vanishes, but in its place are uncomfortable sensations of intemperance. We are too tired to finish the movie and fall into bed, assuming that the effects will clear by morning.

My mind whirling, I fall asleep quickly. Sometime during the night, a slow rhythmic bouncing awakens me. I open my eyes to see Charles sitting on the edge of the bed, teetering and swaying from side to side.

"Are you OK?" I ask.

Leaning over to reach for a glass of water on the night table, he says, "Yes, I just need some water."

He sways from side to side as he inches his hand forward, trying to make contact with the glass. Each time he reaches forward, he rises up from the bed slightly, misses the glass, and then bounces back with a light thud.

I start to laugh, and he giggles, too. His efforts resemble a perfectly executed mime performance, except that he is not acting!

Reaching over, I guide his hand to connect it to the glass, and he tilts his head back and takes a long drink.

"I hope we don't feel like this in the morning." I am surprised that the effects of that tiny sliver of brownie haven't waned.

"So do I," he answers.

We wake up around eight and find to our consternation that we are still tipsy and that our speech remains slurred. Charles helps me with my morning colostomy routine, a slow-motion experience that today seems to be endless. Luke makes a pot of strong Darjeeling tea, and we sit on the patio, eating grapes and melon and drinking glasses of steaming tea through tiny hardened bricks of saffron-laced sugar. Luke and Charles have sourdough toast and wild black raspberry jam.

Luke decides that a long walk will help, so while I get ready, he and Charles wash the few dishes. Since the chemo, I am nearly always cold and have difficulty getting and keeping warm.

**Hints to help you beat the odds . . .**
**losing heat through your head . . .**

Because the scalp is highly vascular, a great deal of heat can be lost through the head. If your hair is thinned, or vanished altogether, assemble some hats of varying warmth to have available for different occasions.

Wrapping a navy woolen scarf around my neck, I wear a thick cotton sweat suit and a blue fleece Patagonia ski hat. The chill of the dream returns to me: the freezing gray water, the steely skies. And the urgent return to the warmth of the sand and the Greek woman who waited for us.

Luke and Charles place themselves on either side of me, and we walk downtown, looping through narrow streets and stopping at sidewalk

**Suggestions for allies . . . bring on the hats!**

A hat is always a welcome present for anyone experiencing hair loss from chemotherapy. Choose one with the goal of helping the person make a fashion statement, dramatic or whimsical, rather than covering up a source of embarrassment.

cafes to rest. Without eyelashes and eyebrows, wearing midwinter fleece in the heat of summer, and peering at the world through dark reflective lenses, I stride carefully down the street supported by my two strong men. I notice an occasional astonished glance. A cluster of teenagers draw aside, suddenly silent, watching the three curious sojourners pass by.

Still giddy when we reach home, we are amused at our predicament but also frustrated by our helplessness. Charles settles me on the chaise in a shady spot in the garden, drops a wide-brimmed straw hat on my head, and leaves me to doze under the rustling maple leaves. Luke wraps up the remaining brownie squares and shoves them into the back of the freezer. Unwilling to throw them into the trash bin, he nevertheless can't imagine any of us wanting to repeat our experience anytime soon.

With each cycle of chemo, my white count falls rapidly, making me particularly vulnerable to infection. I am instructed to take my temperature daily, to avoid raw vegetables and fruits without peels, and to avoid crowds. These restrictions encourage time and space to examine the turmoil of my physical experience and to appreciate the quiet enormity of the changes to my interior world.

Exhausted, it requires tremendous effort to engage socially. My energy is so limited that I ration it carefully, needing most of it just to move from one day into the next. Especially during the first week or ten days after a cycle of chemo, I am exceptionally tired and plagued with mouth sores and

**For your information . . .**
**checking your bone marrow function . . .**

Your blood will be checked regularly with a CBC to see how well your bone marrow is working. An insufficient number of red cells may make you tired, an insufficient number of white cells increases your risk of infection, and an insufficient number of platelets reduces your blood's ability to clot.[7]

**For your information . . . anemia . . .**

Anemia, caused by the temporary reduction in the production of blood cells by the bone marrow, can be a side effect of 5FU. The anemia can increase your risk of bruising, bleeding, and infection and significantly exacerbate your fatigue. New blood cell production falls from about seven days after the treatment has been given, usually reaching its lowest point, called the nadir, at ten to fourteen days after chemotherapy. They will then increase steadily, generally returning to a normal range within twenty-one days.[8]

nausea. I become, during those times, more often a listener and an observer, a bystander to social exchange rather than a participant.

I also crave time and space to be alone: time to witness the interplay between my body and my heart, time to contemplate the new world to which I am being transported. The potency of the drugs, of the disease, of this experience, give me a curious and remarkable sense of power, a deep knowing of what I can and cannot do, without the overlay of expectations of and obligations to my overtaxed superego. There is a power, too, in spending these long hours in intimate communication with myself, in finally getting to know myself, not the carefully constructed mask of social dialogue and community associations. A new potential is arising out of the wreckage of terminal illness, a gold nugget shimmering in the cold ash.

**Hints to help you beat the odds . . . reporting side effects . . .**

It is important that you keep your doctors and nurses advised of your response to the chemotherapy drugs.

Report fatigue, dizziness, rapid heartbeat or respirations, shortness of breath, headaches, or irritability. Contact your doctor or hospital immediately if your temperature goes above 38°C (100.5°F), you develop any unexplained bruising or bleeding, or you suddenly feel unwell, even if you have a normal temperature.[9]

# *Chapter 9*

# If the Bed Has No Stones, the River Has No Song

## DREAMING HELPLESSNESS

### *Autumn 1996*

*I am flying down the slope in the late-afternoon twilight, the corn snow spattering my goggles and stinging my face. With reckless adolescent bravado, I rush to complete the run. Anticipating taking off my skis and joining my older companions, my mind is leaping ahead to the warmth of the wood stove at the end of the trail when my ski hits a depression in the snow and flips me into a tangle of limbs and equipment. Twisted by a ski tip lodged in the snow, my knee is blazing with pain.*

*Suddenly I am leaving the operating room. A masked man points to huge bandages on my injured knee and solemnly admonishes me to keep the leg straight for healing. In the hospital bed, trying to ignore my throbbing knee, I sit up, watching people pass by my door. Later in the evening, I scoot down in the bed, but the sharp angle of the mattress, which hours earlier had been comfortable for sitting, gives me only a small square for stretching out. Reluctant to call for help lest I disturb someone, I slouch down, curling my trunk into a tight ball to allow room on the bed for keeping my leg straight.*

*All through the night, my bones and muscles ache from the cramped position, but I do not call for a nurse or even flag down an aide passing by in the hallway. They all seem so busy, and I don't want to bother them for something so minor.*

Knifelike pains just under my ribs awaken me from the dream. Scared by the intensity and the sudden onset, I wonder, *Would another tumor declare itself so abruptly and so forcefully?* In my fourth cycle of chemotherapy, accustomed to the side effects and discomforts that go along with the drugs, I am alarmed by the sudden unfamiliar gnawing under my ribs. Switching on the bedside lamp, I blink into the flickering light, finally closing my eyes to soften the glare. Leaning into the pain, I try to curl around it, to contain it. Charles quickly sits up.

"What's the matter? Are you OK?" He rubs his eyes. "What happened?" He puts his arm around me, then loosens his grasp. "Oh, sorry—I don't want to hurt you."

"It's OK. It's here." I cup my right hand under my rib and point with my left index finger.

"What do you think it is?" He looks at me questioningly, assuming I am able to answer any medical questions. But obstetrics is a long, long way from oncology, and the breadth of my ignorance is wide.

"I don't know."

"Well, what do you think it *might* be?" he persists.

*Could it be metastasis to the liver?* I wonder. *Would it creep up unawares, with no subtle symptoms warning of a crisis swelling under the cloak of the commonplace?*

"I don't know," I gasp, "but this pain is indescribable. Maybe gallbladder?"

The aches in the dream were so easily explained and could have been so easily remedied had I chosen to call for help, for someone to simply lower the head of the bed. This pain, on the other hand, is coming out of nowhere, without warning, without explanation.

Charles wonders, "Is that the right place for gallbladder trouble?"

"Um-hmm." Getting up and stumbling to the window, I see rooftops shimmering in the mist of early morning and hear a bird peep sleepily from the nest in the olive tree. Leaning over, I rest my elbows on the windowsill.

Perspiration from nighttime hot flashes have soaked my nightdress, and I struggle to pull the damp cotton knit off over my head. Charles brings a clean one and holds it up to me as I once held shirts up for my toddlers to thrust their tousled heads into.

My speech is punctuated by the short gasps that rise from the intensity of this unfamiliar pain. "I think I want to try a shower."

"I'm thinking we should go to the hospital," Charles ventures.

"No, not that." I try to sound reassuring. "This will pass."

"But I think you should be examined," he pleads. "We have no idea what this is." I hear the frustration and fear in his voice.

"But I'm *afraid* to go to the hospital." Tears burn behind my eyelids. "I just want to try a shower now."

"I know you're afraid."

"Please just let me stay here and take a shower," I beg.

I know I have neither the strength nor the will to resist. I need him to help me, to support my staying home. Suggesting a compromise, I agree to go to the hospital in the morning if the pain has not eased. "By seven, the doctors who know me will be there, so it won't be so scary."

"OK," he agrees reluctantly. Once again, he yields to my wishes that spring from both the fear of going back to the hospital, and the embarrassment of needing and asking for help. The dream suddenly flashes back to me, my night of agony that could have been quickly remedied had I been willing, or felt entitled, to ask for help.

My sleepy knight leads me into the bathroom.

"I'll stay right here." He cautions, "You might start to feel faint in there."

I sway back and forth as the warm water washes over me. *If I take a Vicodin*, I caution myself, *that might cover up a pain that's warning me of danger. If I don't take a Vicodin*, I reason, *I don't think I can stand this much longer.* I sit down on the shower chair and lean forward, moaning into my hands. "Oooh, I just can't find a comfortable way to be."

"Do you need help?"

Looking up, I see Charles's face pressed against the glass, rippled and dreamlike through the drizzle of steamy water on the clear pane.

"I'm OK."

His face disappears back into the dream. I have to think of something, something that will draw my attention away from this torment. Like women in labor, I need the distraction that will allow me to focus on something outside of the turmoil in my body.

As the shower beats down on my back, I look at my hands, studying the transformations of my fingernails, enthralled by their mysterious inner life. The pearly silhouettes gather in parallel arcs radiating out from the moons and mark each cycle of chemo as the rings on a tree trunk mark the passing of each year.

> **For your information . . . nail changes . . .**
>
> 5FU may cause your nails to become brittle, chipped, and ridged. As your nails grow out, once treatment has ended, they will return to their prechemo appearance.[1]

Appalling as the genesis of these rings may be, there is a certain beauty in them, and last week I asked Charles to photograph them. The print shows my hand against the pale peach wall, fingers fanned out like the rays of the moon, but the curious washboard ridges are visible only to eyes that have seen them in real life and know what to look for in the photograph.

*How puzzling that the drug sent to attack errant tumor cells at the same time superimposes on my nails a physiological device for recording the recurring cycles.* I wonder, *What part of my body does the chemotherapy not affect?*

My attention away from the tiny washboards at the ends of my fingers, I push myself up off the chair. Charles materializes at once on the other side of the door and looks at me through the wash of water skidding down the glass. "Are you ready to get out?"

Turning the shower valve off, I step carefully onto the mat. "I'm also ready for a Vicodin."

Charles hands me a soft towel. "Do you know where they are?"

It's so hard to talk. Even thinking is hard. *Why is he asking me this?*

"Are they in the cabinet?" he persists.

"I'm sure they are." I throw the towel over my back and lean on the tile counter.

I can hear him picking up bottles, checking the labels, and then putting them down.

I take a breath in and say quickly, before the next pain mounts, "A white plastic bottle—squarish."

I sway my bottom back and forth, back and forth. Finding it hard to bear any level of pain now, I can feel myself begin to panic as the stabbing under my ribs continues. I could call the advice nurse, but I can't stay still long enough to wait on hold, and the effort of explaining my pain, to say nothing of my medical history, tires me just thinking about it.

"Do you want one or two?" I can hear the muted clatter of pills as they tumble toward the neck of the bottle.

"Two." He puts the tablets into my palm.

Pouring water into a thick glass mug, he holds it to my lips. "Thanks," I gasp.

Now I just have to tolerate the pain until the drugs take effect. Twenty minutes, maybe thirty. Then I can sleep another hour or two before starting the day. Charles holds out a clean nightdress for me and slips it over my head.

Gently taking my elbow, he steers me toward the bed.

"I think I'll be more comfortable if I just keep moving." My words come out between short gasps.

Walking toward the living room, I stop at the window. Raising my bent arms above my head, leaning my forearms against the glass, I peer out into the darkness. As my eyes adjust, I can detect the tumble of water racing toward the sea, shimmering in the light of the full moon.

Standing behind me, Charles gently rubs the small of my back, at the same time urging me to let him take me to the hospital. Knowing I have an appointment with the oncologist in the morning, I would prefer to wait for that scheduled visit rather than see a stranger in the ER now.

Hours later, lying on the exam table, I describe the pain to Dr. Liu as he presses on my belly. "It was more or less colicky." I pause, grateful for his careful listening. "In fact," I continue, "even though I don't feel it right now, it was awful while it was happening." *Here I am, relating the night's agony in understatement.* I wonder, *Did the child in the dream greet the morning nurse cheerfully, never admitting what a miserable night she'd passed?*

"Well, let's send you down for an ultrasound."

He looks at me. "It may be gallstones, but . . . I am more worried about the possibility of peritonitis."

**For your information . . . diagnosing gallstones . . .**

Many gallstones, especially silent stones, are discovered by accident during tests for other problems. But when gallstones are suspected to be the cause of symptoms, the doctor is likely to do an ultrasound exam. Ultrasound uses sound waves to create images of organs. Sound waves are sent toward the gallbladder through a handheld device that a technician glides over the abdomen. The sound waves bounce off the gallbladder, liver, and other organs such as a pregnant uterus, and their echoes make electrical impulses that create a picture of the organ on a video monitor. If stones are present, the sound waves will bounce off them, too, showing their location. Ultrasound is the most sensitive and specific test for gallstones.[2]

He presses on my abdomen, looking for hot spots, and decides that it's safe for me to go home after the ultrasound. "I'll check you again in the morning before starting your chemo," he says. "And come back before that if the pain gets worse or if you develop a fever."

The pain persists during the night, and after a Vicodin at midnight, by two in the morning it vanishes.

"Well, you do have gallstones," Dr. Liu tells me the next day. He shows me the ultrasound report and underlines with his finger the words "multiple large stones." He tells me that when operating, surgeons can sometimes see scarring on adjacent organs created by the inflammation of the gallbladder. I imagine the organs around my gallbladder being bruised and tired from the pain.

**For your information . . . gallstone formation . . .**

Gallstones form when liquid stored in the gallbladder hardens into pieces of stonelike material. The liquid, called bile, is used to help the body digest fats. Bile is made in the liver, then stored in the gallbladder until the body needs it. At that time, the gallbladder contracts and pushes the bile into a tube—called the common bile duct—that carries it to the small intestine, where it helps with digestion.[3]

"I'm sending a referral for you to be evaluated by the surgeons."

The pain resolves, yet I sleep fitfully the following night. Unable to get warm, I put on a knitted red angora wool cap, a flannel nightdress, cotton knit pajama bottoms, wool socks, and Charles's baggy, gray sweatshirt. Despite the layers, my hands, arms, shoulders, and thighs are chunks of ice. And my nose another dollop of frost. I have become a snowman. Yet any minute, a hot flash will make me throw off this warm bundling and open the windows to the cold night air. Wild gusts howl outside, and the wind chimes clang a warning.

When I see the surgeons, they worry that an operation while I am so depleted by chemo will carry major risks. Yet waiting presents the risk of my having a full-blown gallbladder attack that requires emergency surgery, augmenting the already known hazards of an elective procedure. Dr. Narayan confers with his colleagues about the possibility of a laparascopic cholecystectomy, but they conclude that the scarring created by the extensive surgery in July makes complications likely.

**For your information . . .**
**emergency versus scheduled surgery . . .**

There can be inherent risks of emergency surgery as opposed to scheduled surgery. Nursing and medical staff may have to be pulled from elsewhere in the hospital or called from home. There will not be time for the patient to make preparations such as refraining from eating for twelve hours prior to surgery or emptying the bowels for GI surgery.

They make a plan to remove the gallbladder at the same time that they reverse the colostomy, a surgery under consideration for spring, after my last cycle of chemotherapy. Meantime I adjust my diet to exclude, in as much as possible, all fats. It seems to be effective, but my allowable foods are radically limited.

A few weeks later, in mid-November, after brazenly eating twelve roasted almonds, I have another gallbladder attack that lasts hours. Unrelieved by the prescribed two Vicodin, I am able to sleep only after a warm bath and another dose of pain meds three hours later.

In the morning, both of us enjoying the quiet lull after the turmoil of last night, Charles brings tea and honeydew melon out to the patio, sits down next to me, and begins, "You know the class I'm taking, the class in medicinal uses of herbs?" I nod, and he goes on. "The instructor has a formula, an herbal formula, that he says dissolves stones—kidney stones and gallstones."

Determined to avoid taking any herbs or tonics that might interfere with the action of the chemotherapy, I nevertheless appreciate his suggestion. After a brief pause, he adds, "Would you be willing to see him?"

"Not now, at least not yet," I decline. "I really just want to leave the chemo to do its job. I don't want to mitigate its impact with anything else."

"I figured you'd feel that way, but if you change your mind . . ."

"Thanks." Across the creek, the leaves are falling from the persimmon tree, leaving the fruit dangling from bare branches like shiny golden globes. Relieved by the distraction of the garden, I say, "We need to start picking the persimmons before the birds get them."

"I don't want you to get up on that ladder though . . . Luke and I can pick them when he comes down."

"We can slice them and dry them."

"Good." Charles looks at his watch. "But right now I think is about time for Miranda to get here for your lesson." Since late August, I have been taking singing lessons from a voice coach who comes to the house and patiently teaches me scales and exercises and Italian art songs. She presses me to sing even when the mouth sores are tearing into the tender membranes lining my throat.

I remember my childhood craving to become an opera singer. My brother and I were taken to opera, symphony, and theater, but as for career choices, the arts didn't appear on the list of possibilities. Contributing to the social good of the greater community was a value we learned through watching our parents, who were deeply involved in social policy issues and political action. Yet despite that potent influence, for my first two years of college I majored in theater, acting, and stage design.

**Hints to help you beat the odds . . . follow your bliss!**

In the words of the great scholar Joseph Campbell, "I say, follow your bliss and don't be afraid, and doors will open where you didn't know they were going to be."[4] This is the time to actually do whatever you have yearned to do but haven't. Whether it's opera, baseball, traveling, or simply slowing down to *be*, this is the time. *Carpe diem!* (Seize the day!)

I left shortly thereafter to marry, and when we moved from Montreal to New York with our young family, I would push the stroller past rehearsal halls, listening to divas and would-be divas practicing scales, watching the outdoor back stage of the Provincetown Playhouse on MacDougal Street from our fire escape and dreaming of having the fortitude to one day plunge back into the world of theater and opera. Yet it was not to be. I had grown more timid and couldn't imagine balancing baby and playschool schedules with rehearsals and voice lessons. More than that, however, was the unspoken expectation to give back to my community.

Ten years later, when I started my third year of college, I switched my major to the classics: Greek and Latin. It seemed a more academic pursuit than dramatic arts, if not more altruistic. Were I asked to trace the trail of obscure logic that brought me to the conclusion that there was an intrinsic social worth to studying fifth-century Attic Greek, I would be hard pressed to do so.

The ink on that diploma was barely dry before I announced my intention to return to school, this time to become a certified nurse-midwife. So now, after years of welcoming slippery new lives into my gloved hands, of listening and offering counsel to fellow travelers suffering various maladies of hearts and minds and spirits, I am answering my craving for song. Miranda, blessed with a powerful and rich voice and eager to share her love of music, is my guide.

In late November, she urges me to attend the Naked Voice, a workshop in San Francisco led by Chloe Goodchild, a voice therapist from England. I agree, so on Friday night, she and I stay at the Adelaide Inn on Isadora Duncan Lane, an area surrounded by massage parlors' blinking red neon signs inviting passersby to come in for a hot tub and massage, and by hookers wearing short shorts and strutting back and forth trolling for lonely men. At the end of the narrow lane, the inn's door leads into a small lobby dominated by life-size stand-up paper dolls of Elvis Presley and Marilyn Monroe. The man at the desk gives us the key, and we lug ourselves and our bags up the narrow, carpeted stairs.

Against my better judgment, we have dim sum for dinner at a restaurant called Tan Kiang, and I hope that the fat of the shrimp and the dough wraps won't start the gallbladder irritation. The night passes without an attack, and I plan to give my GI system a rest the following day by limiting my intake to steamed vegetables.

"Oh, I want to go right back to that wonderful place we went to yesterday," Miranda exclaims happily the next day. "I can't wait to sample more of those delicious little mysteries!"

How can I dampen her enthusiasm with my overly cautious dietary concerns? Without disclosing my reservations, we return to Tan Kiang, and I eat only enough to avoid drawing attention to myself. Once again, the child of the dream comes back, the child who suffers pain all night long because she doesn't want to disturb anyone to get help. And here I am again, grown up, with the same unresolved issues keeping me from doing what I need to take care of myself.

**Hints to help you beat the odds . . . speaking up . . .**

You need to speak up about what you need. Family and friends cannot read your mind, and they undoubtedly want to make choices that will not compromise your well-being. They want to be helpful, but they need some direction from you.

When the workshop ends at six o'clock, Miranda suggests we meet Charles for supper at a café on the coast. When we arrive at the restaurant, Charles is already speaking to the chef about a no-fat meal for me, and we are assured that the chicken breast, pears, and steamed vegetables will be entirely without added fat.

I crawl into bed as soon as we arrive home. I have barely fallen asleep when my outrageous defiance of the gods is answered by the onset of the worst attack I have known. I can't speak through the intensity of the pain and can only groan and grunt and crawl about the house, trying to get comfortable. Charles stays with me, holding me, rubbing me, comforting me. He insists on calling the advice nurse, who tells him that I can take two Vicodin every three hours. The medication only takes the sharp edge off the pain. A blustery rainstorm helps distract me as I lean against the dining room window and watch the creek roaring wildly by. Curling up on the sofa some time after midnight, I am able to doze.

The following night, I have another attack starting around two AM, and this time the Vicodin eventually takes care of it. I doze during the early morning hours, but by noon, the stabbing cramps return. I am exhausted from the pain, the lack of sleep, and the relentless regularity with which these assaults are occurring.

That night, following a few hours of respite, the pain resumes and, despite medications and comfort measures, persists until early morning. Charles insists we go to the hospital, but I fight back, refusing to leave home.

"They talk about a gallbladder attack so bad you'll need emergency surgery." His voice rises in panic. "Isn't this what they're talking about?"

"I don't know!" Finding it hard to think, I am panic stricken by my inability to problem solve.

Starting to abate around seven, after a few hours of quiet, the pain suddenly escalates with an intensity that leaves me, as well as Charles, frightened. He picks up the car keys and drapes a jacket around my shoulders.

"No, please, I want to stay here."

"But we have to do something! You can't keep going like this!" The desperation in his voice dwindles as a new idea occurs to him. "Do you want to see Mark, the herbalist who says he has a nonsurgical cure for gallstones?

"Yes," I concede, "please, as soon as I can."

It is Sunday, but Charles leaves a message at the office. Feeling sad and scared and frustrated, I am also feeling dizzy and have difficulty staying up more than five or ten minutes. The pain abates by evening, and I sleep through the night.

At nine thirty the next morning, the stabbing pain under my ribs starts again, and by the time I get to the herbalist's for a ten o'clock appointment, I cannot sit still. He is late, but an office attendant, after giving me two herbal tablets, presses points on my feet and hands, providing relief for as long as she maintains the pressure.

Mark arrives around eleven o'clock and inserts numerous acupuncture needles, which he then hooks up to electricity. Despite having taken no allopathic medications, the pain becomes bearable. At his direction, I take two more herbal tablets and wait in the waiting room while he treats another patient. A short time later, the pain returns in full force. The assistants again apply the pressure points, making it bearable, but I am beginning to panic. He tells me to continue taking the herbal tablets every two hours as long as the attack lasts.

At home by midafternoon, the agony continues. I take Vicodin and at four o'clock, two more herbal tablets. Charles applies pressure to the points on my feet; I take two more herbal tablets at six o'clock, and by seven o'clock, desperate, I take another Vicodin. Still in pain forty-five minutes later, I take yet another pain pill. Wondering if the herbal formula has prolonged or exacerbated this attack, I decide not to take any more. With Charles hovering nearby, I doze on and off. He is an immense comfort to me, a healing presence. By nine o'clock, the pain fades to a mild ache.

Exhausted from the relentless attacks, we sleep soundly through the moonless night, dense, gray clouds gathering low in the sky. Waking in the morning, the absence of discomfort is noticeable. Relaxing into my painfree body, delirious with relief, I get ready for my appointment at the oncology clinic.

When I describe the pattern of this last week's recurrent attacks and particularly the violent one that occurred yesterday, the nurse specialist surmises that the building intensity of that pain probably signaled the passing of a stone. She checks the ultrasound results and confirms that there are "many large stones." Like the surgeons, she fears my ability to withstand emergency surgery should it become necessary. She makes a follow-up appointment with the surgeons to review the risks and benefits of elective surgery.

Grateful for these long hours of respite and feeling "guardedly joyous" with each day that passes without the return of pain, Charles agrees with my inclination to take no more of the herbal remedy as long as the attacks stay in abeyance. Realizing just how much of my life energy vanished in the turmoil of that constant pain, I wonder, *Had I known the rewards would have been so enormously satisfying, might I have made different choices earlier?*

Remembering my child self in that dream, I wonder why it is so hard to ask for help when I need it, so hard to take care of myself when doing so might inconvenience or disappoint someone else. Had I admitted to Miranda my hesitation to return for dim sum that Saturday, and my concerns that the food might be the catalyst for another attack, she would have been more than happy to adjust her sights to a supper of simpler food. Yet my need to not disappoint her must have been greater than my need to reduce the risk of another attack. In short, my fear was outweighed by my perversion of social convention and by wanting to avoid drawing attention to my need.

**Hints to help you beat the odds . . . speaking the truth . . .**

Be direct about saying what you need. Don't be the legendary Spartan youth who maintains his composure while a fox under his jacket gnaws at his belly, eviscerating him.[5]

Subsequent to the many hours and days consumed by the chaos of gallbladder attacks, we eagerly grab normal experiences anywhere we can. The garden, our peaceful refuge, is also the source of various foods. Gathering the pomegranates that split in the rainstorm, Charles brings them in and follows my directions for squeezing out juice that shimmers like liquid rubies. He pours it into clean jars, seals it, and stores it on the long, wooden shelves in the garage.

That evening we play Scrabble in front of the fire, the stream racing through the darkness on the other side of the windows. For the first time since the crisis of the last attack, I take more herbal pills, one before and one after a dinner of crackers and small bits of smoked salmon. Joan Baez's old hits ("Diamonds and Rust," "Jesse, Come Home," and "Forever Young") draw me back twenty years, when I was a young mother with two children full of strength and promise and laughter. I recall the hopefulness of the times, and the woefully mistaken belief that I, too, would be forever young, energetic, and healthy.

# *Chapter 10*

# Fading Strength

## DREAMING PARADOX

### *December 1996*

*On the table are two celadon bowls with graceful curves that would fit nicely into cupped hands. The steaming oatmeal that fills them is strewn with chopped apples and roasted hazelnuts. I hold another bowl containing a magical healing substance, which I have been directed to sprinkle over what is already in the bowls. Not knowing what this substance contains, I reluctantly add it to the bowls' contents.*

*Charles finishes his quickly and only a very few minutes pass before he grabs his stomach, exclaiming, "I am suddenly having really strong cramps!" Although I feel nothing unusual, I am eating more slowly and have consumed less than half of the cereal.*

*Charles falls to the floor moaning, and I realize that I have poisoned him with the magic potion, the potion that supposedly heals.*

*"Oh, my God," I cry. "What's happening to you?"*

*"I don't know," he groans, closing his eyes, "but I'll be OK."*

*I am afraid to tell him that I think that the potion may actually be toxic.*

*"I can't believe I gave this stuff to you . . . it was supposed to heal! But . . ."*

*"It's probably cleaning something out of me," he gasps, "and, when I recover, I'll undoubtedly be the healthier for it."*

*Feverish with dread, I lie next to him and hold him close.*

Have I brought to our table the poison of my dream? Reaching for Charles in the night, I feel the warmth of his body, the sturdy aliveness of it. Sensing my touch, he wraps his arms around me and whispers, "I love you." Relieved to be separating from the dream, to find him healthy and close to me in our familiar bed, I tell him, "I love you, too." This is my zone of safety, my place of comfort. Knowing full well the illusory nature of this refuge in his arms, I am aware that these times are unpredictable and without guarantees. The chemo is taking a dreadful toll on my body, yet I want to complete the next and last cycle.

Early in the morning, some time after the dream, I am awakened again by blisters in my mouth and the sting of cracking on my lips. Rubbing my eyes, they burn, feeling as if they have turned inside out.

The pyramid of symptoms is about to topple me: For the last several days, all the side effects are unusually pronounced. My mouth, throat, and esophagus are now so tender that I cannot even get much water down; every time I swallow, I feel as if glass shards are being thrust down my throat. My recent lab results continue to reflect a depleted immune system. For several weeks, I have been nearly quarantined, admonished to stay away from all but intimate family, and cautioned to eat only carefully cooked food. Reviewing this breakdown of my body, suddenly the dream returns: the dream potion harming Charles, despite the expectations that it will heal, the chemo damaging my body in scurrilous ways, despite its prescription to restore health.

**For your information . . . diarrhea . . .**

Diarrhea is a common plague of patients undergoing chemotherapy, as the cells lining the gut are rapidly dividing and thus particularly susceptible to the cytotoxic agents. A potentially grave side effect of diarrhea is dehydration. Rapid and excessive fluid loss or dehydration, as well as an electrolyte imbalance and malnutrition, can be a serious condition. It is possible that these side effects will force you into the hospital to receive hydration and electrolytes by IV.[1]

Nauseated, bent over with cramps and diarrhea, I feel too miserable to get up for any prolonged period and instead wear thin the path

**Hints to help you beat the odds . . .**
**when you have diarrhea . . .**

- Eat a low-residue, high-protein, high-calorie diet.
- Avoid spicy foods, beans, dairy, caffeine, alcohol, and tobacco.
- Increase your fluid intake to eight to twelve glasses of water a day; clear liquids such as apple juice, ginger ale, tea, and broth guard against irritation in the bowels.
- Eliminate milk products if they seem to be an irritant.
- Avoid foods that are difficult to digest, such as cabbage, broccoli, cauliflower, and corn in order to give the bowels a rest.
- Eat bananas, potatoes, and meats to maintain normal levels of potassium, which is needed for muscles, including the heart, to function properly.
- Be aware of and report diminished urinary output.
- Practice good hygiene, especially after each episode of diarrhea; ask your physician or nurse practitioner about using a "sitz bath" after bowel movements.
- Rest and reduce activity during bouts of diarrhea.[2]

between the bed and bathroom. I manage to get down a teaspoon or two of helim, a smooth and nourishing Persian gruel that is also comforting. It stays down, but the nausea escalates, and I accept Charles's offer of pot from the carved brass pipe. Two puffs are sufficient to take the edge off the nausea and allow me to sleep without feeling the sickening rocking of a storm-tossed boat on high seas.

**Hints to help you beat the odds . . .**
**dealing with nausea and vomiting . . .**

- Try using relaxation and guided imagery to avert nausea and vomiting before they start.
- Eat foods at room temperature.
- Eat small, frequent meals throughout the day.
- Rinse your mouth before and after meals.
- Drink cold, clear liquids.
- Avoid spicy, greasy, or pungent foods.
- Avoid eating for two hours before chemotherapy.[3]

Still feeling weak and dizzy, I am unable to go to the pottery studio this morning. Last week, Charles, reluctant to let me drive because of my weakness and fatigue, waited outside while I worked, afraid to leave me in case of another crisis. I assured him that I would be all right and promised I would call him if I needed him, yet was relieved that he insisted on staying.

Then, as now, the nausea overwhelmed me at unexpected moments, leaving me shaky and bewildered. Stopping often to sit or even lie down on the wooden benches on the deck, I work slowly on the angel series. The second angel's wings and gown had cracked badly, and her halo had slipped down to her right cheek. Her body was breaking in a progression similar to the dismantling I feel in my own.

Looking down now, I notice that the tiny pink washboards of my fingernails are changing as well. The crenellations of the last few months were largely cosmetic and didn't impair the strength of the nails themselves. Now, however, they are weak and friable. They break at the slightest touch. Even the surfaces are rough, and there are repeating thin arcs of dried nail clustered about the moon.

Several days ago, Luke arrived, bringing high spirits, delicious cooking, and wonderful stories. He and Charles harvested the first crop of persimmons, and then began slicing and drying them. Though I was unable to join them, it was a relief to be distracted by the earthy needs of the garden. Too tired to stand up, let alone help in the kitchen, I have been languishing on the sofa or, when it's warm enough, outside on the chaise.

Today, I will be waving good-bye to Luke. Having him here is so deeply healing, yet during this visit I have been too sick to be very responsive and have found myself at times hoping he isn't disappointed that I'm not more fun. Wanting to be as well as possible, I push myself to rally until he leaves, when I will let myself collapse. Taking breakfast on the patio, I find that I must recline rather than sit at the table. It's pleasant just being in their company and listening to their chitchat, even if I am not contributing to the conversation.

Midmorning, my Uncle Max and Aunt Pat come to say good-bye to Luke, and we all congregate in the front yard for the send-off. My aunt hugs him good-bye, and after promising, "I'll check back on my way home," she sets off to the neighborhood swimming pool for her daily laps.

Starting to walk out to the car with Luke and Charles, I am stopped by dizziness and giddily slide down to lie on the warm bricks. Waving off their concern, "I'm just a wee bit tired it seems!" I shoo them on their way. Before the car is out of sight, my uncle looks down on me.

"Now what's happening to you, honey?" His voice echoes the frown of concern.

"Just tired, I guess." Trying to sound offhand, I not only don't want to call attention to myself but also don't want to believe that anything serious is the matter. These last months it seems as if the people I love have given up their own lives in order to help me through mine, yet I want to not need them any more. I want them to be able to resume their lives before they become impatient and fed up with my endless and voracious needs. And I don't want to be sick, sicker than I already am. My Scottish grandmother's admonitions come to mind: "Keep your chin up"; "Pull yourself up by your bootstraps"; "God helps those who help themselves"; "A good laugh and a long sleep are the best cures."

He looks skeptical. "You look more than tired to me."

Trying to reassure myself, I offer, "I probably just need a nap. . . . But I'm a little tipsy when I stand up," I admit.

"Well, let me help you get back inside." He leans down and begins to lift me up. "Is Charles coming right home from the airport?"

"Yes. He should be back in an hour or so." Hobbling back into the house on his arm, I add, "And also, Pat said she'd stop by here on her way home from the pool. I'm just tired from the chemo."

"Are you done with that yet?" He helps me lower myself to the sofa.

Speaking through the sharp pain of mouth sores, I answer, "No, but close; my last cycle begins at the end of the month!"

"I'll be so glad when you're done with this."

"Me, too." I hesitate before saying, "Just think, if this is what it's doing to the parts of my body that I can see and feel, imagine what it's doing to those cancer cells!" In my mind's eye, I see the dream potion tearing through my tissues, ferociously gobbling up any wayward cells.

"Well, that's right . . . it must be really blasting them!" He sits down in a chair facing me. I can tell that he's questioning the prudence of leaving me alone.

"I'm OK," I tell him, "I promise you I'm OK . . . and I don't want to keep you from your gardening any longer!" It takes a lot of effort to speak this much, but I am trying not to betray the extent of my discomfort.

After a pause, he seems to have made up his mind. "Well, I think I'll just hang around for a while myself." His tone of voice invites no argument.

In minutes I am asleep and awaken later to hear him speaking softly with Pat. Seeing my eyes open, she asks hesitantly, "Do you have the energy for Scrabble?"

Before I can reply, Max remands, "Of course she doesn't! She can hardly lift her head off the pillow." I want to be able to play, but the energy required to move tiles from the holder to the board suddenly seems Olympian.

"Right now, I'll just do a few things in the kitchen." I can hear Pat starting a load of laundry, putting away clean dishes, and taking out the garbage. The hum of activity is comforting, and they are right, I realize—it is helpful to have them here, to not be alone right now. Max is outside weeding the garden when Charles comes home.

**Hints to help you beat the odds . . . giving up control . . .**

One of your challenges might be to surrender control of your household during the time you are indisposed. For some, it is nearly impossible to give up the reins, but if you can turn over some of those chores to someone else, it allows you to further focus on your own healing.

"Well, I should have known you two would be here taking care of things!" Charles smiles. "I don't know how we'd manage without you."

"Oh, you would!" Pat laughs, uncomfortable with the most modest expression of gratitude. "But now I think we'll go. Let us know how she does . . . we're here if you need us."

I doze on and off until late afternoon, when I get up to go to the bathroom, not because I need to go, but because I assume my bladder must be full by now. I take two or three steps, feel suddenly faint, and slip down into a chair. I haven't the strength to call for Charles, who is in the kitchen. It seems a labor just to get breath, and there is none left over for speaking. Standing up after a minute or two in the chair, I topple right back into it. Still feeling faint, I slide down onto the floor, and crawl back to the sofa. *Is the toxic potion of my dream seeping into the physical mass of my body?* I wonder. *Has the healing part evaporated entirely?*

"What happened?" I hear Charles behind me as I am stretching out.

"I'm just feeling faint . . . I'm not sure why. But . . . could you call Clara? I think if she could take my blood pressure . . ." Speculating that my inability to eat and drink has led to dehydration, and that the dehydration has led to low blood pressure, and that the low blood pressure is making me feel dizzy and light-headed in any but the total recumbent position, I am finally putting together the pieces of this puzzle. And of course, no intake of fluids means no output of fluids.

While we are waiting for my cousin Clara to arrive, I ask Charles to get my stethoscope and blood pressure monitor from my work satchel. Arriving shortly after Charles's call, Clara hears only silence when she listens through the earpiece. When I am standing, when I am sitting, and when I am lying down, she hears only a faint, irregular pulse with her fingers on my wrist but discerns no blood pressure reading at all. Concerned about my depleted fluid volume, I am also relieved to have an explanation for this array of symptoms.

**For your information . . . orthostatic hypotension . . .**

Orthostatic hypotension can result from decreased intravascular fluids, which, in turn, can be a result of dehydration. Symptoms of orthostatic hypotension generally occur after sudden standing and include dizziness, lightheadedness, blurred vision, and syncope (temporary loss of consciousness).[4]

"Well," Clara offers, "I think your suspicions are correct."

"But it has taken me so long to get there! It's so obvious now, but it should have been clear days ago." I am embarrassed not to have discerned the meanings behind the symptoms.

"Shouldn't we take you to the hospital now?" they ask in unison.

Knowing it's after hours, I weigh the possibilities in my head. "No, not tonight."

"What do you mean, 'Not tonight'?" Exasperation adds an edge to Charles's voice.

"Tonight the only option is the ER, and I'm afraid of it." I realize my body is telling me clearly that there is something wrong, yet I fear that presenting at the ER might be more likely to harm than heal. The dream flashes by, the dream of the potion that promises to heal, yet assails Charles with grabbing stomach pains.

"I know you're scared, honey, but I feel as if we need help." I can hear fear in his voice as he speaks.

I recall that maxim "The first step to health is to know that we are sick." *I recognize I am sick*, I think to myself, *I am not deluding myself about that anymore. It's just that . . . my memories of those tortuous ER visits are vivid.*

"As soon as morning comes, I'll call the advice nurse . . . I promise. And I'll be able to see my own doctors instead of strangers or even worse, that Dr. Metzger in the ER!"

"Is he the one that kept sending her home?" Clara asks Charles.

"He's the one," Charles affirms. "I feel sick when I think about it." He turns to me, "OK, we can wait until morning . . . but promise me you'll tell me if you start to feel worse."

"I promise."

Tired yet restless, I am unable to sleep. I read for a while and at 3 a.m. roll out of bed and crawl to the kitchen. Swinging the basket of remaining persimmons down to the floor, I settle onto the cool tiles to peel and slice the fruit, laying them out on the drying racks and sliding them into the oven. Every minute or two, I tip to my side and stretch out, pleasingly invigorated as the blood finds its way to my head, fortifying me to once again sit up, peel, and slice. I work in this stop-and-start fashion until 6:45, when I hobble back to bed. Satisfied and tired out by the activity, I am able to doze until eight o'clock, when I call the advice nurse. I give my pertinent health history and list recent signs and symptoms:

- a week of chemo completed on November 1
- since last Saturday, dizziness as soon as I stand up
- inability to either eat or drink because of stomatitis
- severe nausea until yesterday
- last identifiable meal six days ago
- inability to drink more than about six ounces of water daily
- inability to sleep for last three nights
- watery diarrhea for the last four days
- beeling of inability to get adequate oxygen and having to labor to breathe.

Astonished that I have waited so long to call, her voice is sympathetic, "You must be feeling terrible! You need to come in to the ER for rehydration."

"I've had some terrible experiences in the ER." Expecting a protest, I wait before continuing, "I'd rather see Dr. Liu than a doctor I don't know."

"Well, let me see if I can locate him." Her willingness to hear me, to listen, helps me to relax, assuaging my fear.

> **Hints to help you beat the odds . . .**
> **telling your story . . . again . . .**
>
> Instead of assuming that you won't be heard, or that the person on the other end of the telephone hasn't the time to listen to you, go ahead and tell your story—be succinct but also complete in the telling.

"I'm going to put you on hold while I try to find him. OK?" Her kind voice is a balm.

Very quickly, she returns. "Well, Dr. Liu is not coming in today, but I spoke with the oncology nurses, and they want you to come in to be seen by the oncologist on call. Does that sound OK to you?"

"Oh, yes. That's fine. I just don't want to go to the ER."

"I understand."

"When shall I come in?" *Why do I ask this*, I wonder. *When I know the answer?*

That part of me that is so afraid of overstating my case recoils at the possibility of dramatizing the commonplace. When I was very young, and prone to bellowing out the injustices that curbed my wont, my mother, Tashie, called me Brunhilde, the tempestuous Wagner heroine, and urged me to settle down, dismissing my outrage with reminders that I was being overdramatic. Yes, I know now that I am sick and in need of professional intervention. Yet knowing that, I also hear a voice challenging me, *Aren't you overreacting to this? Are you really that sick?*

"Come in as soon as you can." The friendly voice brings me back to the present moment.

"OK. Thanks. Really, thank you for being so nice." By now, I am used to my own doctors' kindness and consideration, but I am still surprised when a stranger extends herself and seems to understand and acknowledge my terrors. Perhaps this kindness is the good part of the dream potion, the part that heals.

Stumbling to the bathroom, I am totally shocked at the image in the mirror. Like many terminal cancer patients, I am gaunt and pallid. Alarmed, I cry out and tears slide down my dry cheeks. Charles, also crying, holds me close. Driving across the mountains, I feel scared at how sick I feel, how almost "not alive." *Am I dying?* I wonder. *Is this how dying happens? Just fading away, getting weaker and smaller and more transparent?*

*But what about the magic potion? The healing potion? Is the magic turning on me, becoming its opposite?* The dream image of Charles writhing on the floor makes me shudder, but I am reassured to see his robust reflection in the mirror.

Once in the oncology clinic, I slump down in the chair, my head on Charles's shoulder. *I want that magic dream potion to heal me*, I think to myself. *I need some magic to save me.*

Opening my eyes, I see the nurse hurrying down the hall toward me. She takes my hand in hers and coos sympathetically, "You really look green!" She starts to help me up but stops herself. "I'm getting you a wheelchair . . . I'm amazed you managed to get up here from the car park!"

She wheels me down to the exam room, where I gratefully lie down on the table. Sitting close to me, Charles holds my hand and strokes my brow, soothing and comforting me.

The new doctor introduces himself, shakes hands, and asks me to tell him why I came in. He is patient and listens carefully as I describe the symptoms. I never feel rushed. He then asks, "Is there anything more? Do you have any questions?"

When I say no, he looks me squarely in the eye and says, "We need to bring you in to be taken care of."

"Do you mean I need to be admitted?" I ask.

Speaking clearly and forcefully, he says, "Yes, you do."

I ask about trying rehydration on an outpatient basis, and he replies, "You really need to be admitted . . . there are too many things going on, and if we compromise now, we may end up with a much more severe problem later."

My fear of being an inpatient is balanced by my fear of the consequences should I continue to resist. "I'm ready," I admit, "I understand." As the seconds pass, I realize I am grateful to have this decision taken out of my hands and begin to anticipate feeling better with fluids. Tired of self-care and self-diagnosis, ready to surrender control to this doctor and this institution, I scrawl a wobbly signature on the admission papers.

After about an hour, I am wheeled up to an inpatient oncology room, given a gown, and tucked into bed. An RN makes three painful attempts to start the IV, wiggling the needle around each time. Knowing my veins are collapsed from the dehydration, I try to be patient and brave. When I run out of both patience and bravery, I ask her if an IV team might help; she decides to call in a colleague.

A second nurse succeeds on the first try and opens the line to run a liter in fast (a "bolus"). When it finishes, a nurse from the new shift starts another liter, this time at a much slower drip of 125 cubic centimeters an hour. Knowing my orders include a bolus of two liters before slowing the drip, I ask for the second, but she says I have already gotten the two.

"No, I have received only one," I insist, surprised at my own persistence. Eager for the IVs that will wash me out of this desert wasteland, my mouth has the same cottony dryness that marked the dehydration associated with my original bowel obstruction.

She checks the chart, and the day-shift nurse has written that I got two liters before the change of shift. Desperate to get more fluids fast, I swear that I have not. She believes me and switches the rate to an open line. Later she comes in to say that the day nurse, reached at home, remembered that she wrote "two" when she *planned* to start the second liter but that her charting got ahead of her actual care, and she left before starting the new bag. I am exonerated but more than that, I start to feel better as the fluid sweeps through my arid body. The magic dream potion is healing me. When the resident comes in a few hours later, I ask him to increase the rate further, as my mouth is still dry, and my bladder empty. When he opens the line, I am flooded with relief.

**Hints to help you beat the odds . . .**
**speaking up when your ally is not there . . .**

Speaking up for ourselves can be a challenge, especially to women, who have been socially groomed to be compliant. Yet now, although having an advocate is ideal, you might have to push yourself to speak up to make your needs known.

Someone takes my blood pressure. The lower number, the diastolic, is thirty-seven at first, and then in the forties on the second measurement. The low blood pressure is another indication of the fluid depletion.

At about eight thirty, seven-plus hours after the start of the IV infusion, I finally urinate. The fluids being pumped through me are rains pummeling the thirsty earth after a long drought.

By midmorning, after several liters of fluid, I am feeling better. Unable to eat and uninterested in food, I am nonetheless fascinated by the food shows on TV and watch the cooking channel the entire day, jotting down recipes and listening to various chefs describe the latest combinations and culinary conceits.

A small green bowl on the TV screen reminds me of the dream, of the magic food that I thought would heal but which seems to poison. *Is my body being poisoned by the chemicals that are prescribed to save me from the invading cells?* I wonder. The nature of chemotherapy for cancer suggests a resounding *Yes*. Yet the question is, *Is the magic potion balanced in such a way that its healing properties can offset concurrent injuries to healthy cells?*

By the following afternoon, steady on my feet and no longer lightheaded, I am on my way home. Once again, I am astonished at the magic of fluids and remember all those articles urging us to drink more water.

**For your information . . . the importance of water . . .**

Functions of water in the body include:[5]

- regulating temperature
- moistening tissues such as those in the mouth, eyes, and nose
- lubricating joints
- protecting body organs and tissues
- helping prevent constipation
- flushing out waste products
- helping dissolve minerals and other nutrients to make them accessible to the body
- carrying nutrients and oxygen to cells.

Knowing that the mouth sores may again lead to dehydration, I am nevertheless comforted in knowing that the remedy is relatively painless, and the relief is rapid. In the days that follow, I am astounded and impressed at how quickly my body continues to heal.

A week after my discharge, Luke and Vanessa come back for a few days for an early Christmas celebration. Feeling cold even in the warmth of the heated house, I wrap myself in woolens and thick fleece and take the chill off my bald head with a knit woolen hat. Noticing that Luke is wearing shiny blue swimming trunks and nothing else, I think it's one of his silly jokes and ask him, "What's up?"

"What's up? You ask!" He laughs, slapping his knee. "What's up?! This place s a steam bath! It must be ninety degrees in here!"

"It is?" Once accustomed to a cool house and open windows, I have forgotten that this house, in deference to my chronic chill, is now kept sealed and heated like a Finnish sauna.

Two days later, Andrew, Rebecca, and the kids arrive. After a round of hugs, the kids charge in to the playroom, greeting their toys like long-lost friends. The wooden train set, the orange velour lion, the purple velour elephant, and the furry brown bunny puppet are all greeted with delight. The dress-up trunk is opened, and Rose pulls a bright-pink tutu over her head, while Nico drapes a tiger patterned fabric over his shoulders, holding it together with a wide silver knight's belt studded with glass rubies.

Tonight Luke cooks blue mountain stew and French bread, and Max, Pat, and a bevy of cousins join us for supper. Lying back on the sofa, I delight in watching the generations mingling and reconnecting. Cynthia starts working with some origami papers, and before long, we have an array of miniature frogs and lobsters and cranes hanging from the tree. *Who will be hanging ornaments on this tree next year?* I wonder. The word *next*, as in next month, next year, assumes a new dimension, a suggestion that whatever "next" is, I might not be here to experience it. Letters from the symphony, opera, and theater, urging us to reserve tickets for the next season, remind me that planning ahead requires an assumption of continuing to *be*, an assumption in which I have lost confidence.

Looking around the room at all these faces that I love, I wonder whether I am carrying this disease for all of them. These colon cancer genes live in me somehow, and because I have them, perhaps neither Luke nor any of the cousins will have to be troubled by them. *You don't have to have this cancer because I am doing it for you!* I hope this can be true, that none of them will have to ever hear this diagnosis.

Luke and Vanessa leave a few days before Christmas, to get home to their children. Hours later, Andrew and Rebecca arrive with Nico and Rose. On Christmas Eve, Rebecca helps Nico set out cookies, tangerines, and hot cocoa for Santa Claus. After Rose is tucked into her crib, Nico dictates a letter:

> Dear Santa,
>
> How are you? We are fine. I hope you are fine. I hope your reindeer are not too tired. Here is some popcorn for them. And cookies for you that we made with Mommy. The cloth is to wipe the soot off your face. I love you Santa. From Nico.

I read *The Polar Express* to Nico while Rebecca finishes some Christmas projects, and then *The Night Before Christmas* when he is tucked in and eager for the night to pass. Before falling asleep myself, I take up the flannel patchwork quilt I am making for Rose and sew a few stitches.

Christmas morning is filled with magic, and my heart is overflowing with love and thanks for the blessings of family, for their presence in my life. Rose finds a big wooden dollhouse under the tree and leans down to look inside it, saying to herself, "Oh, my house! This is my house." She runs into the playroom, coming back with her arms full of wooden figures that were once Zoë's and Andrew's. She puts the cowardly lion into the little wooden bathtub because he needs a bath and puts the tin woodman into the bunk bed because he is very tired. Then she takes all the furniture and the dolls out of the house and proceeds to climb in as she proclaims, "This is my house, and I am going to live here!" Squeezing her head and shoulders into the living room area, she is unable to get further in and pauses, reminiscent of Alice in Wonderland, having eaten the cake that makes her grow and trying to fit herself into the tiny door leading to the magical garden.

Under the tree, Nico finds bookends painted with rainforest frogs, snakes, and dragonflies; a lizard switch plate; and a large carved wooden frog to put on his bedroom wall. Thrilled, he clutches the irregular shape to his chest, crooning: "Oh, I love my fwog! I am so happy! I just love him!" Watching him dance with the frog, and hearing the appreciation and exuberance in his voice, I savor every minute.

Still holding the frog in one arm, Nico picks up a large roughly wrapped parcel and hands it to Rose. "This is for you, Rosie! I made this for you!"

He helps her tear the paper off to reveal a large gingerbread man made from a common paper grocery bag. Two pieces have been cut into the shape of a gingerbread cookie and then sewn together with green wool yarn. Stuffing puffs him out a bit, and a cranberry-colored velvet bowtie rests at his throat. Bright-brown button eyes glance at the excited children, and three more grayish buttons mark the center of his chest.

"Oh, my gingerbread man!" Rose exclaims, as she picks him up and starts dancing. "I love my gingerbread man!" she chants as she nestles her head against the crackly brown paper. Moved by the enchantment that brings the gingerbread man to life, I am reminded of the magic potion of the dream. Not only do I need the *magic* of the dream potion, but I also need the *belief*, the faith that will allow the transformation of the dream into reality.

Seeing the fairy-tale toy he worked so hard to create come to life in

Rosie's arms, Nico smiles broadly, and then joins her dance, the frog hugged to his chest.

"Oh, my froggie," Nico murmurs happily.

"Oh, my gingerbread man!" Rose exclaims joyously, holding him out in front of her, waltzing at arms' length as she admires him.

They are tired tonight after the excitement of Christmas, and Rebecca reads to them and sings them to sleep early. I lie down with them, thankful for their sweet beings, thankful for every minute they are with me. Feeling their chubby little arms wrapped around my neck, I pray to live for them, to be with them as they grow up, to love them always. The thought of not being here next year, of this being my last Christmas, hurls a black stone into the pit of my stomach.

Later, when Rebecca is cooking dinner and I, in my slow way, am helping her, Charles comes in and suggests, "Think there's something a little funky going on with Stella?"

I haven't noticed it until now, but once he intimates that Stella might have had an accident, I can suddenly detect the telltale aroma. "I think you speak the truth!" I laugh as he helps me up off the stool.

We go into the bathroom and find that the colostomy seal has broken all around. Perhaps the paste might be losing its effectiveness. He helps me clean up and apply a new flange and bag.

"I can't believe how wonderful you are about all this," I tell him. "Not only do you tell me when Stella's *acting* up—you help me *clean* her up!" Putting my arms around him, I mean it from the bottom of my heart when I say, "I am *so* lucky." We go back into the dining room, where Rebecca is just putting serving dishes on the table, and Andrew is opening a bottle of Montepulciano.

"How lucky we are to have each other," Andrew coincidentally begins, raising his glass, "and to be together now."

Feeling my eyes tear and my throat thicken, I can only nod and smile. Although I know that saying good-bye to them tomorrow will be hard, any regret is balanced by my feeling deeply blessed to have them in my life and to be so thoroughly included in theirs.

This morning, when Andrew and Charles discuss the timing for getting to the airport, Rose says, "I'm staying with Nana."

"I would love that," I tell her, "but you would miss Mommy and Daddy and Nico." If only they lived next door, I think, the children could visit whenever they wanted to.

"Then you come home to San Diego with us!" she insists.

"And I want to show Nana my new bed!" Nico joins in. "When you come to San Diego, you and Papa can share my new bed!"

Being wanted like this raises my cool core temperature, I am sure, better than any central heating can. They don't seem to care that I have neither eyebrows nor eyelashes, and they don't seem to notice the occasional rustling sound under my sweat pants.

When Andrew, Rebecca, and the children leave for the airport, I am in a funk without them. I feel very sad, wondering how many Christmases I have left and whether I might live to see these precious children mature and grow. Knowing so little about what lies ahead, I feel as if inside me lives a time bomb that is ticking off the minutes before a cataclysmic explosion.

Two days after Christmas, I go in for the blood work required before starting my sixth and last cycle of chemo.

**For your information . . . drawing labs . . . again . . .**

Prior to starting each cycle of chemo, labs will be drawn to determine whether your body can tolerate more drugs. They will be examining your bone marrow function as reflected in your levels of red blood cells, white blood cells, and platelets.

I can feel knots in my veins, and in many places, they are tender to the touch. The redness on my left hand persists and reaches up past the wrist. Before we arrive home, there is a message left on the answering machine saying that the complete blood count (CBC), needs to be repeated next week before I can have chemo. By now accustomed to having chemo postponed a week to allow more time for recovery, I can barely recall the alarm and panic I felt last August, before the second cycle, when they told me I couldn't have chemo because my white cells were too low. At the time, it felt as if the magic with which I had imbued chemo was being taken away and with it my chances of survival. Now, however, it just seems a reasonable precaution.

On Monday, my white blood cell count (WBC), has come up to an acceptable level, and I begin my last cycle of chemotherapy. Nervous at the prospect of no longer being on chemo, I ask Dr. Liu, "What happens now? Now that chemo is almost over . . ."

My last chance is coursing through my veins right now, the last chance to infuse my body with the dream potion of healing. My heart pounds in excitement and dread. *Which magic is flooding me?* I wonder. *The elixir of healing? Or is this the potion that kills?*

"Well. I'll see you in two months." He laughs kindly, lifting me out of the dream. "Unless you need to see me sooner than that."

"You mean, if something bad happens?" I can't bear to say the C-word right now.

"Well, yes."

"Nothing bad's going to happen!" I insist. "I'll get well and healthy." Trying to convince myself, I can hear my own desperation.

He is quiet, continuing to prepare my arm for the IV.

"Right?" I prompt him. "I'll get well, don't you think?"

"I hope so," he says softly, "but I really don't know."

This is not what I am looking for.

"But I am relatively young," I press him, "and healthy."

"Age has no bearing on outcome." Surely knowing what I want to hear, he surprises me with his reluctance to paint a bright picture. "We really don't know why some people do well and others don't."

**Hints to help you beat the odds . . .**
**healing may not include curing . . .**

A cure is a treatment or series of treatments that removes all evidence of disease and returns a normal life expectancy to the person cured. Healing can refer to the physical, as the healing of a bone; to the emotional, as the healing from childhood traumas or divorce; or to the spiritual, as when we move toward inner peace and a sense of connection with others and with nature.[6] When your doctor won't make promises to *cure*, that doesn't equal desertion. He or she may still support you and guide you in your *healing*.

We are both silent before he repeats, "We just don't know."

The mystery of this journey suddenly shimmers in those words hovering in the air around me, and I can feel that he is opening my heart to not knowing. There are mysteries we will never understand. Why diminish them with second-guessing?

**Hints to help you beat the odds . . .
treasuring the moment . . .**

However guarded your future, whatever the unknowns, savor the moment you are living now. Instead of counting your remaining days (an impossible task anyway!), live them fully. Even when you go through periods of despair, remind yourself that there may still be good days ahead, periods of remission, when you can luxuriate in feeling well.

On Friday, four days later, the chemo is administered by the same kind physician who admitted me earlier this month for rehydration. After we exchange greetings, my friend Sophie asks him, "Can you tell my friend some good news now?"

"Good news?" He seems surprised and a little confused by her sudden question.

"Yes. We need to hear some optimism about . . ."

"About her prognosis?" he interrupts. "I can tell you that I have tons and tons of patients with your same diagnosis and they're doing fine!"

"Good!" Sophie sits back in her chair and relaxes. "We need to hear that."

*Yes*, I think to myself, *perhaps we do need to hear that.* Even knowing it may be a fantasy. I need to hear the belief in my capacity to heal. Is that faith an element of the dream magic?

Surprisingly, I can be in this place of optimism, rejoicing in this doctor's exuberant prognosis, and at the same time I can surrender myself to the mystery and be comfortable with not knowing, or even guessing.

"Thank you for saying that," I tell him.

"Well, I mean it. You're going to be fine!" He smiles cheerfully.

I float out of the room, smiling broadly at the possibilities that have just been opened to me. Is recovery reachable? I don't know, but I do know that I need the people caring for me to think it is, to believe in the possibility of magic.

# *Chapter 11*
# Ciao, Stella!

## DREAMING RESTORATION

### *March 1997*

*Items spilling from a tapestry satchel onto an unmade bed seem to have a special significance for me, as if I am seeking something. A small cube that I have apparently been looking for drops onto the bed and sparkles like a cut crystal. It is one of a pair, and I must find its mate. After I have been looking unsuccessfully for the missing half of the pair for some time, I begin to panic.*

*A kindly person hands me a short-handled wooden rake, and by this gesture, I feel supported in my quest. It is fashioned like a metal garden rake, with thick, straight tines, but all made of widely spaced wooden dowels. I rake this tool across the bed covers in the hope that it might snag the missing piece.*

*The mood is quiet and intent rather than panicky, even though there is the recognition that this thing I need might be lost forever. At last, the rake pulls toward me in its tines a crystal cube identical to the first one. Sighing with relief, holding the missing piece in one palm and its mate in my other, I feel I have just made a narrow escape.*

The end of chemo is hard for Charles as well, but for other reasons. I have believed that as long as I am on chemo, the cancer cells will be crushed before they have time to grow and multiply. Now that the six cycles are completed, what will keep them at bay? Charles, on the other hand, worries that he'll lose his grounding without his role of caring for me. Now chemo is over, and soon the colostomy will be but a memory. He awakens early and reaches out to hold me. "I don't know what I'll do when you are well," he begins wistfully. "Right now I take care of you and feel useful doing so . . . but when you are well . . ."

His voice trails off, and tears fill his blue eyes. Feeling connected to him in a new way by this disease that pulls us together, my heart swells with love.

By March, six weeks after the last chemo treatment, my hair is starting to grow back in lonely spikes that stand at attention along the center point of my scalp. On the sidewalk, I cast a pinhead shadow that reminds me of the nursery babies who are born with long hair that nurses gather on top of their heads with a wet brush, creating a fine, spiky mohawk. The peach fuzz that appears in patches elsewhere has a stiff quality that suggests it continues to hold on to the chemo. I am eager to shave it all off, to start again, to remove remnants of my toxic siege. Feeling that I need a clean start, a new beginning, I want to let go of the old hair, I want to mark a new beginning. Aunt Pat agrees to give me a buzz cut, and I am relieved to see the wispy tangles drop to the floor. A cleansing is taking place.

These are my last days with Stella. Surgery is scheduled for the end of the month. I have mixed feelings about this operation that will sew shut the colostomy. My bowels will be reattached to resemble the configuration prior to my illness, minus the eight or ten inches removed in the initial surgery. The dream flashes back to me: the anxiety of finding only one of the two crystals, and then the relief of finding the second and reuniting the pair. I have also befriended Stella: Coping with her is a known; wondering whether my bowel will work after nearly a year of dormancy is the unknown.

Although chemo is finished, I continue to feel its effects. Exhaustion plagues me, my joints ache, and my skin continues to feel tender and friable. I am still dripping: dripping nose, dripping eyes, drooling lips, though that is not as constant as the weeping eyes and nose. Continuing to both sing and sculpt, I am acutely aware of my good fortune in being able to devote my hours and days to healing my body and nourishing my spirit.

**Hints to help you beat the odds . . . engaging in activities . . .**

Embarking on a new hobby or starting a new activity, such as enrolling in an adult education class, can be life affirming and help you reestablish your sense of self-worth.

During the pre-op visit, while checking the scars on my belly, both Stella and the long, vertical Ho Chi Minh trail, the surgical resident explains the planned surgery, the reattaching (reanastamosis) of the colon. He helps me into a sitting position, my legs dangling to the side of the exam table, and passes me a clipboard to sign the consent. Handing me a pen, he notes, "Also, we'll be taking out your gallbladder so you won't have any more problems with it."

I stop reading and look up. "But I haven't had any more problems with it. I haven't had an attack since December."

"Well, you had a lot of big gallstones," he insists, "and they don't just disappear."

"But I think they might have." I hesitate before adding, "I've taken herbs for them."

He chuckles kindly. "Herbs don't make them go away though!" Polite in his disagreement, he shifts position in his chair and announces cheerfully, "And as long as we're in there, we might as well take out the gallbladder."

I remember all the tonsils that used to be taken out "just in case," and the uteri and the appendices. "But I don't want a part of me removed unless there's really a reason." I wait in the silence. "If the stones are still there, I'll be happy to have you take it out, but if they aren't?"

"Stones don't just disappear though," he interrupts. The young doctor looks at me with a confused expression. He is being trained to take out organs that are suspicious or troubling. Here is a patient who repeatedly tells the surgeons how grateful she is that they saved her life, yet now she is balking at his recommendation.

"Well, let me speak with Dr. Zang about this."

"I'd appreciate that." In his absence, sitting up straighter on the exam table, I remind myself, *I am only asking questions. I only want to know whether the stones are still there.*

Dr. Zang walks in, and as always, the calm of his presence reassures me. "You've been taking those herbs, whatever they are," he says and smiles. "And now you think they're working?"

"Maybe. I haven't had any attacks since taking them."

"Well, let's get an ultrasound and just check it out." He turns to the young man he is training. "We'll get her on the ultrasound schedule tomorrow morning or maybe even today."

He pushes the button over the exam table, and the door opens. "Yes, doctor?"

"Can you please see if we can get an ultrasound to check on these gallstones? If they can do one today, it would be a big help."

Getting up to leave, he turns to me and smiles. "Well, you never know . . ." His entire demeanor suggests a willingness to listen, an openness to possibilities beyond the expected outcomes.

Suddenly alone, I am excited that I have held my own and relieved that Dr. Zang has been willing to order this test. I shake off the turquoise paper drape and slip my navy linen dress over my head. The nurse returns with good news. "They can see you right now. Take this requisition down the hall past x-ray, and give it to the receptionist."

Mei Ling, the ultrasound technician, covers the probe with warm gel and slides it over my midsection, quadrant to quadrant. She asks me to turn to my side and repeats the back-and-forth appraisal of my belly. Saying nothing beyond giving me directions to turn this way or that, she moves the bed so that my head is lowered and again scans the abdomen.

Putting down the probe, she pushes aside the beige duck curtain and sticks her head out into the room. "Alan, can you come take a look at this?"

*Is she asking for confirmation at finding a mass of huge new stones?* I wonder. *Or is she puzzled that the multiple large stones on the photograph of my last ultrasound have vanished?*

A young man with smooth, black hair and a ready smile walks into the cubicle, takes the probe, and swipes it across my slippery skin. Turning to face Mei Ling, his eyebrows rise up in surprise as he remarks, "I can't find anything at all."

"No, I can't either." She clicks a few keys on the computer board. "But look at these pictures. These are from last October." I am feeling vindicated.

"Are you sure these are her pictures?" he asks doubtfully.

"Um-hmm." She turns to me. "What did you say you were taking? Dr. Zang said you'd been taking some herbs for this."

"A combination of different herbs," I tell them.

The two technicians look at each other. "Well, it seems it worked!" they whisper excitedly. Alan puts down the probe, and Mei Ling starts swiping a white towel across my greased abdomen.

"Of course we're not supposed to tell you the results, but . . ." Mei Ling is unable to contain the excitement in her voice. "All those gallstones are gone! This is amazing!" Helping me off the table, she adds, "Go back to Dr. Zang's office now and he'll discuss the results with you."

Walking down the long hallway to surgery, I smile to myself. Dr. Zang greets me, the envelope of the ultrasound studies in his hand. *How did they get here before I did?* I wonder.

"You probably know by now that the stones are gone! Those people down in ultrasound are so excited they can't stop talking about it." He grins. "I want to learn more about this. I have so many patients who have stones, but they are poor candidates for surgery." He chuckles. "And I'm going to present your case at grand rounds on Wednesday."

"So I don't have to have my gallbladder out?"

"No, you don't. Is that a relief to you?"

"It really is. Silly maybe, but I feel as if I want to hang onto any organ I can." After all, the gallbladder isn't there for nothing! Knowing that it stores bile until it is needed to help with fat digestion, I also know that fat digestion may become less efficient with its removal. And who would want to do anything that might hinder the rapid processing of fats?

"The risks are small, and few people have any long-lasting sequelae." He speaks respectfully and thoughtfully. "But we'll leave it in if you want us to."

"Please, let me keep this one."

So the plan is modified: The bowel will be reconnected, but the gallbladder will stay right where it started out when I was born.

Next I see my oncologist, for a final blessing before the surgery. After he examines me, he ventures, "I'll be out of town next week, in Los Angeles, so I won't be able to visit you while you're in the hospital."

Touched at his concern, I hasten to reassure him, "That's OK . . . I just hope you're going somewhere fun and not to meetings!"

He hesitates before saying, "Well, my daughter Jessica has been nominated for an Academy Award, and—"

"Of course you want to be there!" I break in. "I hope she gets it, and I hope you have a great time!" A combination of modesty and pride light up his face and widen his smile.

Andrew arrives the night before the operation. I have spent the day and night fasting and prepping for surgery with unpleasant bowel-cleansing regimens.

**For your information . . . prepping the bowel . . .**

A clean bowel prior to surgery is very important, allowing the surgeons to view the operative site clearly and reducing the risk that you will get an infection after the operation. Your surgeon will give you a diet sheet to follow, as well as instructions for taking several doses of a strong oral laxative before the surgery.[1]

I check in to the pre-op area at nine in the morning, drop my clothes into a plastic bag with my name scrawled on it in black magic marker, and don the white cotton OR gown printed with navy geometric designs. Charles and Andrew spend the day waiting with me in the pre-op area. Regretting not having tucked in my bag the travel Scrabble game, we read the *New York Times* and work on crossword puzzles. Hours pass, and we are notified of delays caused by emergencies and by surgeries taking longer than anticipated. Andrew and Charles take turns going to the cafeteria for food, but fortunately, my appetite has been quelled by last night's bowel prep.

Some time after nine o'clock in the evening, a nurse comes into the cubicle to announce that I am next to go. I worry that the doctors will be too tired to concentrate, and Andrew is concerned when he learns that I will be having a nurse anesthetist rather than an anesthesiologist.

The parallel that immediately occurs to me is that it's like having a midwife rather than an obstetrician: The midwife and the nurse-anesthetist are trained to treat and care for patients whose medical needs stay within fairly normal parameters, whereas the anesthesiologist, like the obstetrician, can continue caring for a patient whose condition requires higher levels of medical expertise and intervention.

Dr. Zang comes in and, in response to our questions, says that he feels totally comfortable working with this nurse-anesthetist and that if an anesthesiologist is required, there are several in the area who can be pulled in the case of an emergency.

We discuss whether to go ahead with the surgery tonight or to reschedule for the following week. Should I reschedule, Andrew will have to get more time off from work in order to return at a later time, and there is the possibility that he will be unable to stay more than just the day of surgery. And remembering last night's phospho-oral laxative and this morning's enemas, my stomach knots at the prospect of repeating them in a few days. We all decide to go ahead with it, and Andrew steps out to the nurses' station to let them know.

An IV is started, a paper cap is put on my head, and my wedding ring is taped to my finger. The nurse anesthetist, a tired-looking young woman, asks me some questions about allergies. Charles and Andrew kiss me good-bye, and I see the familiar cold overhead suns of the OR drawing closer as I am rolled through the wide doorway. Seconds pass, or so it seems, and I am awakened by Andrew's jubilant voice, "Mom, the surgery went great and Jessica won the Oscar!" Grinning my delight, I drift off.

I awaken later to find my hand clasped in Andrew's and a bouquet of periwinkle iris and creamy tulips nodding from a vase on the bedside table. "The surgery went fine," he repeats, "and Rebecca sends love. Charles has gone down to the cafeteria." I feel the tightening around my calves and hear the wheeze of the leggings being pumped with air, and then the rushing release of pressure as the air is expelled. I feel the discomfort of the NG tube once again threaded through my upper GI tract, and I hear the occasional slurp from the suction apparatus on the wall.

"Do you remember what I said last night?" Andrew leans forward excitedly. "That Jessica won the Oscar?"

**Hints to help you beat the odds . . .**
**escaping from your own reality . . .**

Although you will have days of despair and even fury, make an effort to move out of that space and into the ordinariness, as well as the extraordinariness, of lives outside of cancer. It was cause for my celebration even within my own family when my heroic oncologist's daughter, Jessica Yu, won the 1997 Academy Award for Best Documentary Short for *Breathing Lessons: The Life and Work of Mark O'Brien*. Other people's activities and accomplishments can provide refreshing glimpses into the "other world" and spur you on to enter into it yourself when you are able.

"Did you see her?" I mumble.

"Um-hmm. While you were being repaired, we were watching the TV in the waiting room. She looked great and gave the best speech by far!"

"What did she say?" I am curious.

"Oh, something about her dress and accessories costing nearly as much as making the prize-winning film! But with great humor and poise." Still sedated, I contentedly drift off again.

The surgeons check my wound every day, but the NG tube makes it difficult to move my head to see what they're seeing. By tilting up the head of the bed, I find that I can gaze down at my abdomen. Staples mark the site where Stella once reigned, and more staples march from my belly button down past my pubic bone. Noticing that my nose is sore, particularly when I move my head, I reach up to touch it with my finger. It is very tender.

**Hints to help you beat the odds . . . avoiding martyrdom . . .**

If something hurts, or seems otherwise "not right," mention it to your nurse. The problem might be easily remedied or at least explained in a way that eases your worries about it.

Four days after surgery, Andrew is scheduled to leave. The day before his planned departure, the NG tube is still in place. He worries about leaving before it is out and speaks to Dr. Zang, who agrees that there is no reason not to take it out this afternoon.

"Great!" my kindhearted nurse affirms. "You've been waiting a long time for this." I can hardly wait to be liberated from the thick hose that curves into my nostril, down the back of my throat, and into my stomach, where it sucks up anything floating by.

The surgical resident joins in, "That thing's been in long enough! Time for your liberation!"

Turning to Andrew, I joke, "I hate to see you go, honey, but if your departure means hastening this removal, that's some compensation."

My nurse asks me to sit up and supports my back with her hand, while an aide rests her arm on my shoulder. As the resident leans over to carefully peel the adhesive tape that holds down the tube, I lay back and try not to grimace at the startling pain I feel when my nose is touched. The tube is pulled swiftly up through my stomach, my esophagus, and my throat, and tossed into the trash bin. The head of my bed is rapidly lowered, and I am lying flat on my back again. Looking at the faces leaning over me, I see their expressions of interest and expectation change to looks of horror and dismay and finally embarrassment.

"Oh, Mom," I can hear the shock as well as the tenderness in Andrew's voice.

Hurtled momentarily back into childhood, the resident simply says, "Wow!"

My kind nurse gasps and mumbles, "Oh, my God! What happened?"

"Call someone from plastics," the resident directs the nurse at his side. "Do we have a Polaroid camera on the floor?" he says to the space behind him. I can hear more people coming into the room and occasional muffled gasps.

"Well," I ask expectantly, "what *did* happen?"

Andrew leans over and strokes my head. "It looks as if there's some necrosis Mom," he explains. "The whole left side of your nose is black. The tape must have been too tight."

**For your information . . . necrosis . . .**

Necrosis describes tissue that has died when not enough blood flow reaches the area. The cause can be trauma, radiation, or chemicals.[2]

My kindly nurse whispers, "Oh my God! I am so sorry. I'm so sorry," and retreats to the back of the room.

*That tired anesthetist*, I think, *she was probably just too pooped to pay attention.*

Charles, holding my hand, turns away from my face and asks Andrew, "What's necrosis?"

*But a tired anesthetist can make worse mistakes than this*, I continue my musings, *like too much anesthesia . . . just relax*, I remind myself, *don't overreact.*

"It means the tissue has died—the pressure of the tape has shut off the circulation."

Alarmed by the growing dismay on the faces leaning over the bed, I am further unnerved by the sudden hubbub of activity. Only Andrew's voice remains steady and calm, yet I can also see the worry on his face. Charles looks anxious, a child struggling to wake up in the middle of a nightmare. Reaching up to touch my nose, it feels numb, as if injected with Novocain. Andrew reaches for my hand and brings it down to rest on the bedcovers. "It's best not to touch it, Mom."

A doctor I have not seen before leans over me. "I'm Dr. Willis. Mind if I look at your nose?"

**Hints to help you beat the odds . . .
having someone there who can ground you . . .**

Amid a wild swirl of intense activity, it is possible that you can stay relaxed and grounded in the company of one strong ally who can remain calm and reassuring despite the crisis. That is the ally you want to have with you for especially difficult procedures or conversations.

"Go ahead." I smile to reassure him. *I lie here with a half-dead nose*, I mull, *yet for some reason I am trying to bolster the moods of the people around me.*

"See here, it's notched, too," the new doctor explains to the nodding heads staring down at me. "The tape has pulled the NG tube, and the pressure has made a clean cut clear through the outer nares." He straightens up and asks no one in particular, "Has someone called plastics?"

He turns toward me. "We've asked someone from plastic surgery to come down and have a look. Half of your nose appears to be necrosed, that is, the tissue is dead, and so we may have some repairs to do later." *Repairs? More surgery? This is too much to take in.* That Andrew and Charles are here as my witnesses allows me to relax and let them do the remembering and noticing.

**Suggestions for allies . . . listening for both of you . . .**

At times like these, you can be immeasurably helpful in paying attention so that you can later help clarify what is happening.

"I need to take a photo of your nose," the voice behind the camera apologizes. "Do you mind?"

"No. Not at all." My gracious accommodation astonishes even me. *Not that I should be rude*, I think to myself, *but here I lie, nose blackened and torn, facing perhaps more corrective surgery, perhaps disfigured for life, yet I am trying to make everyone feel comfortable and welcome, reassuring them that I am all right.* The flash bulb goes off three times for three different angle shots. I turn to Andrew. "What does it look like?"

"You don't want to see it, Mom. It's pretty gross. Black." *He's right*, I think, *I don't want to see it, don't need to see it.*

He pats my arm and smiles. "I really think it'll be OK, Mom, but it's pretty shocking."

*I don't need to see it*, I continue with my thoughts, *I know what it looks like.* I already have a picture in my mind, a recollection of my Aunt Nan during the months before she died. *The melanoma that killed her started in her nostril, her left nostril.*

I can hear muffled voices outside my door.

"Eliza," the surgical resident is speaking to me, "we're going to have a specialist have a look at your nose." He smiles and continues, "Just a precaution."

"That's fine." Anything's fine. *Right now I am busy remembering my aunt and her nose. The surgeon scooped out the disc of melanoma, and her nose dropped into her face.*

"Hello, Eliza, I'm Dr. Patchit, chief of plastic surgery. Just came up to have a look at your nose. Do you mind?"

"Not at all."

"Can you feel me touch here?" I see his finger zero in on the center of my face but feel nothing.

"No."

"Feel this tapping?"

"No."

The resident starts to explain to the consulting surgeon, "See, there is also this tear; the tube cut through . . ."

"We need to film this," interrupts Dr. Patchit.

*As time passed*, I remember, *after chemo, radiation, and too many surgeries, Aunt Nan's face started to look like a jack-o-lantern softening into November.*

"Was the NG tube painful for you?" asks Dr. Patchit.

"It's always uncomfortable." *I'll bet none of these people has ever had one*, I think to myself, *or they wouldn't have to ask.*

"Where did it hurt you?" he continues his line of questioning.

"My throat mostly. Also my nose."

My nurse steps forward from the shadows and asks, "Did you tell anyone?"

A new person with another camera walks into the room and interrupts, "Excuse me! Eliza, I need to take a photograph of your nose! Do you mind?"

"Please," I invite her, "whatever you need." Then I turn back to the questioners and admit, "I can't remember."

My nurse persists, "Why didn't you tell me?"

**For your information . . . NG tube taping standards . . .**

The tape securing the tubing to the nose will generally remain for twenty-four hours. At that time, the nostril should be inspected and cleansed and the tube retaped.[3]

*By the time she turned herself over to hospice care,* I recall, *Aunt Nan's face was collapsing in on itself, the sunken hollow in the center revealing just a suggestion of what her nose had once been.*

"Well, everything hurt." It's true. The NG tube, the IVs, the abdominal wound. So much hurt that very little stood out, and if I complained about everything, I would do nothing but complain. Why talk about pain when there's nothing to be done about it? Why complain when I believe that everyone's working diligently to help me and all the other patients on the floor?

**Hints to help you beat the odds . . .**
**complaining versus informing . . .**

Letting your nurses and doctors know when something is painful is information that can help them diagnose a problem or complication, as well as provide them with information that can help them make you feel better, whether with reassurance, comfort measures, pain medications, or other assistance.

The plastic surgeon brings me back to the conversation at hand. "You really need to tell the nurse when something hurts."

*Don't they realize that something always hurts now?* I wonder.

The doctor tells the nurse to call the pharmacy for an antibiotic cream, which he instructs me to apply to the area four times a day. Handing me his card, he suggests that I make an appointment with him a few weeks after my discharge or sooner if I feel the need. Andrew follows him out to the hallway, where they confer briefly. Charles leans down and holds me, pressing his cheek to mine. "I'm glad Andrew is here right now because I wouldn't know what to do."

"I am, too." I stroke Charles' hair. "And thank God he suggested getting this thing out now!" Charles stands up and turns to Andrew, who has come back into the room.

**Suggestions for allies . . .**
**remembering your own need for support . . .**

In the face of all you are doing for the person who is sick, it can be difficult to remember to also attend to your own needs for support. When you feel that you need another ally there to support you, or to give you respite from caregiving, take the steps necessary to make that happen.

"It is scary to look at, isn't it?" Resting his hand on Charles' shoulder, Andrew tries to reassure him. "But the notch will heal, like any other deep cut, except very slowly, because of the necrosis. That's why plastics came racing down."

The image of my aunt floats back to me, her nose reduced to a cluster of bumps and lumps in that sad hollow of a face.

I look at the faces looking warily at mine. "It must look pretty dreadful!"

Andrew laughs warmly. "Let's put it this way, Mom: Wait a few days before you look!"

I can see the strain in his face and hasten to reassure him. "I'll be OK." I really believe I will be. *Or*, I wonder, *will I have no nose by the end of the week? Or half a nose?*

As the room begins to empty, Andrew sits down on the chair by the bed. "I am glad I stayed."

"And I am also. And glad you asked them to take that thing out tonight." Just having him near me helps me heal. I know this to be true. "I am so thankful you're here, honey."

"Me too, Mom. Twenty-four more hours of this and . . . well . . ."

He doesn't have to finish his thought. Twenty-four more hours of the tight tape and necrosis might have been confirmed. My nose might have decayed without hope of healing.

The dream comes back to me: the missing pieces. Not only the missing piece of colon, now the missing piece of nose. Finding the ends of the colon and sewing them together. Finding the ragged edges of nose, unable to feel them, reluctant to see them. Remembering the blackened hollow in Nanny's face, the scourge that finally killed her. Remembering the calm of the dream, the urgency without panic, I wonder whether my present calm is coming from the quiet grace of the dream. The powerlessness of my present situation comes hand in hand with an acceptance that quiets the heart and with a faith that quells anxiety.

# *Chapter 12*
# No Exit

## DREAMING ENTRAPMENT

### *April 1997*

*Charles brings me to a house, a house that sits on a small, untidy city lot. Roughly finished, it is square and plain. He lets me in with his key and immediately turns to leave, promising that he'll return later.*

*I stand alone in the kitchen, feeling abandoned and afraid. I go to lock the door, but there is no door handle, no lock, and no hardware of any kind. There is no way even to keep the door closed: It makes light squeaking sounds as the breeze pushes it slightly one way and then the other. I turn to find another door or window but find only blank walls. When I come back to the door with no handle, it has disappeared. Standing in a room with no means of escape, I am horrified to have been left in this situation and dreadfully frightened. I feel so vulnerable, so unprotected, so decidedly alone.*

Eight days after surgery, Charles brings me home. During my recuperation, my mother is here to help, tempting me with nursery food like custard and rice pudding, keeping the flowers fresh and watered, smoothing clean sheets over our bed, and generally doing the tender ministrations I remember from childhood. I assume that when my appetite returns, and my diet expands, my bowel patterns will resume a normal routine. As my mother relieves Charles of some of his responsibilities in caring for me, she also offers to him the nurturing and attention that were suspended when my energies and capabilities were eclipsed by my own needs.

**Suggestions for family . . . help for the helpers . . .**

When someone is diagnosed with cancer, the disease spreads, to some degree or another, throughout the lives of everyone who loves that person. Remember, you can't take care of this person you love without also taking care of yourself. In addition to following a healthy diet and exercise program and getting adequate rest, you also need respite and emotional support. You may need to widen your circle of allies so that the burden of responsibility can be spread out.[1]

My big challenge upon returning home is to have a bowel movement the old-fashioned way, without the colostomy. It was only on the last day of my hospital stay that I ate solid foods, so now the big test is about to begin: Will my body serve me as it once did? This morning, my friend Susan, knowing my anxiety regarding the vicissitudes of my GI tract, sent the following email:

> Well . . . ? We've been lighting the poop candle for you, and Sarah even said a prayer for your pooping when she said grace last night at dinner. We're thinking of you!
>
> Susan XOXOXOXOXO

Sarah, my five-year-old goddaughter, keeps me plied with drawings and notes of remarkable brevity, the most common being "I love you." Only hours later, I am able to respond:

> Sarah's prayer and your poop candle just worked! EUREKA! Yeah for you! Yeah for Sarah! Yeah for candles! Yeah for prayers! (Yeah for Colace and oatmeal too!) I miss you . . . la la la . . . Thank you Sarah! Thank you Susan!
>
> Love,
> Eliza

**Hints to beat the odds . . . remembering that humor heals . . .**

Although there is much about living with colon cancer that is far from humorous, there are comic moments also and opportunities to turn the macabre into dark comedy or even silliness and jest. Lightening up with a laugh or a giggle will lighten your burden at the same time.

Two weeks later, when I return for my postop visit, sensation is returning to my nose, and the puckered edges of the notch, once held together by tiny butterfly bandages, are now pulling closed by a deep purple streak of scar tissue. The blackening that so alarmed the staff has faded, and I have no inclination to undergo further surgery to repair the scar. The abdominal wound is marked by a blaze of deep lavender from my naval to below my pubic bone, and on either side, where the staples have been removed, bluish pinpoints march in parallel lines.

The surgeons expect me to be jubilant now that the colostomy is gone, but I have not yet adjusted to Stella's absence. There is no pain, yet a certain discomfort and trepidation arise in the adjustment to using parts of my body that have been dormant for nearly a year.

**For your information . . .**
**psychological as well as physiological etiology . . .**

Although my anticipation of pain and of "something not working right" were factors in my anxiety after the takedown, it is also possible that the vague discomfort I was noticing was a symptom of the stenosis (narrowing) beginning to happen.

Five weeks after surgery, I am having intermittent cramping, not unlike the pattern of symptoms that started this siege nearly a year ago. Trying to shove the pain into the background of my awareness, I keep my lunch date with my cancer-club friends. Despite my efforts to seem relaxed and well, the cramps intensify. I excuse myself and decline their offers to drive me home. The advice nurse makes an appointment for the following morning for me to see Dr. Liu.

X-rays show no blockage, and Dr. Liu suggests it might be a twist or a sharp bend in the colon, similar to a kinked garden hose. Or the locked doors, I think, remembering my dream. Trapped. No way out. He suggests I drink a bottle of citrate of magnesia, thereby blasting the kink into straightening itself out. One bottle and many cramps later yield no relief, so Charles brings me back the following morning. Dr. Liu suggests I try another dose. The second bottle causes more severe cramping, and finally, late at night, my bowels open and release their vast contents, leaving me tired and drained, physically and figuratively.

The cramps continue off and on for the following four days, but they are mild and less frequent. On the fifth day, I awaken to realize that I have slept the entire night and that my gut is quiet. This siege is reminding me that there is something about my body that I can no longer trust. I cannot blithely decide to start aikido or weed the garden or dig a hole for some herbs, or even plan lunch with friends, with any assurance that my body will withstand the challenges. So many things are now beyond my reach because of the most human of impediments: a body that is wearing out, a body that is no longer dependable. And then I realize how I took it all for granted for so long, how I never thought to be grateful or thankful or appreciative of all that this sturdy bunch of cells does at my bidding. And this unpredictability: Isn't this the human condition? The concept I had readily ascribed to theoretically I am now having to integrate into my body and my life.

My gut quiescent today, I accompany my mother to visit some distant cousins. When I go into the kitchen to ask whether I can help with the tea tray, my cousin says, "Your mother just told me what you are going through." She hastens to continue before I can respond. "I want you to know that I had the same thing, and I am just fine!"

I am shocked, as I had understood that she had had breast cancer. Only now, it seems, learning that I have colon cancer, does she disclose the true nature of her disease. Once again, I am struck with the shame of this plague, the penchant for identifying one's cancer with anything but the colon, the organ of waste removal.

The day before Mother's Day, we go to another cousin's open studio, about an hour-and-a-half drive from home. While admiring her exquisite porcelains, I sample a few almonds and some brie on a slice of baguette. Within an hour, my stomach is churning and my bowels are grabbing, whether from the food or from menstrual cramps, I am not sure. Unwilling to succumb to illness once again, I concentrate on the beauty around me and say nothing. Before starting the long drive home, we meet a group of cousins for dinner. The thought and smell of food is repellant, but not wanting to dampen the party spirits, I order a cup of pureed bean soup and a small salad.

**Hints to help you beat the odds . . .**
**learning lessons can be hard . . .**

Listen to your body! It is giving you important information, but it is information lost unless you pay attention to it. When you have been critically ill over a long period of time, it can be tempting to cover up further illness so as to spare those closest to you from having to dive back into that dark place with you. Our yearning for normality can overshadow our own common sense and push us to act foolishly.

After about four teaspoonfuls of soup and a few stabs of lettuce, the cramps become more severe, and I start an orbit that loops from the table to the bathroom to the table and so on.

Driving home, I lie down on the backseat, trying to curl around my aching belly as if offering comfort. The cramps are so like those that assailed my body before the cancer was removed that I try to figure out how I could possibly have grown another tumor in these short weeks.

"Are you OK, honey?" Tashie reaches back from the front seat, groping for my hand.

Too tired to meet hers or to speak, I groan, "Um-hmm."

I start shaking with chills, my teeth chattering and my whole body bouncing with the cold.

"She's cold, Charles, she's shivering. Is there a blanket in the trunk?" Tashie's hand, once resting on my thigh, now thrown off by my body's jittery dance, hovers above me.

**For your information . . . shaking with chills . . .**

This feeling of intense cold, when my body would shake with shivers, seemed to occur when my body was challenged with a rapidly building crisis.

"I don't know," Charles replies. I can hear that he is having difficulty thinking about my needs at the same time that he is navigating Bay Area Saturday-night traffic.

Desperately cold, I muster my strength to speak shorthand, "A moving blanket. In the trunk."

At the next stoplight, Charles jumps out of the car, hauls a dusty quilted blanket from the trunk, and quickly folds it around me. "Should we go to the hospital?" he asks anxiously.

"No. No, I just want to go home," I insist, even though the pain is escalating fast, and the chill uncontrollable. Afraid to go to the hospital, I also figure that this is the "kinked hose" syndrome again and that a blast of citrate of magnesia will cure me. *The magnesia that will open the doors of my dream,* I muse, *the magic that will release me from this place of no escape.* The cramping slows somewhat after a successful trip to the bathroom, and I am able to doze fitfully.

"I really think we should be going to the hospital." Charles is restless, pacing back and forth by the bed. It is three o'clock in the morning, long before dawn, and the cramping is escalating.

"I'll be OK," I assure him.

"That's what you always say!" He is exasperated and extends his hands in a gesture of futility. "And there are times in the past when, if I listened only to you, you might be dead now!"

"But I *am* OK, and I will be OK." *What makes me so sure?* I think to myself. But I don't want him to be worried, so try to minimize my anguish. I can feel the force of his quiet annoyance, and perhaps fear, at my refusal to go to the hospital.

In the morning, hoping to blast through the kink fire-hose style, I take two tablespoons of milk of magnesia and a small glass of prune juice. We have been invited to a Mother's Day brunch but, still feeling tenuous, I urge Tashie and Charles to go without me.

**Hints to help you beat the odds . . .**
**recognizing bad judgment . . .**

I made a number of poor decisions here, which I urge you not to replicate! Instead of hiding under a cloak of denial, and then trying self-medications that might have disastrous consequences, receive and act on the messages your body is sending and let others around you *help* you, including helping you think clearly so that you can make good decisions.

"I think one of us should stay here with you, honey." My mother stands next to the sofa and reaches down to run her warm hand over my fuzzy scalp. Finding my red angora hat on the floor, she pulls it gently down over my ears.

"Thanks, Mama." It feels so good, so soothing, to have my head covered in this softness. *How did she know?* I wonder.

"I'll stay with you," Charles walks into the living room. "I don't need to go to this brunch anyway."

"No, please, both of you go," I want them to enjoy themselves. "I promise I'll be all right." I also need time alone with my body to try to figure out what is going on.

They reluctantly leave, and I am alone in the quiet. Curling up on the sofa, worn out by the pain, I have no words in my lexicon to describe this exhaustion. *What is happening to me?* I cry to myself. I just don't understand.

**Suggestions for allies . . . staying with your hunches . . .**

If you are uncomfortable leaving your sick friend alone, don't be talked out of it. Stay with her. Your observations are probably more accurate than are her protestations.

Trying to doze, I am roused repeatedly by the stabbing sensations in my gut. These cramps remind me of the agony of that night last July 2. Frightened by this realization, during a lull I call the advice nurse, even though I wonder whether I'll be able to speak clearly enough for her to understand what I need.

"I've had surgery for cancer, colon cancer."

"When was your surgery?" asks the voice on the other end of the line. "I know this is hard for you . . . take your time."

Soothed by the patience and understanding in her tone, I try to remember. "The last one was in late March."

**Considerations for hospital staff . . .
transmitting empathy . . .**

The slightest indication of warmth and patience speaks volumes to the person listening and sets the stage for a mutually satisfactory exchange between care provider and patient.

"And now this pain is your biggest problem?"

"Yes."

"Are you vomiting?"

"No."

"Are you nauseated?

"Yes."

"Do you have a fever?"

"I don't think so." Remembering the chills during the long ride home, I add, "But last night perhaps I did."

"Just give me a minute here." There is a long pause, when I can hear only the whirr of her computer.

"I've made an appointment for you to be seen at the oncology clinic tomorrow morning. Meantime though, if your symptoms get worse, come in to the ER."

"OK." Starting to put down the receiver, I hold it to my ear again and say, "Thank you . . . very much."

"You're welcome. I am sorry you're feeling so bad." Hanging up the phone, I realize how little it takes to make me feel better, how her kindness has comforted me.

Not long after that phone call, my stomach starts to roil and grab. Crawling to the bathroom, I just get to the tile floor before starting to throw up yellowish-green fluid. Charles and Tashie come home to find me lying on bunched up towels on the tiled bathroom floor.

"I need to go to the hospital," I tell them. "I am desperate."

"Oh, I knew we shouldn't have left you alone!" I can hear the anguish and helplessness in Charles's voice, a vocal wringing of the hands.

"I was OK then," I mutter between gasps.

Charles tries to help me dress, but the pain and the vomiting make it difficult. Clothes feel abrasive to my skin. There are so many internal stimuli, a heaving stomach and a tortured gut, that even the slightest external irritation is unbearable. I finally find a soft turtleneck, and then throw on the blue-and-white cotton jumper. I am crawling to the door when my body is seized with vomiting, and I am appalled to sense that the enormous pressure on my abdomen has caused me to wet myself.

"Stay right there, honey, I'll get you clean clothes." Charles returns with a basin of soap and water and washcloths and towels. While Tashie finds dry clothes, he helps me wash and change.

Settling in for the forty-five-minute drive, I sit on the front seat with a towel under me and the stainless steel puke bowl on my lap. Amid fierce

**For your information . . .
symptoms of a bowel obstruction . . .**

Symptoms of a bowel obstruction may include:[2]

- Abdominal fullness
- Abdominal distention
- Abdominal pain and cramping
- Nausea and vomiting
- Failure to pass gas or stool
- Diarrhea
- Fecal breath odor

cramps and violent episodes of vomiting, I construct mind games to trick me into thinking we are closer than we are: after this exit, we'll start our climb through the mountains; after this curve, we'll reach the summit; and so on.

Charles drives up to the emergency entrance and races inside to get a wheelchair. The admitting clerk says that I will see the RN next, and my agitated mother exclaims, "But she can't wait, she needs to see someone now!"

Seeing a sick child with the nurse, I know I need to wait. I also see that this wait is torture for my mother who, sighing audibly, looks accusingly in the direction of the nurse. In less than five minutes, I am wheeled to the RN's cubicle, where she takes a brief history and records vital signs. She yells to the space behind her, "Give me a good bed; we'll have this patient for several hours." Turning back to me, she says, "They'll be coming for you right away." Pausing, she adds softly, "I hope you feel better."

I nod my thanks as a young male nurse comes out of the double doors. "You can wheel her through now," he gestures to my mother. Apparently irritated that the nurse doesn't take over the wheelchair himself, she looks at him disdainfully, and I know she is about to order *him* to push the wheelchair. Planting herself behind me, she pushes me through the door

**Considerations for hospital staff . . . speaking kindly . . .**

It just takes a few words said in a kind tone to relax and reassure a patient who is anxious, tense, and fearful of what is happening inside of her.

**Hints to help you beat the odds . . . absenting yourself . . .**

An occasion like this might be an appropriate time to visualize yourself in a quiet, peaceful place. Although your ally loves you with the passion and fury of a mother bear, that shrill demand for instant care can be embarrassing. So take yourself to a sublime headspace, and let others work out the details of their communication on their own.

being held open by the nurse who, seeing Tashie's youthful vigor, undoubtedly has no idea that she is starting her ninth decade.

Marching ahead, my mother announces defiantly to anyone within her range, "This time my daughter is *not* going to be sent home before she's been properly tended to!"

We haven't even gotten into the exam room when she demands loudly that the nurse call Dr. Liu or Dr. Zang, insisting, "They want to be called."

This nurse, overwhelmed by my five-foot-nine mother towering over him and issuing commands, repeats, "I'm a nurse; the doctor will come."

"I want you to call them NOW!" she demands.

Another nurse comes in, and they help me onto a bed and into a hospital gown, at the same time responding patiently to my mother's shrill directives. A mother myself, I ache for her fear and alarm watching her child teeter on the edge of a dark abyss, but I have no energy to reassure her.

A kind-faced doctor walks in and rests his hand on my shoulder as he asks, "What's happening?"

"Can't you see what's happening? She's in terrible pain!" Wanting her just to step back and be quiet, I remember the agitated mothers of women in labor demanding, "*Do* something! Anything!" and sometimes, "*I* never went through this when I had *her*!" Hearing the tears start to thicken her voice, imagining them clouding her deep-blue eyes, I try to understand her own pain.

The ER doctor manages to maintain his composure against my mother's touchingly desperate and frustratingly abrupt demands. Suddenly she seems to realize that this man is trying to help me, and she steps back, arms folded across her chest.

"I am Dr. Ektahadi, the surgical resident." The very handsome Persian man smiles sympathetically and extends his hand. "I know you're in

**Considerations for hospital staff . . .**
**empathizing with the family . . .**

It is a difficult task to maintain your composure, patience, and compassion when confronted with this kind of furious and agitated demand for immediate care. Try to remember, in the midst of it all, that these people are afraid that something catastrophic is happening to this person they deeply love. This fear may be compounded by a remembered incident of perceived (or, in fact, real) inferior care by the healthcare system. Your patience and calm at this point can quickly shift the communication to one of mutual respect.

a great deal of pain, and I want to help you, but first I have to examine you. Is that OK?"

"Yes."

While examining me, he orders the nurse to start an IV, and then orders medication for the pain and nausea.

This doctor is another angel in the firmament of my narrowed world. Gentle-handed nurses keep me clean and hold my head as it tosses uncontrollably with the insurrection that has seized my body. Retching, moaning, and feeling embarrassed at the commotion I am causing, my sense of time collapses. The pain starts to subside as the narcotic sweeps through my tissues.

My mother is listening to every word, occasionally breaking in with her opinions and cautionary tales. It is a testament to Dr. Ektahadi's poise and compassion that he takes no offense at her ultimatums and hovering vigilance but instead listens to her, considers her counsel, and explains his plan. Propelled by fear into frantic efforts to control, her response is in direct contrast to Charles, who is silenced and nearly paralyzed by his terrors.

Dr. Ektahadi orders an NG tube. I hear the words *NG tube*, and grotesque as it might be, I feel grateful anticipating the relief it will provide when it begins to drain the air and fluids from my distended stomach. But Tashie panics. "NG tube!" she roars "Look at her nose, look at where that last NG tube cut her nose!"

Gesturing, "It's OK," I moan, "I need it." It is when I shift positions to accommodate the insertion of the NG tube that I realize that the IV is lodged in the antecubital space, the inside bend of the elbow, requiring my arm to be straight at all times. *Of course*, I remind myself, *The dehydration has collapsed my veins. They were probably lucky to get a vein at all!*

The doctors ask if I want them to call Andrew. "Yes, please," I nod and drift off.

Dozing through the hum of activity around my bed, I feel a hand on my shoulder and hear Dr. Ektahadi's voice. "I spoke with your son, and told him you are here and what's happening with you." Recognizing my mental blurring from the drugs, he waits while I take this in. "I also spoke to Dr. Zang, and he'll be here to see you in the morning." Rocked in a cradle of compassion, I feel safe and therefore free to drift off to sleep. Not safe in that my body is no longer threatened, for I am well aware that this crisis is grave. But safe in that I am surrounded by competent and caring people who will help me through the hours and days ahead.

Alerted by the quiet voice of my sweet and tender son, I open my eyes to see him approach my bed: How he got here, where we are, or what time it is does not concern me. There are no words to describe my sense of comfort and peace at feeling his touch and hearing his voice. All night he is here, resting in one of those reclining chairs, ready to jump up the minute he hears me stir. I throw up a few more times, or rather retch, as there is now little to throw up. I am parched . . . I have lost track of where my lips are; my mouth has become a space bound by rough torn parchment paper, totally dry.

Dr. Zang comes by and says that I most likely have a small bowel obstruction, probably due to adhesions. He agrees to increase my fluids to 150 cubic centimeters an hour. Dr. Ektahadi checks my belly, which remains tight and rigid.

I hear a voice instructing me, "When we tell you to, you must hold your breath for about twenty seconds," and realize that I have been shuttled to x-ray without my waking. The voice echoing through the speaker saying "Take a deep breath in and hold it . . ." keeps me awake for a few seconds before she says, "Relax now, and breathe." Hearing these instructions repeated several times, wondering why they don't just take the pictures, I hear the same voice say, "You're all done!"

Sleeping again through the journey back to the surgical ward, I awaken in my room to hear Dr. Zang expressing his surprise at finding that the obstruction seems to be not in the small bowel as he had thought but in the colon.

The pain persists, despite the IV hydration and the NG decompression, and the CT scan confirms the involvement of the colon. Dr. Zang arranges for a diagnostic colonoscopy.

Dozing on and off, I am aware of being wheeled down to the fourth

**For your information . . . colonoscopy defined . . .**

A colonoscopy allows an examination the entire large intestine, from the rectum up through the colon to the beginning of the small intestine. Colonoscopies enable the physician to identify inflammation and abnormalities such as bleeding and polyps and are thus used to screen for signs of cancer. The physician can remove abnormalities such as polyps using tiny instruments passed through the scope. The removed tissue is then sent to a lab for analysis (biopsy).[3]

floor to the GI procedure room. While Andrew stays in the waiting room, Dr. Zang perches on a high stool to observe the proceedings. I am contentedly sedated, feeling nothing, and am conscious of only a few comments breaking through the haze. Watching on the screen, I can see the staples binding the two ends of colon together. The point of constriction transforms the cylinder shape into that of an hourglass and prevents the tube passing any farther. Through the doctors' commentary, I hear repeated the words: "Inflate . . . stop . . . release."

Then I fade to that sleepy place again and find myself in my room with Andrew and Dr. Zang.

"The site where the ends of colon were stapled together has constricted to the size of a pinpoint, and this stenosis [narrowing] has created a mechanical obstruction," Dr. Zang tells me later. "We could see this when the lighted tube was threaded through the rectum and into the colon."

"What made that happen?" I ask.

"Well, we're not sure. It is an unusual complication of stapling." He pauses before continuing. "At the site of the stenosis, a balloon was inserted in the narrowed space, and then inflated to stretch the lumen, to enlarge the opening."

**For your information . . . stenosis at the stapling site . . .**

A rare complication of reanastamosis is the narrowing of the intestine at the site of stapling. In some cases, the stenosis can be corrected with a single balloon inflation; in others, the inflation must be repeated serially over a period of time.

> **For your information . . . proper terminology . . .**
>
> The proper term for the procedure I refer to as "balloon colonoplasty" is "flexible sigmoidoscopy with balloon dilation."

"Sounds like balloon colonoplasty!" I like having a name for the procedures I experience.

He laughs. "Well, I've never heard that term, but it describes it pretty well!"

"And it makes it sound less peculiar."

Andrew breaks in, "What are the chances that this stenosis will recur?"

"Well, we'll have to repeat this procedure again, maybe more than once. We're planning a second one for tomorrow, and we'll see how it looks."

Against the backdrop of Andrew's and Dr. Zang's voices, I drift off to sleep. The sun is low in the sky when I awaken, and I can hear the sound of dinner trays being slid back into their slots on the carts.

I still feel terribly dry, as if my body just cannot catch up, even with the accelerated IV rate. Concurring with my impression that I continue to be markedly dehydrated, Andrew gets a resident to order a bolus, a rapid infusion of fluid, of 500 cubic centimeters. Despite the various medications, the cramping and retching continue, and diarrhea is further stressing me. Clutching a dull-pink plastic bath basin to my chest, and dragging my IV pole with its array of small and large bags swinging jauntily from steel hooks, I hobble back and forth between bed and bathroom.

The next morning, Dr. Zang comes in before his first case. "You were vomiting again last night," he comments, looking for confirmation.

I think a minute and, unable to remember last night, reply, "No, I don't think so."

Andrew reminds me, "Mom, remember, you vomited *a lot* last night!"

Of course. How can I forget? Now all those memories come flooding back to me, the hurried trips to the bathroom, the unspeakable tiredness . . . it takes so much energy. Despite my allegations that I am feeling better this morning, Dr. Zang and Andrew stress that the rest that my body needs will be possible only by getting a total break from the pain and nausea, and to do this, a more aggressive stance must be taken with the drugs. Stronger medicine is ordered and administered. Feeling my body relax and my muscles slacken, I realize, *He knows what I need better than I know myself.* How is it that I am so out of touch with what I need?

**Hints to help you beat the odds . . .**
**an ally can help you remember . . .**

Both pain and the medication to address it can affect your thinking process, another reason to rely on your ally to validate your impressions or, if appropriate, subject them to a reality test.

Andrew sits facing me, working on his computer, and I lie here feeling peaceful and finally comfortable. He softly taps on his computer keys as I drift in and out, absorbing his warmth and comfort, and feeling unspeakable relief that the pain and nausea finally seem to have passed.

At eleven thirty he packs up his bag, kisses me good-bye, and leaves for the airport. How lucky I am . . . to have that remarkable person in my life.

Charles comes in the afternoon and stays until quite late. Seeing how hard this is for him, I understand better his difficulty being here in the hospital, in this land of foreign culture and foreign language. Both Andrew and I work in similar settings and feel relatively at home here, yet most of the words Charles hears are totally incomprehensible, and a great deal of what he sees is an impenetrable mystery. Watching him wave good-bye at the door, hearing his step fade down the hallway, I fight back tears.

Toward Wednesday morning, the cramps start again. The decision is made to repeat the colonoscopy, not tomorrow as planned, but today. The lumen has narrowed to seven to eight millimeters, and the balloon is again inserted and inflated. This time the opening can accommodate the tube being passed through, and I can see the inner passageways of my bowels on the screen.

Before being discharged home five days later, I am given an appointment slip for the procedure to be repeated in two weeks, at the end of May. Another in mid-June reveals that the lumen has stayed reasonably open, and the decision is made to wait six months before repeating the procedure.

Yet toward the end of June, less than two weeks after the recent colonoplasty, I can sense trouble stirring in my gut.

Rushing about trying to get ready for a road trip to the Wallowa Valley, I am not feeling at all well. It is hard to resist lying down every time I pass by a bed or a sofa. Tired and slightly nauseated, mild cramps come and go. I make salmon and chard for dinner, but am unable to eat.

When Charles asks what is wrong, I tell him, "I just feel punk. I am not sure what is wrong."

"I really hope it's not another one of those . . ."

He doesn't need to finish his sentence for me to agree with him, but then I think, *I never even thought of that possibility*. And then the lightbulb goes off in my head. The bowel movements have been getting narrower and narrower, pencil-like, suggesting the narrowing of the intestinal lumen. And for the past four days, none at all. Determined to make this trip as planned, I also understand that once we are on the road, we'll be in remote areas where medical care might be meager and of unknown quality. It is essential that I discover what is amiss before we leave. Persuading myself that I can get through the night, we decide to make the hospital our first stop on our trip north.

Driving to the hospital, I am musing on the different experience it is to be seeking help before something turns into an emergency. I feel so unsure of what is going on inside me, yet some part of me knows that this is not normal.

**Hints to help you beat the odds . . . averting a crisis . . .**

Seeking professional help before your symptoms reach crisis proportions eases the situation for you, for your providers, and for your family and allies. The challenge is in making the distinction between symptoms that will resolve spontaneously and those that require intervention.

We arrive a little after seven and take the elevator to the procedures floor. In the midst of asking me questions, the RN interrupts herself and stares at me. "Don't I know you? Haven't I been your nurse?"

Then another nurse comes back, and they both look at me and say, "Of course we know you. You're a midwife, right?" They have been kind and reassuring from the beginning, but now they are even more so, pressing my hand comfortingly. Just minutes later, Dr. Collins comes to see me and asks me to tell my story: no bowel movement since Saturday, rectal bleeding Saturday night, watery diarrhea Sunday, occasional moderate cramping.

"How about the bowel movements before Saturday?"

"Little." I felt embarrassed to be once again discussing the appearance of my stools.

"Like pencils?"

"Like pencils, yes."

"Sounds like it's closed down again. I'll get to you as soon as possible, and meantime the nurses will start an IV and get you prepped."

I hesitate before asking, "About travel . . . we have this road trip planned—"

"No problem." She dismisses my concerns with an encouraging clap on the shoulder. "We'll take care of this, and you'll be just fine!"

**For your information. . . . the colonoscopy procedure. . . .**

You will lie on your left side, and pain medication along with a mild sedative will be given to you through an IV. A colonoscope, a long, flexible, lighted tube, will be inserted into your rectum and then up into your colon. This specialized scope transmits an image of the inside of the colon, an image that you may be able to see on the video screen unless you are too sleepy. The procedure itself takes from thirty minutes to an hour, and you will need to rest at the facility for one to two hours until the sedative wears off.[4]

By seven thirty I am in a hospital gown, lying on the procedure table, and getting an IV started. When Dr. Collins comes in, I am already turned over onto my left side. Placing her hand on my hip, she says, "That's me behind you, we're ready to start, everything's going to be fine."

The next thing I remember is her saying, "We're through, it went fine, we opened the stricture . . . and have a fun adventure in Oregon!" I go into the recovery room, and two hours later, we are on our way north. The plan includes returning every two weeks for this balloon colonoplasty rather than waiting for the obstruction to cause pain. Charles and I are both feeling a certain joyousness that this hospital visit has been relatively brief and minor. By August, two months later, I am returning on a monthly basis for dilation of the stricture.

Every two months, I see the oncologist and repeat the CEA levels. I stop worrying about the lab results, as they have been consistently normal.

The oncologist checks me every six months. Pleased that there is no evidence of disease, he congratulates me on my good health.

He shakes my hand and is about to leave the exam room when I ask

**For your information . . . the CEA . . .**

The carcinoembryonic antigen (CEA) assay is a test that measures the level of CEA in the blood. CEA is released into the bloodstream from both cancer cells and normal cells. When found in higher-than-normal amounts, it can be used as a tumor marker for colorectal cancer.[5]

him a question that has been bothering me: "I feel a bit worried about my ovaries still being there, about getting ovarian cancer."

He looks up at me. "Any special reason you're worried?"

"Not really, I just have this feeling that I want them out." Thinking for a few seconds, I tell him, "I don't want *anything* left inside me that I don't need for survival!"

He laughs and offers, "Well, you can see one of the gynecologic oncologists for a consultation, but it's likely they won't want to go into your abdomen again unless they really need to!"

"Maybe not, but I'd like to hear what they think." What a flip from just a year ago, when I worked so hard to persuade the surgeons to leave my gallbladder inside me. At that time, I didn't want anything removed unnecessarily. Now, I want everything that's unneeded taken out.

"I'll send a referral, then, to Dr. Kinjo, and his nurse will call you to make an appointment."

"Thanks so much."

Dr. Kinjo's evaluation in May reveals neither ovarian nor uterine disease and, because of known extensive abdominal scarring, a prophylactic oophorectomy (removal of the ovaries) is not advised. The plan instead is to continue relying on the serial CEA levels to monitor a possible recurrence of cancer activity.

**Hints to help you beat the odds . . . spiritual succor . . .**

Finding your spiritual center, whether through a religious community or through your own spiritual explorations, can help you cope with your illness and all the attendant changes. For some, it might be a daily practice of meditation or yoga; for others, it might be church attendance. Hopefully, atheists might be open to trying yoga and/or meditation.

My April appointment with Dr. Liu falls on Good Friday, so I decide to go to the cathedral before my appointment at three fifteen. The building is an old, wood-framed domed structure, and the rhythmic buzz of the liturgy and the swell of music pouring through me wraps me into a quiet prayer for grace and strength. Sitting next to me, Charles studies the structural patterns of the dome.

Full of music and the quiet that comes from stepping outside my routine, we leave for the clinic. Shown to Dr. Liu's exam room, I sit down and turn to the magazine rack before settling in for a good read while waiting for him to come in. I pick up the February issue of *Atlantic Monthly*, and behind it is a stack of letters, copied on white recycled paper. I pick one up and read, "To our patients: Since Dr. Liu will be leaving the practice . . ." I am stunned; I read and reread the words and feel the floor slip out from under me. He is so essential to my being well, it seems impossible to believe that I can carry on without him. Only a minute or two pass before I hear a *tap-tap-tap* at the door. "Hello, hello, Eliza." Still in shock, I say nothing in reply and sit there like a stone, waiting. His pixyish face peers around the corner, eyes twinkling, smile warm. Terrified that I might cry, I remember nothing of what he says. He sits down on a stool facing me and asks how I have been.

"Fine . . ." I blurt, "but I see that you're leaving, and I am . . . I don't know . . . I'll miss you . . . I can't imagine getting through this without you."

He stares at me and says, "What is different about you? You look changed! What is it? You look so different!"

"I don't know," I shrug.

Shaking his head, he repeats, "You look so changed somehow."

But all I can think about is his leaving.

As he continues to look at me, a puzzled expression knits his brows. Embarrassed, I can hear in his voice that whatever the changes are, they are not flattering. I feel I have somehow let him down.

Pulling myself together, gathering all the poise I can muster, I ask, "Why are you leaving?"

"I want a change . . . something different."

"Do you know what you'll be doing?" My heart is in my throat as I speak.

"Perhaps some volunteer work . . . some traveling . . ."

But rising anxiety leaves me unable to pay attention to what he is saying.

"I'm sixty-one," I hear him say. "Young for retirement, but ready for a change."

We talk about the changes in the practice of medicine, the corporate takeover. I understand his frustrations.

"You know, I leave work, I go home, I open the door to another world entirely." He says. "I want to do more in that world. My wife works in history, in art . . . it's another world that I haven't had time for."

"But now you will." I am concentrating on not crying, on trying to be a good sport, and happy for his plans.

**Considerations for medical staff . . .
when a critical team member leaves . . .**

The relationship between a cancer patient and her doctor can be intense. If the patient is doing well, there may be a belief that any alteration will threaten the status quo and that that doctor, and no other, can heal. When that practitioner leaves, it can cause panic.

"Yes." He smiles and continues, "And you need to choose another doctor. Do you have a preference?"

"I don't know the other doctors, really . . ."

"Well, they're all good . . . it's more a matter of personalities than anything and the different places they trained."

"Who would you choose for a member of your family?"

"Really, they are all good . . . it's a matter of personality, chemistry."

"Well, all else being equal, I think I'll go with another *Chinese* doctor!"

**For your information . . .
the magical thinking of childhood can return . . .**

When, against all odds, you are able to recover from what might have been catastrophic, it is easy to slide back into the magical thinking of childhood or bargaining with the gods. *If I do (fill in your own oath), I will be well. If my doctor is (fill in), I will stay well.* Even when you can identify what you are doing, and laugh it off lightly, there is often a kernel within you that holds on to that belief that magic is possible.

He laughs and agrees, "I'll make an appointment for you with Dr. Feng in four months."

For a brief moment, caught up in conversation, I have forgotten my sorrow at his pending departure.

He asks me how my family is, and I mention that Andrew and his family are moving to Wisconsin. I can't think of anything else to say. Most of my energy is absorbed by trying not to cry, trying not to be a big baby. I always ask him about his family, especially about Jessica, but not this time: I can't collect my thoughts.

He looks at me for a long minute, studying my face, and says, "You look so different than you always have: Is it your short hair? What's different?"

"I've probably gained weight!" I blurt out. I hear in his voice that I seem less . . . something.

Shaking his head, he says, "No . . . something else." Reaching for his lab forms, he suggests, "Let's get a thyroid level just to check it. And while we're at it, I'll send in a mammogram request." With our appointment becoming businesslike and task oriented, the lump in my throat softens. "And we'll do a bone scan, see how your bone density is."

"What do you think of Fosamax?" I ask. "I mean, if I need something like that."

"Of course, they all say these drugs are safe, but the newer drugs have only been around for a few years, so what do we know about what their effects might be down the line!"

He goes on to ask me when I had my last tetanus shot. When I can't remember, he decides to give me a booster today. These details of general patient care are reassuring in their ordinariness.

**Hints to help you beat the odds . . .**
**reclaiming the ordinary . . .**

The most ordinary events in your daily life can become forces for grounding you, for steadying you on your path. Initially, it may seem appalling that, in spite of your intense suffering, people around you continue to shop and go to work and take their kids to piano lessons. In time, though, especially as you begin to be able to participate in these activities and conversations, activities can steady you, strengthening you to withstand the buffeting of the winds of so many changes.

"I'm really going to miss you . . . a lot."

"You're going to be fine." He leans forward laying his hand lightly on my arm. "I really think you're going to be fine."

Picking up my chart as he stands, he says nonchalantly, "You wait here, and I'll send somebody in with your tetanus shot."

In a few minutes, a woman comes in to the room, holding a syringe, a gauze pad, and an alcohol swab. She checks my name, asks me if I have any allergies, and swabs my exposed shoulder. After administering the shot in my upper arm, she marks a little slip of paper, presumably with the dose given and her initials. She instructs me to move my arm a lot, to avoid keeping it stationary, and to have a happy Easter. Then she is gone.

In the silence, I realize that Dr. Liu has said good-bye, that he is with another patient now, and that I am not going to have another chance to say farewell. I button my dress, pick up my purse, and walk into the waiting room. Tears are brimming in my eyes, and I hand Charles the letter announcing Dr. Liu's pending departure. He asks me what else was said, but I can't answer him. He asks other questions as well, but all I can do is try not to cry.

**Hints to help you beat the odds . . .**
**accepting heightened emotional responses . . .**

A diagnosis of cancer carries with it so many losses, such as good health, role definitions, belief in the future, confidence in watching your children and grandchildren grow into adulthood, and the humdrum stability of life before catastrophic illness. These losses can diminish your reserve to withstand further loss, and you might collapse into childlike weeping on occasions that might not have provoked such a response before your illness. Allow yourself to feel the intense sorrow connected with these losses, the small ones as well as the major ones.

The next morning, I awake determined to see Dr. Liu again, to say a proper good-bye. I tell the voice at the other end of the line that I need to schedule another appointment. Kindly refraining from inquiring as to my reasons, she schedules me for the following week. Beginning to feel better about seeing him again, about the thread not yet being broken, I also begin to convince myself that somehow I will be OK even in someone else's care. By the time of my appointment, I am relatively poised and confident that his departure will not bring about my demise.

The next week I have an appointment with Ellen, an acupuncturist and friend.

"What's happened to your face?" she asks. "It's crooked—the left side's different from the right."

"That's what Dr. Liu said last week." The floating anxiety and despair I am feeling inside seems to be written on my face.

"Have you seen it, too? It's amazing!" She leans forward, studying my face in the shaft of light coming through the high window.

"I do now. But I didn't see it until Dr. Liu mentioned it, and then I looked in the mirror."

"Well, what's happening with you?" She starts rubbing my back, and tears slide down my cheeks. "Are you feeling depressed?"

"I guess." Suddenly I feel the heaviness push down on me. "I feel as if I'm not living in this body, as if I'm watching it, yet completely detached."

"Something's really got a hold of you!"

"Well, I don't feel myself, that's true." I am relieved that both she and Dr. Liu recognize what I have been feeling: that some essential part of me is lost, or perhaps I just cannot connect with it.

By and by, I can see the crookedness in my face begin to ease, and at the same time, the gray boulder pressing on my chest begins to crumble and fall away. Life begins to assume a familiar rhythm. I continue to gain strength and increase my stamina, and the disease becomes less central to my life. This is not to say, however, that the losses have been regained, nor the deficits filled. I am left with a mind that is less keen, a diminished resilience to stress, a body that is quick to tire, and an aging of my tissues that has not yet corrected itself. Time and a return to my preillness routine will be the catalysts, I am sure, that will help me reshape my life to its former configuration. Only later do I realize how naive the assumption is that I will ever return to "normal."

# *Chapter 13*
# Hanging On

## DREAMING ICE MOUNTAIN

### *June 1997*

*Carrying Rose, who clings to me like a monkey, I am climbing up a steep conical mountain. Covered with ice and snow, the peak as well as the sky is deep white, a white that echoes traces of blue in its depths. A tempest rages, blowing ice chips and snowflakes into my face and eyes and threatening my precarious balance.*

*Her legs hug my hips; her arms loop around my neck. I cross the wide lapels of my thick overcoat to wrap around her. I feel her little fingers gripping my shoulders and her exhalations warming my neck. Recognizing the hazards of our climb, I am moved by the child's confidence that I will keep her safe.*

*There is a compelling but unarticulated need to reach the top of this mountain. A rope strung along either side of the trail allows me to maintain my balance as I slowly climb. As I take each step, I grab the rope, placing hand over hand. Yet to do so means releasing my grasp of Rose, and I am terrified that letting go even with one hand might allow her small body to be blown out of my arms and into the tempest swirling around us. Or that she might teeter forward or backward, causing me to lose my balance, and we would both tumble helplessly into that cold, colorless space below.*

*Each step requires a difficult decision, a renewed weighing of risks, yet we move upward, finally reaching the top, where a trail leads directly into a huge lodge. The cavernous square room is carved of ice, with thick ice columns supporting its high ceiling. There are neither furnishings nor people. Although relieved to have reached safety, I am unsure now what is expected of me.*

As I begin to awaken, the wind of the dream whistles through me, the chill reaching into the warm bed. Shuddering to think of carrying Rose through that perilous country, I am unable to shake myself from the images, from the thought of any harm coming to her tender, young body. How is it that I am bringing this openhearted, lively, loving child into a glacial and perilous landscape?

The dream loosens its hold on me as the sky ripens into early summer, and the sunlight throws saffron silhouettes on the pale wall behind the altar, outlining the prayer wheel, the onyx loon, the ceramic angel, and the magic wand. It is nearly a year since that first surgery of July 2. As I try to reclaim some of the normal aspects of my life before cancer, I am also acutely aware that nothing is the same, that the world has shifted in the way that a kaleidoscope, given a gentle twist, displaces into entirely new patterns.

My first day back at work is a short shift on a Tuesday, six hours instead of the normal twelve. Driving through the mountain roads, taking the fork that leads, not to the hospital where I have been a patient, but to the hospital where I am on staff, I am both excited and apprehensive to be starting back. Moving through the web of a waking dream, I feel as if I am living in someone else's body, or as if I am someone else living in my body. Parking my car under an elm tree at the far end of the parking lot, I walk through the glass doors to the lobby and notice that there are unfamiliar chairs and loveseats arranged around new tables, which are spread with small stacks of daily newspapers and magazines such as *Sports Illustrated*, *You and Your New Baby*, the *Watchtower*, *Field and Stream*, and *Good Housekeeping*.

Watching me step off the elevator on the fifth floor, the skeptical security guard hunched over a tattered magazine asks to see my identification. She is new since I was last here, yet already she's settled in.

"So?" I hear a challenge in her voice and in the manner in which she throws back her shoulders to sit taller in her chair. Her efforts to become larger by that gesture remind me of the advice that, should you come upon a mountain lion while biking or hiking, stand tall to give the illusion of grand stature. She peers at the card identifying my department and staff position. "You're one of our midwives?" Relaxing her shoulders and sitting back in her chair, she smiles. I am no longer a mountain lion for whom she must appear larger than life. Her attitude has evolved quickly from suspicion to inclusion.

"Yes." I hesitate before adding, "But I've been away a while!"

"A while?" She leans back in her swivel chair and slaps her knee lightly. "I'd say longer than that." Leaning forward, she continues, "Why, I've been here since last September, nine months already, and I've never seen you, never!" Her voice lifts to suggest a question.

"That's because I've been gone since before then." It feels odd that she, who has worked here for months, is the old-timer, and I, who have worked here for years, am the rookie. And the irony is that not only does this woman see me as a new arrival, I myself feel both uncertain and tentative.

"Well." Her welcoming smile is reassuring. "Nice to have you back."

Walking down the postpartum wing, I pass the open doors of patient rooms, the doctors and midwives leaning over charts on the movable carts, aides passing fresh water pitchers, and a nurse with a ring of heavy keys slapping against her thigh, who is passing out medications. One woman, newly delivered and hugging her swaddled baby tightly to her chest, is being wheeled into her room. It all looks so very familiar, yet I cannot imagine reentering this world and resuming my professional role.

The midwives' call room door is partially open, and I see that it has been transformed into a postpartum two-bed ward. One mother is leaning over her baby cooing, and the other is stretched out asleep, her mouth relaxed and slightly open. Beyond the window are violet-tinged hills dotted with the wide, lacy umbrellas of spreading oaks. I press the round metal plate that triggers the sensor that opens the doors to labor and delivery and walk in.

"Oh! Eliza's here!" calls a nurse from down the hall. "Eliza's back!" They cluster around the nurses' station, a bouquet of bright faces poised to greet me.

"We knew you were coming today!"

"You look so well."

"Well, we heard you were, and hoped you would be, here!" another voice interrupts.

"Oh, you look healthy and wonderful!"

"So Thursday we're bringing lunch, a potluck, to celebrate."

In their excitement, in their urgency to welcome me, they talk over each other, each sweetly tolerant of the other's interruptions. Although at first I try to respond to each one, it becomes confusing, and I feel comfortable just taking in the love and tenderness.

Taller than most, I look down at the excited faces, warmed by these greetings. "What shall I bring to the potluck—" I start, guessing what their responses will be.

"But that's the point—*we're* bringing lunch for *you*!" Laughing, they happily spar for my attention. I am moved by their kindhearted reception.

"I have a problem though," I begin. "The midwife call room seems to have disappeared."

"That's right, it has; it's a patient room now." A nurse points beyond the double doors leading to the newborn nursery. "Your call room's over there now."

"Does anyone know the combination for getting in?"

"No, but Dinah's there already—she's waiting for you, and she'll tell you."

With the agreement of my department, I have requested and been granted the opportunity to work alongside a colleague for these first days back, rather than directly managing patients without a period of reorientation. Moving as a body, the nurses guide me toward the new call room, announcing, "Dinah, Eliza's here!"

**Hints to help you beat the odds . . .**
**eliciting helpful responses . . .**

Some people want to return to work with as little fanfare as possible. Some want to be open about their diagnosis and invite questions about their condition. Others want to be treated as if nothing had happened, as if the old normal is being reestablished. It's best to assume that your coworkers are unsure as to how to respond. As you reenter the work environment, you can guide them in the direction that works for you.

Feeling like a celebrity with all this devoted attention, I also feel dislocated, by the true relocations of rooms, new staff, and altered surroundings, but also by virtue of my feelings that I can only describe as the opposite of déjà vu—that is, sensing that I perhaps have *not* been to this someplace that I know I actually *have* been to.

"Oh, Eliza, welcome back. I am so glad you're here." Dinah steps into the hall, arms open to enfold me, and pulls me back into the room. "I was wondering where you were."

"I was, too! I went back to the old room and found patients there, and then went onto the floor . . ."

"Oh, of course. I forgot to tell you that the call room is changed. It happened so many months ago, and I forgot you've been away that long." She looks at me as I put down my bag and take off my jacket.

"What's it like being back?"

"I'm not sure yet . . . but strange. I feel a bit like Rip van Winkle."

She laughs and sympathizes. "Of course it feels strange. You've been away and a great deal has happened in your life that has transformed everything, even the way you see the world around you."

"I don't even feel like the same person I was then." Smiling, I look up and add, "And maybe Rip van Winkle's experience isn't the analogy I'm looking for—he fell asleep and not much happened to him except he got older. Actually I feel more like Alice after eating one of those cakes that transformed her utterly, to the point she couldn't even climb back into the world that had been hers!"

The dream comes back, and I am climbing that steep ice mountain while holding tightly to the little girl pressed against my chest. Is that treacherous storm echoing the turmoil of this disease and its treatments? The landscape that threatens annihilation with the slightest misstep?

"Alice became bigger than that world had been, Eliza. And think how vastly enriched and variegated *your* world has become." She speaks in her characteristically measured cadence, with a formality that I welcome in this age of hasty conversations and distilled sound bites. "So much you've experienced—a lot of which I'm sure you'd rather not! But those experiences have made you . . . I can't even begin to guess how the lenses through which you look at the world have been changed by your illness."

I plunge back into the dream, traveling through that hostile and treacherous blizzard, holding tightly to the glowing essence of Rose. Each step taken is at risk of losing the life-affirming dream child. And traveling through the hazardous landscape of dread disease, I must hold tightly to the life force, the impulse to live. How can I honor this mandate, this decree of a dream?

"Sometimes I think I'll never even be able to get back to that place I knew before that night last June, when the futile labors of my belly sickened me." I notice that my speech is beginning to reflect that certain formality and richness I associate with Dinah's.

**Hints to help you beat the odds . . .**
**finding understanding . . .**

An experience with cancer can be so life changing that you may find that you see your life and those around you as if viewed from another planet. Nothing seems the same, even those things that are essentially the same—they are *perceived* differently, through different lenses. When you find someone that can empathize with that transformation, despite not experiencing it directly, it can be comforting to be understood and heard.

"Oh, Eliza!" Dinah throws her arms around my neck. "I am so glad you're back here at least, and the nurses have been so eager for your return . . . but I know it's not so simple for you."

**Suggestions for allies . . .**
**helping to name and validate the changes . . .**

When your loved one begins to reenter life as a now-well person, he or she may look fine, and it may be tempting to resume life where it left off, to pretend nothing ever happened. This may work for some people, but others may be reassured by your recognition that intangible as well as tangible things have changed in their lives, and that although there may not yet be words to articulate it, there is the awareness that a sea change has occurred.

"No," I admit with a smile. "For one thing, I just hope I can be good enough to merit this place of . . . " Stopping, I struggle to find the right word. "Honor, maybe, of being so valued . . ."

"Well, let that be the least of your worries! Right now let's just have a nice quiet day."

"I'm glad I'm not here alone for this first day—I mean, the only midwife." Our unit is blessed with sharp and quick-thinking nurses, yet the midwife still is the primary labor manager, the decision maker, and I am not ready to resume this responsibility. "That would be too hard."

Changing into scrubs, I am tying my shoelaces when she says, "You let me know what you want to do today. You can do as much or as little as you want." I so appreciate her articulating this without making me feel incompetent or cowardly.

Walking out to the floor arm in arm, I respond, "I don't know how I feel yet, but thanks . . . I really appreciate it."

The gaggle of nurses is there to greet us once again, and Dinah puts her arm around me, announcing, "See what a wonderful present I have brought you? Our own Eliza is back!" It is hard for me to feel deserving of all this ebullient enthusiasm. Will I be the competent midwife, the graceful birth attendant that they remember?

**Hints to help you beat the odds . . .**
**thanking the people who help you . . .**

It is important to express your thanks to the people who have been especially helpful to you, whether they are friends, family members, colleagues, doctors, or nurses. A short note or card with a simple thank you will be appreciated. One day when you have the energy, you can host a thank-you party for your key supporters.

Checking the board that lists the patients, Dinah tells me each one's history and current status. Listening to her report, I am startled to realize how distant I feel from evaluating a cervix, managing a labor, ordering a medication, cutting an episiotomy, or enjoying that awesome experience of welcoming a newborn as it sallies forth through the watery portal into waiting arms and hearts.

For the last twelve months, I have been the patient. In fact, yesterday, I was the patient, and today, less than twenty-four hours later, I am the provider! And I am limited to clear fluids today in preparation for the colonoscopy scheduled for tomorrow, when I will be the patient once again. And twenty-four hours after that, I will be back in labor and delivery. *Role confusion*, we called it in graduate school.

**For your information . . . role confusion . . .**

Role confusion refers to uncertainty about one's place in a community or family. When illness strikes, roles such as breadwinner and caretaker may be surrendered, and one assumes the role of patient. And as the patient begins to reenter the world of before the illness, role confusion may be exaggerated: *What is my role now? What is my place here?* Navigating through and clarifying role changes is one of the challenges of being a patient.

When staff from other departments come by, men and women I know only peripherally, they are distantly polite but clearly unable to fit me into their panoply of familiar faces. In their eyes, I can read their frantic silent notations, "I *know* I know her, but I just can't place her!" Perhaps the swirls of short hair gripping my scalp are disorienting or the loss of extra pounds. I sense a difference in my relationships, acutely aware that the tenuous thread that connects us to each other can so easily and unexpectedly break.

Shadowing Dinah for the next several hours, when we step out into the hall to confer, she suggests, "Why don't you take this delivery? It should be uncomplicated, and she's *very* nice." Her eyes sparkle with encouragement. Yet despite her generous support and encouragement, I feel in an alien land, a land that I should know but that no longer feels familiar. Until today, I thought I would slide back into work with confidence and delight and am puzzled by my hesitation and self-doubt.

I trust, though, that just being at this delivery will whet my appetite, that I will be itching to "get in there" and handle the next delivery myself. For months, I have been anticipating my return to labor and delivery, to feeling the vigorous life beneath my fingers as I guide the slippery bodies out into the world. Perhaps that yearning speaks to the dream, to my clasping the small child to my breast. Yet now that I am here, there is an element of my being a stranger in this landscape of which I once was an integral part. Slipping back into the role of participant now seems awkward at best.

While making rounds earlier, we introduced ourselves to this laboring mother and the attentive father-to-be. Now the nurse pokes her head out the door and nods to us, gesturing that they are about ready.

**Hints to help you beat the odds . . .**
**more about returning to work . . .**

Depending upon how long you have been absent from work, as well as other circumstances particular to your situation, your return to the workplace may go smoothly, or it may challenge your sense of competence and self-confidence. Hopefully, your superiors will be patient in allowing you the time and space you need to reestablish your skills, regain your confidence, and make a satisfactory adjustment.

After scrubbing our hands and arms up to the elbows, we pull on our paper boots, tie flowered paper caps on our heads, press quilted paper masks to our noses, drop plastic splatter shields over our faces, and walk in. Neither parent seems troubled that all they can see of us now are our eyes behind the clear shields.

Two pairs of sterile gloves are set on the delivery table. The nurse fastens the ties of our gowns behind our backs, and then gestures toward the size seven (my size) gloves, "Just in case . . ." Her eyes twinkle above her mask.

Keeping my hands crossed at my waist, I shake my head and whisper, "Thanks, but not this time." I can feel their eagerness to get me back on track, to help me rediscover "my grain in the wood." Being back in the context of birth seems so familiar, so comfortable, so deeply compelling, yet at the same time, I am finding it difficult to simply reenter that world from the space I now inhabit.

"They're here if you want them . . . if you change your mind!" Her grin wrinkles the smile lines at the corners of her deep-green eyes.

The baby's wrinkled scalp becomes more visible with each push. Dinah cautions the mother to pant lightly as the head eases out and turns slowly to the side, Dinah's hand underneath for support. This baby is neither hurried nor reluctant, gliding easily and smoothly out into the world, blinking into the light with a baffled yet peaceful expression. Dinah gently swings her onto her mother's naked belly and clamps and cuts the cord.

"Touch your baby," she urges the mother and father. "She's yours." The father bites his lip, leans over, and laying his cheek lightly against the baby's head, his back shudders with silent sobs as he wraps his arms around his wife. Watching this family evolving before my eyes, I am struck with the privilege of caring for women becoming mothers, for men becoming fathers, for babies becoming sons and daughters. Longing to return to that role, I also dread discovering the possibility that I can no longer be the midwife I once was, that somehow when they slashed through my belly looking for the tumor, they might have slashed through my mental prowess at the same time, leaving my mind as well as my body altered. Eager as I am to reenter my professional role, I also sense a palpable relief that, at least right now, I am not responsible for anything at all.

Memory of the dream returns, the little girl Rose, vigorous and resilient, and I begin to think that it is *she* that I must remember and honor, the part of me that can be strong and capable and full of zest for living well.

A woman with a history of two normal births comes in, and I think, *No problem.*

"Here's your woman, Eliza!" Dinah invites me to take the delivery.

"Yes! Yes!" the nurses clamor. "She'll be perfect for you."

"But remember, you don't have to," Dinah kindly volunteers. "You have time, time to wait until it really feels right."

"I think I can do this," I venture. Sitting down to review the chart, I am surprised that some details of charting have changed. Different forms only, but jarring nonetheless. The patient's medical history is essentially normal, and this pregnancy has been uneventful.

The triage nurse comes out of the exam room. "She's six centimeters, Eliza, and the baby looks great!"

I stand up, but my feet feel glued to the floor tiles. Turning to Dinah, I admit, "Actually, I don't think I am ready." It is at this moment that I realize with certainty that, today at least, I want my role limited to that of spectator only. Lacking confidence, I am disinclined to reenter the natal field or to make any care decisions on my own.

"That's fine," she interrupts. "You'll know when you are." She stops and then continues, "Would it be easier if we just decide now that today, all day, you'll be the observer? And we won't even offer you any more deliveries?"

Ordinarily, it would feel like giving up, except that Dinah has communicated this proposal in such a way as to leave my dignity intact. "That sounds good . . . because when I turn you down, I feel like a failure each time. This way I'll get the failure part over with right now!" It is Dinah's empathy that allows me to feel comfortable in confessing my self-doubt.

We both laugh at the irony of my remark, and then Dinah's face turns solemn when she admonishes, "But Eliza, this is not failure!"

Once again, I hover in the background while Dinah delivers another girl. This time, though, the plan has been settled and agreed upon, the plan that I will continue to observe only, easing the pressure of deciding from one hour to the next if my confidence has returned enough to take charge.

The anxiety of resuming my professional role has been compounded, I am sure, by feeling hungry and tired and headachy, because of having not eaten since yesterday in preparation for the colonoscopy tomorrow.

Although I am scheduled to stay on labor and delivery for six hours, five is all I can manage, so at one o'clock I leave for home. Grateful that the midwives have been so accommodating in carving a schedule for me that gradually expands to full shifts, I realize that working up to those full twelve-hour blocks will be a slow process.

**For your information. . . . preparing for your colonoscopy. . . .**

When you schedule the colonoscopy, mention any medical conditions or medications that you are taking. For one to three days prior to the procedure, you will be asked to follow a liquid diet, which includes foods such as fat-free broth, strained fruit juice, water, plain coffee or tea, diet soda, gelatin, and popsicles. (However, avoid all red foods, such as red Jello, red popsicles, etc.) You will be instructed to take a specified oral laxative the night before the procedure, and then to repeat once or twice at specified intervals. Because of the sedation, you will not be able to drive after the procedure, so you will need to arrange for someone else to take you home.[1]

Walking out into the sunlight toward the parking lot, I am disappointed in myself, that I have not folded back into the staff as a fully fledged member, but rather have stumbled through the day, an outsider standing tenuously in the inside circle. Driving home through the looping curves of the mountain road, I think of the dream child of intense aliveness and vitality in a landscape of hostility and threat, the stalwart babe winding her arms around my neck as I anchor her to my heart. Traveling through that hostile and treacherous dream blizzard, holding tightly to the glowing warmth and essence of this little girl, each step taken is at risk of losing the life-affirming dream child. And traveling through this hazardous landscape of dread disease, I must hold tightly to the life force, the impulse to live. How can I honor this mandate, this decree of a dream?

# *Chapter 14*
# The Inward Journey

## DREAMING CRONES

### *July 1997*

*On a slim, silvery racing bicycle, I am pedaling down a narrow country road. Wearing gray shorts and a light shirt, I feel free. Turning onto a trail through pinewoods, I am blocked by an old red bicycle thrown across the pathway. Nearby, a child of about eleven or twelve years is picking berries with her mother. When I ask her to move the bike so I can pass, she warns me that there are witches in the woods, and they will harm me if I go further. I tell her I believe her about the witches being there but that I do not fear their reputed malevolence. Unable to convince me of the danger, she drags her bike away, and I nearly fly down the winding trail.*

*Many shallow brooks switch back and forth across the trail, leading me to believe that it is actually one stream that I am crossing at different places. Turning a corner in the trail, I see before me a wide and deep muddy river and am alarmed by its size. It is urgent that I get across this place, the last crossing I have to make. It is too deep to wade. The strong current makes swimming risky. My heart sinks with fear when the morning excursion that started out with such joy becomes terrifying. Turning away in despair, I take a few steps and see that just upstream, the river hits a shallow spot with lots of islets. I walk easily from one stone to the next and am soon across the divide. The path resumes, and a short distance away, I come upon three witches sitting at a small wooden table in the pine forest. They all have wild-looking gray hair framing wrinkled and kindly faces. Sitting down at the table, my back slightly to the path, we begin to talk. I sense an immediate understanding from them and realize that they can teach me many things.*

Months pass, and as my strength gradually returns, I notice that at the same time, my spirit and resolve seem to be fragmenting in the swirl of obligations and activities. Reminding myself to live the lessons I have learned, I seek out the stillness in the day and set aside time to be with myself, listening to the silence and also to those old crones at the table, perhaps, and to my own voice speaking softly through my dreams.

**Hints to help you beat the odds . . .**
**slowing your reentry . . .**

In your eagerness to get back to normal, it is tempting to take on too much all at once, perhaps exacerbated by your wish to demonstrate your recaptured health to those around you. Slow down and take time to make thoughtful choices about where and how you want to spend you energy and hours. This may be a time to, again, reshuffle your priorities.

Seeing myself as a stranger in an unknown province, I study my surroundings, almost like the dreamer watching the dream. Books, Internet links, and the media, like aerial photographs of a landscape, provide information about the topography of cancer and metastatic disease and the associated treatments and procedures. Time and again, I reach for stories that are funny, entertaining, and remote from grave illness. At other times, I welcome books of poetry and prose directed to the inner world, the spiritual self, and the long journey home. The Internet poses an irony, as there is a part of me that wants to learn nothing more than I am already forced to know through experience and the other part of me that historically has relied on the acquisition of knowledge to overcome seemingly insurmountable hurdles.

In recent years, the media have covered cancer extensively, especially those lodged in the organs of sex and sensuality, breath and thought. Not so with colon cancer, lodged in the entrails that carry toxic waste from the body. Colon disease grabs headlines only when famous people are felled or when celebrities such as Katie Couric bring it to the TV screen. I have fallen into the habit of reading the obituaries, with special attention to age and cause of death. When my quick scan is stopped by the words "colon cancer," or just plain "cancer," I shudder at the lives truncated before fully lived, at the children and grandchildren left with the empty places at the dinner table and painful swellings in their hearts.

Studying a map of this new country, I notice the city streets, the plazas and parks, the rivers and waterways, the government buildings and civil monuments. And beyond the city are the narrow country lanes, the farmland, the rolling hills, the flat prairies, and small villages: cottages gathered about the reassuring spires of wooden clapboard churches. Doctors and nurses are my cartographers, mapping out the alternate routes, describing possible hazards and dangers, and recommending one or two routes they trust. Most are eager to help prepare me well for the journeys and side trips that have been necessary along the way; a few have been insufficiently interested to bother offering advice or counsel.

Studying the faces of compatriots whom I join in this new land, like perusing snapshots of the populace of different areas, I get a more intimate view of the nature of one part of the land as distinct from another. The widening circles of support continue to astonish and buoy me and range from those in my structured support group at WomenCARE to the Cancer Club, a group of friends who happen to have cancer and who meet monthly to chat and keep each other afloat. These groups of women are able, through their shared experience, to furnish details of their personal travels through that province, to describe the specific photographs of certain areas to which I might be traveling, and to assure me that there are several routes for getting to the same place. They can suggest where the road may become a dirt trail, with vague markings to guide me; where it might suddenly revert to cobblestones, making solid footing precarious; where it might suddenly span a tumultuous body of water, requiring me to find a bridge to safety. Like the women in the dream, they know this region and its hidden surprises and shadowy threats firsthand and can help me feel safe as I navigate my own way. There is great comfort in being with fellow travelers who share the same terror and have felt some of the same doubt and anxiety. It is a group with whom none of us has to be brave or to pretend to have forgotten. One of the women, a young lawyer whose only child is just three years old, says one day, "It's just so hard not knowing how our stories are going to end."

An enormous source of support continues to be family and friends who may not have shared this experience of cancer but who bind me closely to them with their unfailing love and support, even when my humor has vanished and any charm or grace is hard to perceive. Cancer is not an attractive disease, and colon cancer is probably one of the least so, yet a well-placed joke or hug would nearly always break the tension of some of the worst moments.

**Hints to help you beat the odds . . .**
**tickling the funny bone . . .**

A quote from Groucho Marx: "A clown is like an aspirin, only he works twice as fast." Laughter really is a wonderful medicine; it stimulates the release of endorphins, a substance in the brain that helps control pain. Hospitals use humor therapy to ease pain, reduce stress, and promote relaxation.[1] Comedies and humorous books, as well as clown shows, of course, can provide comic relief even in the hardest times. (Remember to splint your abdomen with a pillow when you laugh!)

Buttressed by this foundation created by family, friends, and support groups, and by doctors and nurses, as well as the media, I nonetheless recognize that there are difficult questions that have been posed by this experience and that I cannot address them without witness or answer them without assistance. A year after diagnosis, after the chemo is completed and the colostomy is reversed, I initiate regular contact with Judith, a Jungian therapist who has been my guide in times of stress and sorrow.

"I am sobered at how quickly you skim over your story," she remarks after I deliver a hurried synopsis of the last year. "I am struck by the utter seriousness of your experience," she continues, "yet I see how easy it is for you to turn your attention elsewhere."

Pale-green maple leaves brush against the windowpane in the silence that follows. She looks at me, clears her throat, and resumes, "Your succinct statements carry a nuclear load! You graciously express these

**Hints to help you beat the odds . . .**
**psychotherapy and support . . .**

Having cancer is a major stressor, when all your coping mechanisms are called into play. A psychotherapist can help you understand your responses throughout this period, help you explore the meaning of this experience, and help you identify ways to enrich and deepen the quality of your life.

intense feelings, these profound sorrows, yet rush on as if to hurry yourself out of the dark places you've been."

I shift my feet and lean forward. "It's back to that place of not wanting to overstate, of feeling a certain embarrassment at yet another disaster upsetting the precarious stability of my world."

In the quiet, I feel her eyes on me as I look through the window at the splatter of sky through the lacy patterns of maple leaves.

Shepherded through the province by her gentle presence, she helps me interpret what I am seeing and steers me away from places where I might trip or take a wrong turn. She helps me figure out why one way feels better than an alternative route, why I am comfortable in some parts of the region and not others, and how to best avoid the areas that are threatening or scary. In this province where maps and photographs have been useful tools of orientation, Judith helps me to further *understand* the experiences, to find the deeper meanings, and to avoid the pitfall of shoving them into an ignominious past.

Aware that I have an ongoing motif of not expressing painful matters, she urges me to work toward being able to more easily know and articulate what I am sensing. "When we *know*," she says, "but don't *say*, eventually, we no longer even know."

"Well, one thing I know is that I have lost a child, and another thing I know is that I have had cancer. And those two things are what everyone dreads the most—in a way, I become the walking embodiment of everyone's worst fears."

Her barely perceptible nod encourages me to continue.

"I see that fear sometimes when someone stares into my face, looking for, perhaps, the secret that allows me to live with such loss and at the same time horrified should the loss be contagious. It makes it hard sometimes, I think, for people to be with me . . . it's too scary."

**Hints to help you beat the odds . . .**
**coping with the "contagious cancer" myth . . .**

Although less common today, it is possible that you will be confronted by the fear of the contagion of cancer. Friends and associates may avoid you altogether or avoid sharing food with you or bathroom facilities. You can choose to spend your time with other, more understanding people, or you can try to educate and address the fears of those who operate under the belief of "cancer-as-a-contagious-disease."

Some part of me expects her to say, "No, that must be your imagination." But she concurs, agreeing that people who have met great tragedy can be, on a primal level, feared by others. These currents run deep and strong and, most of the time, remain unavailable and unarticulated.

Lifting myself out of this strange melancholy, with near disbelief I remark, "But I'm surviving it—and amazed when I think about it. If I had ever guessed my future, I would have been appalled and totally unable to accept the predictions of fate. And absolutely convinced that I would not have been able to survive these events."

"You're finding now that you have a strength that, in the past, you have resisted acknowledging. You must claim that power and bring it fully into your life now!" Adjusting her silky persimmon scarf around her shoulders, she continues, "And part of that strength depends on your speaking from the deepest part of yourself: the bare bones, the deepest gut truth, what really needs to be voiced."

Reflecting on the meaning of what has happened, she also pushes me to explore the changes that this experience requires. She urges me to consider questions such as, "How do I walk this? What is this new way of being?"

I know I need to seek a balance that will allow me to enjoy family and friends and also safeguard the solitude and sanctuary that allows me to continue to heal and regenerate. Judith urges me to ask the questions that will lead to exploring the choices that might predict healthy outcomes and to seek the answers not only in my intellect but also and especially deep within my body: *How do I know it's a yes? How do I know it's a no? What do I know? What do I want? What is my gut telling me? What is the best for me right now?*

*What is it I know for sure?* I wonder. *What are the lessons of this illness?* Emerging from the ashes of this life I left behind last July 2, I can feel a new story trying to live. *How is my response to threat manifested in my response to this disease?* I ponder, and, *How will my responses be different in the future?*

"You have always been very vulnerable to the psychic contents of other people," she reminds me, "and now, given the surgery, this is especially true: The body has been ripped open, and there has been a rip in the aura as well as in the body. On many levels, you must take back your power."

As she speaks, I think, *How obvious, how clearly she understands.* My innate strength. I am beginning to understand it only as I experience the stripping of that power through the dependence and helplessness imposed on me by this illness. Only by the experience of *not* having it do I finally understand *having* it.

**Hints to help you beat the odds . . .**
**understanding our strengths . . .**

Sometimes it is only by its absence that we recognize a strength. By becoming dependent we recognize the power of independence. By becoming gravely ill we appreciate health. By confronting the finiteness of our life span we treasure each day. The challenge is to remember these lessons learned, even as they fade behind the scrim of returning good health.

Time passes, we meet and talk, and I realize that she is articulating the muddled impressions that have been trailing through my mind. She is helping me organize into an intelligible whole the chaos of images that have been pressing against my psyche for attention.

"It seems not random chance that this cancer lodged in your belly," she cautions. "Listen to that gut now, pay attention to your body's responses to your emotional states." Remembering that any occasion of tension and anxiety triggered sudden abdominal cramps and often diarrhea, I know she speaks the truth. And then I wonder, *Is it because I had become used to a chronically traumatized GI system that it took so long for me to realize that I was in a grave crisis that night last summer? Had abnormal become normal to the extent that I could no longer make the distinction?*

"Your dance with cancer is a redemptive and transformational act. Your voice, your reality, can no longer be overridden or suppressed," she cautions. "You need to live it." How do I defend those dream-child qualities that sustain and promote life? My task, now, is to cling to them, to guard them in safekeeping, to never, ever forget them. This is my work.

There are physical things, such as eating well, exercising, taking daily aspirin to prevent inflammation, and meditating. There are the daily decisions I make, the choices that might promote health and well-being or those that might catapult me back onto a life lived too fast and too densely. And being hurled back onto that spinning carousel, just doing what I need to do to maintain my balance, to not tumble off, will command all my attention and demand all my energies.

**Hints to help you beat the odds . . . paying attention . . .**

You may have teetered on the edge of the abyss and yearned for stability. When you begin to gain ground, to stabilize in your new "normality," it requires vigilance to pay attention to the signals from the inner worlds of your body, mind, and heart. Stay on course, living in the way that you feel sustains inner calm, and try to ignore the siren calls of overcommitment and distraction.

Although wonderful body workers, healers, and fellow cancer sojourners sustained me throughout the first year of diagnosis, surgeries, and treatments, I am doing most of this inner-journey work now. It is almost as if treatment allowed neither energy nor focused attention for *thinking* about the experience. Resisting the distraction of analysis, I was completely engaged in *living* the experience. It seemed a hallowed time, when all my sensory attention was riveted on the vicissitudes of my body, the opening of my heart, and the retreat into the private spaces of my inner landscape. Only now am I beginning to engage in understanding and integrating these experiences into my newly precarious yet abundant life.

Feeling the customary patterns of my days begin to fall into place, I am reminded that constant vigilance will be required to hold on to the lessons learned. It was easier to say, "No, I can't do that" or "No, I can't help you" when I was bald and thin and weakened by a terminal disease than now when I am looking well and eating and working like anyone else. In the height of my illness, there was a part of me that felt protected and cocooned by the constraints the disease imposed upon me. People felt sorry that there were so many things I could not do, but I felt peaceful in the quiet of not even trying.

Now, without the isolating shelter of active disease, I must be awake to the needs of my body as well as the needs of my family and community. To protect myself from the impulsive reaction to agree with requests so as not to disappoint somebody, I try to refrain from committing myself, instead waiting for twenty-four hours before responding. During that protected time, I can consider carefully whether I have the time, the energy, and the inclination to do whatever is being asked of me.

Saying what I need and want is another challenge that is on its way to resolution and perhaps will always be in process. My professional life has focused on the needs, wants, and heartaches of my patients and clients. To shift the focus to my own needs and desires is an abrupt and difficult task. In the world of the spirit, as well, I must explore the meaning of all this and the possibility that I can keep myself healthy and impervious to another assault.

Judith also leads me to the edge of the abyss and encourages me to look down into it, to acknowledge its power to pull me in, and to honor my own powers to resist its terrifying allure. She helps me to savor the heavy sweetness of the Dark Angel, whose shape was cast a long shadow over so many days and nights.

"*And what obligation do you have to the Dark Angel?*" She is articulating a question that has been pressing vaguely in my consciousness, yet I am unable to figure out a response.

"I'm not sure I know," I venture. "Except perhaps to never forget her . . . to remember how close she is . . ." I am fumbling for words.

"I think one obligation to this encounter might be to live what she forced you to do when you were sick, to take with you into wellness the inner authority to rest when tired, to flare when angered, and to be true in your response when cut deeply, rather than standing like a deer with the headlights in your eyes."

"I know too how much I need solitude, how important that time alone has been . . . and how hard it is to hold on to."

She presses me to recognize that I am not entirely at the mercy of the wayward cells, that my own impulse to live is one factor among many that will determine the timing when the Dark Angel, powered by golden wings, swoops down to gather me in her arms for my last flight.

# *Chapter 15*

# Slipping from Wellness

## DREAMING SPLITTING OPEN

### *August 1998*

*Nico and Rose are wandering in and out of the bathroom, chattering and playing as I am bathing. Hearing their peaceful conversation, feeling the relaxing rhythm of their activity, I am comforted.*

*Shockingly, my left breast suddenly starts to bleed under the nipple, while just above the areola, the skin starts to tear open, making a horizontal slit like a winking eye. I can see in the narrow opening some thick blood and gnarled, black tissue. Although horrified, I am at the same time relieved, as I have been feeling that something rotten was lodging in this breast. Wanting to avoid calling the children's attention to the wound, I lay a dry, white washcloth over the gash.*

*Using my fingers to exert pressure above the opening, I am appalled at the size of the knob that begins to ooze out. Realizing that I need to have a place to put this lump, I glance about for another washcloth or paper napkin and settle on a wrinkled page from the* New Yorker. *I lean over and out comes a blackened, deep-red glop the size of a hen's egg. I feel faint seeing it, thinking that somehow my entire breast is falling out, that there will be no end to it, that maybe my entire insides will spill out through this gash.*

*Looking down at the slit, I see what is apparently normal breast tissue, pinkish gray, and in flat layers like shad roe. I am reassured to see it tucked safely in place. The bloody mass is discreet and now seems to have been thoroughly extruded. Although the children worry when they see the splash of blood, they are easily distracted by some bath toys and don't see me wrap the blackened nugget in the paper and shove it behind a folded yellow towel.*

Wrestling to untangle myself from the sticky spider web of nightmare, the sickening egg a vivid image in my mind's eye, I press my breasts in search of the dream lump. Cancer has been receding into the shadowy places in my mind, no longer an active concern. Is this dream pulling me once again into the possibilities on which I have turned my back? Last week, a friend sent me a colorful watercolor, which included the scrawled sentiment, "Most people don't know that there are angels whose only job is to make sure you don't get too comfortable and miss your life."

Or maybe it should say: *Most people don't know that there are angels whose only job is to make sure you don't get too comfortable and* lose *your life.* The image of that hideous lump exploding from what I assumed was healthy breast deflates my upbeat optimism, reminding me that I need to stay *awake*. Vigilant. If I have been getting too comfortable, this lingering dream is pushing me out of that place of complacency.

A counterpoint to this aching dread is a telephone call from Rose and Nico, now living thousands of miles away. Four-year-old Rose, breathless with excitement, says, "Nana, will you send me all the things from . . . from my . . . Nana, will you send me . . . everything from your world?" She is still perplexed as to why we don't live together and proclaims, "We will live together now, all together. Because we are a *family*!" Her reasoning is clear, without complications and without question. Reassuring her is difficult, as I feel truly bereft with them so very far away and will likely cry if I tell her how hard it also is for me.

"It's hard to be so far away," I acknowledge, "but we'll come as often as we can, and you'll come here, too."

"Can you come here tomorrow?" she asks hopefully.

My heart drops when I have to explain, "No, not tomorrow, Rosie. But soon . . . perhaps for your birthday."

"Oh, yay! Nana and Papa will come for my birthday! Yay!" I can hear her drop the phone, and I imagine her dancing with glee.

"Nana?" Nico asks. "Will you and Papa come for my birthday, too?"

"I hope so, Nico. The grown-ups will talk together and figure out when we can come. We miss you a lot."

"I miss you, too." There is a brief silence before he adds, "Nana, you and Papa can share my bed when you come visit . . . it's a bunk bed!"

The innocence, the trust in their voices are sources of both comfort and sorrow. How long do I have in this world? How many months and years remain for me to spend time with them? My arms ache with longing as we say our farewells.

**Hints to help you beat the odds . . .**
**finding emotional nourishment . . .**

Children, with their vigor and innocence and belief in all possibilities, can provide a counterpoint to disease, reminding you of all that you long for and nourishing you with their love and trust that all will be well. If not a child, perhaps there is someone else in your life whose presence nourishes you. The connectedness that evolves is a healing power in and of itself.

It is August of 1998, more than two years after my diagnosis. The balloon colonoplasties, once done every two weeks, then every three, then four, and so on, are no longer needed. My bowels are back to functioning in an acceptable manner, and I have come to terms with the loss of Stella. We have even started a major renovation on our house: adding a second story, which in this earthquake country practically requires rebuilding the first story. Taking on this project is a testimonial to life, to a future, to a belief in my wellness. It is also enormously disruptive, with areas of the house closed off entirely. Surfaces, floors, and clothes are buried in dust despite scrupulous efforts to isolate the essential living areas. There is a nearly continuous din of hammering and sawing and a dizzying array of choices when selecting paint colors, window coverings, faucets, flooring, lighting, and items such as drawer knobs.

The WomenCARE support group, which I attend every other week with eight other women, continues to be my safe haven. Here I can bring up things understandable only by those who have trod this path: small things, like, *This little bump on my rib . . . is it a tumor that traveled over from my colon? The ache in my joints . . . has the cancer reached into my bones?*

To the bigger issues: *What matters? How do I want to spend my time? What are my priorities, now that I have faced the dark angel?* She passed by me this time, yet feeling the chill as the shadow of her wings took my sun away, my days are densely laced with an intense awareness of the tenuous quality of the strand that holds us to this life. Like my friends in the "Cancer Club," with whom I meet monthly, we understand the terror of living with cancer, the agony of chemotherapy, and the tenderness of looking at the sweet faces we love, knowing our time with them may be suddenly cut short.

**Hints to help you beat the odds . . .
finding community in peer support . . .**

Even if you have support from friends and family, a support group can be an important adjunct, a community in which your story will be heard by those who have trod very similar paths. A support group provides a forum where you can disclose worries and fears that might be alarming to family members and close friends.

This summer I am working extra shifts to cover for staffing shortages and colleagues on holiday. Grateful for their kind attentions and generous gifts during my illness, I am eager to accommodate their schedules. The busy workload is exhilarating, reconnecting me with cherished friends and reassuring me that I can still function in my professional role. It also offers respite from the construction site we continue to call home.

Making rounds on my laboring patients, I catch the eye of the lab technician and ask him to draw my CarcinoEmbryonic Antigen (CEA), as I am due for the routine screen. He readily agrees, and I extend my arm as he swabs alcohol over a vein.

As he labels the collection tube before leaving, a midwife turns to me and asks anxiously, "Aren't you nervous when you get those drawn?"

"No." Dismissing her concern I tell her, "It's always been normal, I feel great, and I'm sure it's normal today!" Yet pressing the gauze sponge to the puncture site, I am reminded of the dream, of pressing that lump of black-and-red decay from my breast.

Three days later, August 6, I am astonished to return home to hear on the answering machine, "This is Dr. Feng, I need to speak with Ms. Livingston." There is a pause before he nervously resumes, "Please can she call Dr. Feng at the hospital right away?"

Hearing these words in that tone, my heart drops into my toes and through the floor. I feel as if the substance of my body is draining through to nothingness. I know that bad news is quickly conveyed. Customarily, test results come through the mail, a typed letter with the name of the test, the parameters, and the findings. Then at the bottom is a tiny note of congratulations from Dr. Liu. A phone call, however, suggests a certain urgency in transmitting the information. Charles, in an effort to comfort me, points out that this is a new doctor, and perhaps he has a different way of communicating with patients.

The anxious tone of Dr. Feng's voice translates into panic, carving out an empty hollow in my stomach. Looking at Charles, I see the alarm in his face. Neither of us can comfort the other, yet, as if trying to convince himself, he says, "Maybe it's something else . . ." His voice drifts off uncertainly.

Doubting whether I can survive another crisis without Dr. Liu, my sadness at his absence is rekindled. I hardly know Dr. Feng. The voice on the answering machine, however, conveys hesitation, determination, and kindness all pressed into an amalgam and threaded through the telephone wires. I immediately return his call, insisting to the advice nurse that she get through to him right away. Understanding my urgency, she promises to put a note on his desk.

Shifting from numb shock to silent tears, I curl up on the bed; Charles lies down and holds me; we are like nestled spoons. The dream lingers, tormenting me with vivid images of the reddish-black lump bursting from the deep gash. Has the colon cancer metastasized to the breast?

Within minutes, Dr. Feng calls. Listening to him mentioning some minor health matters, I can tell that there is another reason for his call.

He finally says, "And then there is something else . . ."

I help him out by offering, "My CEA is up."

"Yes, yes, it is. It is 5.1," I hear him say. "It's been around one since your first surgery." In the pause, I can hear his reluctance to continue. The tumult in my chest is making me lightheaded.

"There are other things that can raise it, of course, but we need to do some tests to find out more about what is happening."

We have met only once before, yet I have a clear sense of his distress in having to disclose such news. He clears his throat and continues, "So I want you to have a chest x-ray. You can pick up the requisition from my office any time." Lungs are common sites for colon cancer metastasis; red warning flares pulsate behind my closed eyelids. So maybe the dream lump was coming from the lungs! And traveling through the breast to escape, to leave in its trail only healthy tissue.

"And go to the lab for another CEA, just to confirm these results." Brought back to the conversation by his voice, I remind myself, *Yes, this can be an erroneous lab result—a lab error—a slipped decimal point—perhaps it's really 0.51—perhaps my collection tube got mixed up with someone else's.* A parade of possibilities flash by before I hear, "And we'll schedule a CT scan of your abdomen and pelvis. I have already sent a requisition, and they will call you with an appointment." *And another common site of metastatic disease is the liver*, I remember, as he pauses before continuing, "It may take a few weeks to get you into the schedule . . . I think they're pretty backed up right now."

He waits, his silence inviting my questions, but this somber news has swept me into a churning sea of ominous possibilities.

I can hear a sadness in his sigh as he breaks into the hush. "I am very sorry to have to tell you this. Do you have questions?" Another pause. "Is someone with you?"

"Yes," I whisper. "Thank you."

"Good." He sounds relieved. "Come up to see me in the morning, after you're finished in radiology."

Leaning into Charles's solid chest, I begin to regain my center enough to remember my manners. "And thank you . . . these calls aren't easy, I know."

"Oh, of course," he pauses again, giving me time to formulate questions or concerns, before he signs off. "So I'll see you tomorrow."

I hang up the phone and feel myself sinking into space. Crying, I manage to verify Charles's assumptions.

"I want to go right away to get the chest x-ray." Wanting answers as soon as possible, I also need this task. I want to be able to do my part of the job, and right now, that means getting a chest x-ray.

**Hints to help you beat the odds . . . getting well is a job . . .**

Framing healing in the context of a "job" validates the work involved. It is important to acknowledge the fact that the work of getting well requires time, energy, attention, and focus. Otherwise, you risk sidestepping the reality of the disease and turning your back on the task of healing, completing the small tasks that go into getting better.

Driving to the hospital, we are both quiet; there is not much to say. Waiting in the radiology department, I watch people come and go. An Asian woman in a wheelchair stoops as she gets out for her x-ray, holding her belly and softly moaning. Her tense body and plaintive cry remind me of the abdominal pain that began my odyssey. The tech helping her is kind, a middle-aged gentleman with a Persian accent. While I wait, several people are called, giving me a chance to watch this man's interactions with frightened patients. Struck by his kindness and courtesy, I hope that he will be the one to summon me when my turn comes.

In a row of seats with wooden armrests, I wait with others in my bright-green gown. My status is immediately recognizable by my attire: just days ago, it was the navy scrubs of professional staff or jeans and a shirt and sandals. And before that, the hospital gowns stamped with navy flowers or tan geometric figures, announcing my position as patient at the bottom of the institutional hierarchy. And now, in this room, Charles is the only one in street clothes. The men on either side of us, their long, hairy legs jutting out from beneath gowns like mine, flip through magazines. We become a community, lined up there in our rough cotton robes, waiting for machines to photograph the body parts specified on our requisitions.

Someone around the corner starts snoring loudly, like a small plane shuddering as the propellers slow their spin. A stout man with sparse, wavy, white hair and a large, rounded nose jokes, "I know about this place and waiting, but this is too much!"

Next to him, a woman looks up from her *Harpers* magazine and asks, "Is he really sleeping?"

The man peers around the corner, and grins, "Yup! Like a babe."

"Ee-Lie-Zah!" The kindly Persian man calls my name, pronouncing it slowly and lyrically. Bowing slightly, he informs me, "My name is Ahmed." He takes me into the film room and stands me up against the cold, steel rectangle mounted on the wall, my chin lifted to rest on the curve of gray painted metal. He gently pushes my shoulders forward and tells me to take a deep breath and hold. I hear the *thunk* of a picture being taken, and then his voice: "Relax now."

In those moments, he becomes my light, my hope that I might meet the healing angels who guided me through the complex web of care during my first siege. I begin to realize that a good part of my fear is related to Dr. Liu and Dr. Zang having retired, and Dr. Narayan having relocated, to my sheer terror of someone new opening up my abdomen.

**Hints to help you beat the odds . . .**
**breathing . . . and breathing deeply . . .**

The value of deep breathing, at the core of many Eastern approaches to healthcare, is also recognized by complementary health practitioners in the West. When you inhale, your diaphragm flattens to allow the lungs to expand. As you exhale, your diaphragm returns to its domelike shape. This diaphragmatic breathing, also known as abdominal breathing, is the most efficient way for exchanging oxygen and carbon dioxide. Under normal circumstances, your diaphragm works automatically, but when you are under stress, there is an unconscious tendency to override the process. When this occurs, your breathing becomes uneven, rapid, and shallow, thus reducing the level of oxygen in your bloodstream and brain, leading to fatigue and increased tension.[1] When you feel anxious, tense, and tired, start to relax through some slow deep breathing. If you are too tense, ask your ally to lead you to that quiet place inside the breath.

The requisition is a "stat read," so I am ushered back to my place in the row of chairs to wait. Two people remain in the small space. A few minutes later, someone comes in and tells those two people that they are to leave and go into another room around the corner, where the man was snoring some time ago. Surprised, they get up and leave as they have been directed. I conclude that perhaps I am going to get news that requires privacy. My chest tightens. *Breathe in slowly, take it easy*, I tell myself, sucking in the stale air through pursed lips. *Now exhale, relax your shoulders, relax your chest.*

Just minutes pass before Ahmed returns to lead me down the hall, Charles following. He has a large manila envelope in his hand, and we stop at a small enclosure that was once perhaps a closet, and has now been fashioned into a tiny office.

"Eliza, this is Dr. Butler, the radiologist." A man with tired eyes turns toward us and nods as he takes the envelope.

Dr. Butler puts his hand over the phone he is cradling on his shoulder, snaps the films up on the light box, quickly scans the x-rays, turns to me, and says abruptly, "The lungs look OK, but when are you getting your CT scan?"

"I'm waiting to be notified of my appointment—I understand they're very backlogged." When he frowns disapprovingly, I add, "If you can do anything to speed it up, I'd really appreciate it."

The next morning, I hand carry my x-rays and the radiologist's report to the oncology clinic. Lung fields are clear, with no detectable lesions. The high CEA level is confirmed by the repeat test. Dr. Feng listens to my lungs, percusses my chest and back, and palpates my belly, with special attention to the liver area. He is gentle, and his compassion is conveyed more through silence than through any particular spoken words.

It is nearly two weeks before the CT scan can be scheduled, so I continue working on labor and delivery during this time of waiting. A few days after the CEA results, during a minor suturing after a delivery, I accidentally stab the tip of my finger with a needle. Following the protocols for such incidents, labs are drawn on both the patient and me for hepatitis B and C and for HIV status.

Four days later, tests indicate that screens for hepatitis B and HIV are negative. When the patient's labs come back positive for hepatitis C, I am stunned: In addition to probable metastatic disease, I am now faced with the potential of hepatitis C, for which there is no cure. The labs will repeat the tests to confirm the positive result and will do serial testing for the next twelve months.

Although repeat testing indicates that the patient's hepatitis test is a false positive, during those days of waiting for results, I ponder the many risks of exposure inherent in midwifery. Assuming that my cancer diagnosis represents an overwhelming collapse of the immune system, I cannot trust my body to deal forcefully with exposures to pathogens. Is continuing to deliver babies simply a variation of Russian roulette? Does protecting myself from potentially infected fluids require that I no longer work as a midwife? That would be another loss. Although the ominous hepatitis C results have proven false, it may be unwise to challenge my body to withstand further assaults.

Considering the possibilities, and weighing the potential benefits and losses of continuing in my profession, is making me dizzy. Projecting myself into the future, predicting my situation in some far-off time, is confusing at best. Tethering my imagination to the confines of the present, tending only to my needs of the moment, I limit my planning to the weeks leading up to the surgery. After the scheduled CT scan, we will proceed with plans for our vacation and then return for the surgery, when my medical leave will start. I am aware of a certain peace in yielding the illusion of control, in letting go of speculation and guesswork.

Following several hours of eating nothing, scan preparations start with the introduction of contrast dye, beginning with the ingestion of two liters of a milky, strawberry-flavored concoction. An enema and an IV follow. Told that I will be notified of the results late in the afternoon, by five o'clock I have heard nothing. Calls from Andrew prod the medical group into action, and at around six o'clock, the on-call oncologist rings us at home.

"There is an area around the bladder that concerns me," she says in a lilting Indian accent. "I will order an ultrasound for you tomorrow, to evaluate it further."

Ignoring whatever it is about my bladder that suggests a problem, my mind jumps right to the core of my fear. "My liver is OK then?"

"Well," she says slowly, "it looks OK to me." There is a question inherent in the tone of her voice. Elated that she has not mentioned an abdomen rife with lesions, I also realize that a specialist has probably not yet read the scans, that her conclusions are drawn without the benefit of a radiologist's report.

Nevertheless, I feel my body relax with relief. "Oh, thank goodness."

"Come to the hospital tomorrow for an ultrasound," she resumes. "I'll leave the necessary papers at the desk here for you."

Hanging up the telephone, I am feeling a certain calm, a sense that I can continue to put one foot in front of the other. Standing at the eye of this storm, I am ready to take in what I need and also to surrender to the forces shaping the days to follow.

The next morning, carrying my requisition for ultrasound down to the patient registration desk, I read: "6 cm. Pelvic mass to left of midline, rule

**For your information . . . diagnostic ultrasound . . .**

Ultrasound imaging, also called ultrasound scanning or sonography, obtains images of internal organs by sending high-frequency sound waves into the body. The reflected sound waves' echoes are recorded and displayed as a real-time visual image on the computer screen. A transducer is attached to the scanner by a cord. The technician spreads a lubricating gel on the abdomen, and then presses the transducer, a small, hand-held device about the size of a bar of soap, firmly against the skin to obtain images. The ultrasound image is immediately visible on a nearby screen that looks much like a computer or television monitor.[2]

out fluid." Pelvic mass. What an ominous term. Walking down the hall, I feel hyperalert, my senses open and acute, yet at the same time composed.

The warm gel sliding across my abdomen is comforting in a fundamental way and a striking contrast to all the cool, stainless steel of the equipment. Unlike the technicians' exuberant responses when they found me free of gallstones last year, now they are quiet as they study the screen. The particular pattern of clicks I hear suggests that they are taking several pictures from different angles. They seem concerned with an area low in my pelvis. Although a small adjustment in the tilt of my head would allow me to view the screen, I don't want to see whatever it is that is muffling their words and straightening their smiles.

They finally wipe the gel off my belly and help me up into a seated position. They politely demur when I ask them to tell me what they have seen. Instructed to take the films to the oncology clinic, I am seen by the doctor on call.

Confirming the notation I read earlier on the ultrasound form, she says in an impassive voice, "A pelvic mass down near your bladder is about seven centimeters in diameter and appears to be fluid filled." She shrugs and muses, "Is it cancer? I don't know." So the small egg of my dream is becoming the large tangerine of reality, the dream lump in my left breast becoming the *real* lump in the left lower quadrant of my abdomen. We leave knowing enough to be frightened but not enough to know what we are frightened *of*.

Arriving home, I watch the men silhouetted against the cobalt sky, raising the framing for the second story. As they lift our house into the firmament, I feel as if I am free-falling to earth. What happened to that testimonial to life? Will I ever sleep in that bedroom? Bathe in that bathtub? What irony that am living through the noise and chaos of construction yet may not survive to celebrate its completion.

The following morning, August 19, I have an appointment with a gynecologic oncologist, the same Dr. Kinjo I consulted last May regarding removing my ovaries. His is the only familiar face in the surgery now that Dr. Narayan and Dr. Zang are gone. I am putting all my trust in his skill and wizardry.

He leans back in his chair and begins, "There is a mass on the left ovary, which may be one of three things: a benign cyst, ovarian cancer, or metastatic colon cancer." He clears his throat quickly and then continues. "If it is the last, the chances are that it has spread elsewhere. Given the CEA, a benign cyst is not likely."

**For your information . . . metastatic disease . . .**

When a cancer spreads to a distant organ, the distant tumor will have the same kind of abnormal cells as the primary tumor and will carry the name of the primary tumor. For instance, if colon cancer spreads to the lung, the disease is metastatic colon cancer, not lung cancer. If it spreads to the ovary, it is still metastatic colon cancer as opposed to ovarian cancer. Any treatment protocol will be directed at colon cancer, not lung cancer. Only when the pathology report is completed will the diagnosis be confirmed as either a metastatic cancer or a new primary cancer, in this case, metastatic colon cancer or ovarian cancer.[3]

Feeling as if I am on a runaway train headed for the dark underworld, my thoughts flutter randomly about, touching on the prospects of metastatic colon cancer or ovarian cancer.

My glance falls on Charles, whose eyes widen like blue saucers against his increasingly pale face.

Mustering my courage, I smile as I ask the doctor, "Well, what shall I hope for: ovarian cancer? Or metastatic colon cancer?"

Shaking his head, he looks straight into my eyes and says, "Neither one is any good."

That is not what I want to hear. I need to be soothed like a fevered child, told that everything will be all right. How can I believe I will heal if the doctor doesn't? And how can I heal if I don't believe it's possible? Regardless of my prognosis, of what he knows, and I know but don't acknowledge, I need a space for hoping and believing in the possibility of survival. Lingering in the hallway, I wait, anticipating he'll say something more, something encouraging. In the silence, I remember the dream, the hideous egg of decay, the foreshadowing of this decree of doom.

"I have scheduled your surgery for August 31," Dr. Kinjo informs me, "and chemo will begin shortly thereafter." *In that case*, I think to myself, *with surgery not happening for ten days, we will have time for the family vacation we have planned.*

**Considerations for hospital staff . . . allowing for hope . . .**

Even when signs point clearly to the potential for an unfavorable outcome, it is important not to take away the patient's hope. Simple words such as "We'll figure out a way" can help.

Leaving the hospital, Dr. Kinjo's bleak assessment, *Neither one is any good*, echoes in my head.

Driving home, Charles and I are silent, each in our own world of fear. Rebecca calls, and when I tell her the news, she gathers their children and takes them to the hospital where she can be with Andrew when she tells him what has happened. An image of their lives without me flashes by: They are thousands of miles from any family—who will visit them for birthdays? Christmases? Thanksgivings? Graduations? Charles is not one to initiate contact and has left the management of family intimacies to me. When I am gone, will he suddenly become proficient at initiating contact, at reaching out from isolation, at maintaining the ties that bind?

The next day, I attend my twice-monthly support group at Women-CARE. Although I have told Julie about the new tumor, for the rest of the group, this is shocking news. While we are acutely aware that we live in proximity to a time bomb that can explode unexpectedly at any time, we are nonetheless aghast when it ignites. They listen carefully, offering no platitudes. Exchanges are honest in this group that shares a common if painful history. My terror is familiar, common to all of us, and needs no explanation. I leave knowing that the support of this group of women will be essential in the days and weeks to come.

A few days before we depart for our planned holiday in Oregon, I receive a phone call from an old friend, Carly, with whom I worked in an alternative birth center many years ago. She is now a naturopath practicing in another state, but here on vacation.

Sitting on the patio the following morning, the sun splashing through the bean tree, we catch up on each other's news. I am relieved that, although there is considerable hammering going on up above us, the table saw is idle, allowing us to converse easily. Charles brings us iced tea with honey and fresh mint. When she asks for the details of the health crisis I mentioned over the phone, she listens attentively as I tell her what I know.

When I come to the end of my story, she folds her hands and leans forward. "What is the plan now?"

"Surgery right after we get home from vacation. And then, after that, I don't know." Not knowing seems OK with me.

"Are you thinking about chemotherapy?"

"I'm not sure. I guess we pretty much know it's cancer, it's just a matter of which kind, but . . ."

"I hope you *never* do chemo again!" Charles breaks in, his voice straining with exasperation. "It nearly killed you last time." He turns to

Carly, eyes wide with astonishment, and says, "You can't *imagine* how sick she was!"

"Yeah, that's strong stuff," she agrees. Turning to me, she asks, "Do you feel as if it nearly killed you?"

"I don't know. It made me really sick, but I truly believed in it. I thought that the sicker I got, the sicker and deader the cancer cells would get!" Remembering my trust in those chemo solutions, now it feels like looking back on an innocence that has been totally eclipsed by recent examinations. If it was the magic potion I thought it was, what is this tangerine size tumor doing in my belly? Almost apologetically, I add, "I really counted on it to banish those nasty cells."

"But it didn't work!" Charles's voice rises in frustration. "If it worked you wouldn't have this tumor now!"

"Well . . ." Carly shifts her position, leaning away from the shade of the market umbrella and into the sunlight. It seems clear that she is committed to maintaining a certain neutrality, a nonjudgmental impartiality.

Having known her as an intelligent, skilled, and meticulous labor and delivery nurse, I am eager to get her response to my situation. "What would you do?" I ask.

"Well, I've been thinking about that since we spoke this morning."

In the pause before she continues, I realize how ambivalent I continue to be about treatment choices. Unlike Charles, who is terrified of my undertaking anymore chemo, convinced its only effect was injurious, I am not only, like him, frightened of chemo but equally frightened of the outcome should I *not* get chemo.

"A colleague of mine is establishing a classical Chinese medicine clinic at the college in Portland. He is in China right now himself, so you wouldn't be able to see him before your surgery." She speaks slowly and carefully. "But he has brought from China a very skilled and knowledgeable doctor whose specialty is cancer."

Hope rushes into my belly, radiating heat to my chest and throat. Warmed by the possibilities suddenly unfolding, I hold my breath.

She continues. "He has only been here a few months, but I have been very impressed with his expertise—it's not my field, of course, but already he is respected and lauded by people who have worked with him."

"I would like very much to see him!"

"Good." Carly settles back in her chair, her long, honey-colored hair gleaming in the late-summer light. "I wasn't sure you'd be open to something like this, but I can make some phone calls and pave the way for you."

**For your information . . . Chinese medicine . . .**

Chinese medicine, which originated over four thousand years ago, addresses the balance of the body's different energies, such as *Yin* and *Yang*, and the proper flow of these energies, known as "Qi," throughout the *meridians*. Each meridian is associated with various organ systems in the body. Illness is believed to be the result of an imbalance in the energies, or a blockage along a meridian. This imbalance or blockage can be corrected by stimulating the related *channels* through acupuncture (the use of needles), acupressure (the use of pressure on specific points), and herbal remedies.[4] Although there is, at present, no conclusive evidence that Chinese medicine has a proven effect on disease, PubMed, the database of the National Library of Medicine, has 270,000 citations to journal articles containing information on complementary and alternative medicine, many of which address Chinese medicine.

"We can see him when we drive north, take a side trip to Portland for a day." Charles stands up and grins. "I am so glad to be thinking of something besides more chemo!"

Smiling, Carly offers, "I'll be back there next week, so I could meet you at the clinic if that would be helpful."

Dr. Kou is slight and youthful looking and speaks softly. Feeling my pulse, he then sits straight in his chair and looks at me through his fine, steel-rimmed spectacles, silently studying my face. After several minutes, he rises and goes to sit at a wooden desk, where he leans over a large sheet of white paper, pen in hand. In the damp August heat, we wait expectantly, anticipating a cure coming through his fingers onto the page. More time passes.

Carly speaks up. "Would you like us to leave and come back later?" He nods, and we step outside into the late afternoon sun. Walking through the streets of the city, Charles and Carly talk quietly as we pass voluptuous gardens packed with late-summer blooms in deep purples, reds, and golds. Oak and maple leaves carve kirigami shadows on the sun-soaked pavement. Their conversation blurs into the background buzz of honeybees, the hum of traffic, and the exclamations of kids tossing a Frisbee.

Comforted by the sounds of predictable life going on around us and by the murmurs of conversation, I am nevertheless feeling distant from all that I have known and assumed to be true. There is a dreamlike quality to these days, a sense that the nightmare I am living will explode and leave me beached on the shore of that space between the worlds.

Returning to the clinic, we relax in the waiting room for a few minutes to allow the doctor more time. I pick up a flyer about Qi Gong and read that through this ancient practice, an individual can increase and direct "Qi," one's own vital force, toward healing.

**For your information . . . Qi Gong . . .**

Qi Gong refers to exercises that improve health and longevity, as well as increase a sense of harmony within oneself and in the world. Principles of Qi Gong are described as the mind as the presence of intention, eyes as the focus of intention, movement as the action of intention, and breath as the flow of intention.[5]

Tucking the flyer into my purse, I follow Carly and Charles into the office. Dr. Kou is still hunched over his piece of white paper, which now has intricate Chinese characters marching in wide columns. On his desk are about ten or twelve brown paper bags, the familiar lunch bags of grammar school. Looking up, he smiles warmly.

"Oh, good." He picks up a brown paper bag and reaches in to scoop up dried roots, leaves, twigs, shriveled fungus, and gnarled objects I am unable to identify. Some look like slices of sun-washed bone.

Moving closer to better examine the exotic pieces resting on his palm, I listen to his instructions. He speaks slowly, realizing that he may lose us. He sighs, tired perhaps from the effort of explaining the formula with his limited English. He hands the bags to Charles and turns to me. "Drink one cup decoction three times every day."

Picking up a plastic bag from the desk, I can see that it is filled with dried red berries, smaller and pinker than cranberries. "Ghou Qi berries. Lyceum fruit. Eat five berries every morning."

"Are there other foods you suggest I eat? Or not eat?" I ask.

"Soups are *very* good," he emphasizes. "Easy to digest. Vegetables very good, too . . . and fruits, especially plums."

Before leaving, we make arrangements to return after the surgery. All I have heard during these last two hours is swirling about in my head, filling me with an exhilarating hope.

We drive back to the mountain cabin for two nights with my family before returning home for the surgery. The first thing Charles does when we arrive is soak the herbs and assemble the tools required for following Dr. Kou's instructions. Like a chemist, he devotes his afternoon to the meticulous preparation of the decoction.

There is a poignancy now, knowing how rapidly my life may change. Nico and Rose are playing by the stream, carving tracks in the mud and floating pinecones through the murky water. The dream flashes by, the children playing joyfully in the bathtub while I am hiding from them the sinister event taking place in my body, the extrusion of the fetid egg. I sit down on the riverbank and watch, savoring every minute, delighting in their shrieks of glee and their exuberant engineering plans for expanded waterways.

"Hi, Nana!" Nico stumbles over in his too-big Wellingtons and collapses next to me on the grass and pine needles.

"Hi, honey—it looks as if you two are reconstructing the canals of Venice!"

"Venice!" shouts Rose. "What's Venice?"

"Is that the place where the roads are made of water? Where you paddle boats to get places?" Nico looks at me eagerly for confirmation.

"Do the princesses take boats, too?" Rose smacks a pinecone down into the mud, splattering droplets of water on her cheeks.

"Right, Nico, the people in Venice get about in boats called gondolas or vaporettos." Turning to Rose, I add, "And I am sure the princesses have very special boats, fancy ones, to take them about, to transport them to their balls."

"Or they walk!" Nico adds.

"Or they walk. How right you are." Like his father, Nico seems to absorb information like a sponge, and his curiosity leads him to investigate anything he doesn't understand.

"But princesses don't walk," Rose insists. "They need to be carried! Or ride!"

"Maybe . . . we'll have to find out about that."

Shifting the conversation slightly, I ask, "Do you kids know that Nana and Papa are going home tomorrow?"

"Why?" Nico asks solemnly, as Rose rushes up to me and insists,

"No, you can't go home! We're a family. I want you to stay with us all the time."

"We would like to stay with you all the time, but we need to get back."

"What for?" they both ask at once.

"Well, Nana needs to be in the hospital again."

Crawling into my lap, Nico leans his head against my chest and moans, "Why?" Seeing the pain twisting his sweet face, I can feel an intense ache in my heart. *Why indeed?*

"I need to have an operation; the sickness has come back." He puts his hands over his ears and rocks from side to side on my lap. *Oh*, I wail to myself, *if only I could take this pain away from him.*

"I know it's hard to hear. It's hard for Nana, too. But I got well last time, and I am going to work very, very, very hard to get well again."

Rose wedges herself into my lap, and I wrap my arms around their sturdy bodies.

"I don't want you to be sick, Nana."

"I don't want to be sick either, sweetheart. But I'm going to get well again." *I have to get well*, I promise myself. *I can't violate the trust in these young eyes.*

Knowing their confidence in Andrew's magical abilities as a "real doctor," I tell them, "Daddy's going to come be with me and help me get well." Sensing perhaps that even Daddy's skills may not be sufficient to claim victory over my disease, Nico presses into my chest, burying his face.

"Promise you'll get well, Nana?" Rose asks trustingly.

"I promise I'll work really, really hard to get well!" My reassurance is guarded. Why can't I simply say, "Yes, Rosie, I'm going to get well, I promise!" It's the putrid egg of the dream that reminds me of the dreadful possibilities that will emerge as the surgeons once more open my belly.

Nico jumps up from my lap, hand still clasped over his ears. " I don't want to talk about it right now."

"We don't need to. Let's work on developing your waterways!" The lump in my throat swells with the recognition that this may be the last time the children see me healthy, the last time I can play water games with them. To not disappoint them, to not disappear from their lives, I must generate all the resources I can summon to prevail against this disease. The sweetness of this moment is all the more so knowing it may be the last.

Rose rolls off my lap and grabs a shovel, but Nico runs toward the shelter of the big pine tree. I am relieved to see Rebecca join him and turn my attention back to Rose. Two years younger than Nico, who has been in the world long enough to know the reality of disappointments and losses, Rose still trusts the reassurances of the adults in her world, assuming a happy ending to all stories.

As the sun sinks behind the gray jagged peaks of Three Fingered Jack, a chill sets in, and I gather the shovels and pails while Rose makes last-minute adjustments to the waterways. We join Nico in the house and settle in to read stories in front of the fire. The other grown-ups are fixing dinner, tossing the salad, or setting the table, but I, given my condition, am excused from such chores and free to luxuriate in the warmth and loving sweetness of Nico and Rose. A perk of catastrophic illness that I must remember to appreciate!

Looking at the beloved faces around the table that evening, I study them, committing to memory the details of voice, expression, and gaze. In the tilt of a head, in a gusty laugh, in a solemn contemplation, in an attentive look, I feel sorrow for what I may lose but gratitude for all that I have had. And knowing that they will be with me as I forge through the precipitous country ahead, I am thankful for their support, their strength, and their faith in my capacity to heal.

## *Chapter 16*

# Cutting Fruit

### DREAMING SURGERY

#### *August 1998*

*Making my way along an external hallway hugging a low building on my left, on my right I see an expanse of clipped green lawn and swaying palm trees. I turn to walk through a door that leads into a large room filled with people.*

*A sinister-looking man with pins piercing his body in different places and a jewel-cut stone over one eye, wears a piratelike scarf and a smug sneer. When he approaches me, I start to run, not toward the door open to the outside, but toward the bar area where I have left my purse. I am horrified to see people dressed in black, their faces obscured by long hoods, running monstrous nails through arms, legs, and torsos of the guests, and then affixing their bodies to the wall.*

*Impaled by glittering spikes that yank painfully at my flesh, my arms are extended, my feet float above the ground, and my head falls wearily to one side. Blood streams down my legs and trunk and fills my eyes.*

*As the nailers approach, I am shocked to feel myself drop down to the floor, no longer fixed in place. Hoping to be overlooked, I lean against the wall, hands extended, as if I am still impaled.*

*After they pass, I start running toward the door to escape, but the entire landscape has changed: Where there was garden and grass and trees, there is now nothing growing, only desolate land split by a wide asphalt driveway leading up to the building. Menacing creatures are walking toward me when I awaken.*

Stirring from the ominous dream, I feel in my body the agony that may be ahead for me. Yet I remind myself that I *do* escape from that hideous room of torture, I *am* able to find a way out of the doom and into the sunlight, albeit into a suddenly barren landscape.

Much as I want to live, the possibility of dying cannot be avoided. While making arrangements for my death, such as updating my will and sorting through personal and business papers, I am nonetheless counting on life.

*Am I doing all I can to live?* I ask myself, wondering if in some unconscious way I am giving up, surrendering myself to circumstances that may be more within my control than I imagine. *I am working hard to live!* I insist. I am trying to let go of the anguish, trying to settle my mind and heart in a serenity and quiet in which the damaged cells can heal and thrive. I am eating nourishing foods and walking and meditating every day. And singing and working with clay. Aren't these choices for life?

**Hints to help you beat the odds . . .**
**responding to bad news . . .**

This acceptance of "what is" and "what will be" is a hard place to reach, but it can provide a comfort and serenity of its own. This is only one of many possible responses and may not be possible for you or even what you want. Answer your challenges in a way that works for you, whether it's to fight, to deny, or to embrace them. And your responses may vary in different situations: You may be a fighter one day but rush into denial on another.

There are times when there may be an element of choice in the matter of living or dying, but there are also times when the larger forces take over. This feels, to me, like one of those latter times. Although I am doing all that I can toward affirming life, healing my body from this disease, the Fates have me, and my willingness to surrender to them is essential. In some deep way, I know, all is well.

I consult with Judith, the therapist whom I have continued to see on an intermittent basis. She comments that, during our recent sessions, she has noticed in me a withdrawal from the world and senses within me a deep weariness.

"Is this gearing up for another battle?" she asks. "The retreat to gather reserves before the assault?"

**For your information . . . building on your strengths . . .**

Lawrence LeShan, a psychotherapist who has worked extensively with cancer patients, uses an approach with them that differs from conventional psychotherapies. Instead of asking, What's wrong with this person? How did she get this way? What can be done about it? LeShan asks, What is right with this person? What are her special ways of being and relating? How can we work together to move this person more and more in the direction of living a full and zestful life?[1]

Perhaps, on some obscure level, a part of me has known that the truce of this last year was never more than temporary. Perhaps I have, indeed, retreated into solitude in order to focus on building my spiritual strength to withstand another challenge. And I wonder, *Are the gods revisiting me with disease because I have failed to learn the lessons I need?* A cruel possibility, and one that I hesitate to put into words, as I am convinced that we get cancer not because we need to learn a lesson but that we learn lessons as a consequence of having cancer.

**For your information . . . finding a therapist . . .**

Many people find therapists though word of mouth: from their doctors, from friends, from members of their support group. Whether you choose a psychiatrist, a psychiatric mental health nurse practitioner, a psychologist, a social worker, or other is less important than assessing whether or not this person is a good match for you. For this reason, it is a good idea to interview two or three people and identify the person whose view of the world, and of health and illness, is congruent with your own.

I hear the light scratch of leaves brushing against the wavy windowpane, and then her voice again, at the same time both gentle and urgent. "You are living with an absolute awareness of death. A *knowing* that comes, paradoxically, from *not knowing*."

"Yes," I agree, "but the surprise is that death, even in this proximity, does not frighten me. It feels like a companion, a presence gently touching my cheek." The minute I finish speaking, my mind swings wildly in dissent, and I hurry to add, "That's one piece of it. The other piece is that it's terrifying: I am desperate to keep living, to thwart the encroachment of this maestro of finales!"

I recall the three Fates of Greek mythology: Clotho, who spins the thread of life; Lachesis, who measures the lengths of lifetimes; and Atropos, whose quick snips announce death. It is Atropos to whom I want to yell, "Stop! Please don't do that! Put those scissors away! This is a mistake." And at the same time I want to say to her, "If this is my time, so be it. I will not wrestle Fate." There is a peace in knowing there will be no fight. The purr of an overhead fan ruffles the leaves of yellow dahlias nodding from the glass vase.

After a pause I add, "The roller coaster of my emotions makes me wonder what I think about anything . . . because what I *think* I thought five minutes ago seems the opposite of what I think now . . . in fact, the minute I have one thought, an inner dialogue catapults me to a divergent point of view, and I quickly feel as passionate about the one as about the other." Is this truly a battle I am waging? I think not, yet at times I feel as if I am indeed girding my loins for holy combat—a skirmish that I want very much to win. One minute a woman warrior striving for victory and the next instant floating in a sea of stillness, surrendering to the Fates.

"As I was saying, you are living now on the most intimate terms with death," Judith repeats. "These are sacred times: Honor them and keep within you an image of serenity and peace."

"Most of the time that center still point feels quiet, ready to accept whatever happens," I say. "And then suddenly the Furies will enter me and jostle me onto the battlefield! That feeling of rage quiets in seconds and doesn't linger, but it's there sometimes. More often than not, though, I watch what's happening now, this brush with the Dark Angel, from a point of surprising disengagement, much as I watch unpleasant medical procedures from a distance that removes me from the immediate pain."

When I stop speaking, Judith waits a minute or two before commenting, "Because once you have stepped aside from life, as you have, you live in that space between the worlds. And living in that space, you can be intensely connected in specific situations and with specific people at the same time that your general engagement is waning."

We talk about that in-between world, that peculiar state I inhabit since facing the distinct possibility of dying before I feel finished with living. The shape of my cosmos is again being redefined by this new diagnosis and will be further altered by the revelations of surgery and pathology. As we speak, a serenity is surrounding and penetrating me, a palpable stillness that comforts and reassures. For reasons I am unable to fathom, in this, my moment of what might be utter despair, I am floating in a sea of peace, confident in the triumph of love and awed by the fleeting glory of our lives.

**Hints to help you beat the odds . . .
riding the emotional roller coaster . . .**

It is not only possible but also probable that at times your emotions will take you on a roller coaster ride, including sudden shifts into joy as well as dark plunges into despair. These perhaps polar opposites can reflect the turbulence of your inner life, as well as the stresses and strains on your physical body. They are all valid, they all compose a totality of experience. Try to ride it out with some deep breathing, meditation, yoga, or whatever helps.

Two nights before the surgery, Charles and I drive up to the North Bay and spend the evening with my cousins Cordelia and David. Music plays softly, chants from Taize, and we sit together in a peacefulness that soothes. They have arranged for a friend to give me a massage, and when she arrives, she and Cordelia busy themselves preparing, dropping ironed white sheets onto the massage table, sliding hot-water bottles wrapped in flannel underneath, placing tiny vases of ginger blossoms and scarlet poppies on the low tables, and bringing me water with lemon to drink. As she leaves the room, Cordelia hands me a pale-blue silk robe to put on after the massage. When I decline, worrying that I'll get massage oil on it, she insists, "It doesn't matter; I want you to wear it!" And eventually, I do, happily wrapping my oiled and cosseted body in the billowing folds of silken sky.

From the heady relaxation of the massage, I join the others on the deck overlooking the oak tree–dotted hills. Although there is conversation going on, it is quiet, nearly hushed. Sitting on the porch in the liquid slant of late-afternoon sun, we have iced tea with twigs of mint stuffed into the tall glasses and slices of lime floating on top; purple grapes, honeydew melon, and wild strawberries; and small sandwiches with slivers of cucumber, loose tangles of watercress, or layers of lox, onions, and capers inside.

The sun drops lower in the sky, and I am feeling deliciously relaxed, far, far away from the events that are scheduled to start tomorrow, and also far from the hammering and sawing going on at home. Cordelia fills the tray with empty dishes and announces, "I'm going to start a bubble bath for you—and I'll summon you, madam, when it's ready!" Balancing the tray and trying to suppress a giggle, she bows low and turns quickly toward the house.

The bathroom has a big plate-glass window looking out on the ridge. "You may even see a deer walk by if you're really quiet," Cordelia says as she hands me a glass of sparkling apple cider.

I lean back in the tub and raise my glass. "To you, my sweet cousin. Thank you for—"

Tossing her head, she admonishes me: "Just relax and enjoy it; this is your time, and you've earned it!" She sweeps out of the room, and returns moments later with a camera. Snapping a picture, she exclaims, "You sure don't *look* sick!"

"I don't *feel* sick either . . . that's what makes this so unreal."

We leave for home late that night, and I begin my twenty-four-hour fast for the surgical bowel prep. The next day, Nico and Rose call from their new home in Wisconsin.

"Nana, will you be here for my first day of school tomorrow?" asks Nico.

"No, Nico, I thought I would be, but I'll be in the hospital tomorrow. We planned that I would be there for your first day of school, but I have to be here now so that I can get well!"

"Will you be here for my second day of school?" he asks eagerly.

"No, I'll still be in the hospital, but I'll speak with you, and—"

He breaks in, "Nana, will you be able to come see me in my new school?"

"Yes, I will, Nico, but not for a while." I am crossing my fingers that next month I'll be, not driving to the hospital for chemotherapy, but jetting halfway across the country to see my grandchildren. "When I am well enough to travel, I'll come see you in your new school."

The phone is passed to Rose, who scolds, "Nana, I don't like it when you're sick! I want you to get well *now*!"

"I'm working really hard to get well as soon as I can."

"My daddy will get you well! Daddy will make you well, Nana!" I hear the phone drop, and then the muffled clapping of her pudgy hands.

Rebecca rescues the phone from the floor. "Sorry about that drop! She just gets so enthusiastic and forgets that you can't see her!"

Feeling loved, nurtured, and valued, I doze in the glow of their conversation. Luke arrives later from Portland, and Andrew from Chicago. Andrew will stay just for the surgery and the day following, and Luke for a few days longer.

Waking early in the morning to complete the presurgical bowel prep, as we leave the house, I can't help wondering in what state I will be returning. When I saw Dr. Kinjo for my pre-op visit day before yesterday, I commented, "At least I have only that one tumor."

"We don't know that," he cautioned. "The CT scan picked up only that one, but there may be others we couldn't see."

Winding through the mountain roads, I wonder whether this crisis

**Considerations for hospital staff . . . clinging to hope . . .**

Even when the outlook appears bleak to you, remember that hope, even against the most depressing odds, helps a person to put one foot in front of the other, to continue being engaged with life, to find the strength to continue slogging through. Don't let your discouragement breathe life into your patient's worst fears.

marks the end of my journey or whether it's just a side road, a temporary diversion. Andrew confers with Dr. Kinjo in the passageway, and Luke goes off in search of a cappuccino. A nurse helps me into a gown and hands Charles my clothes and sandals in a big, white, plastic bag. While someone from the phlebotomy team is starting an IV, the anesthesiologist checks in, confirming that I have no allergies, no removable dental structures, and no prostheses. Someone puts a paper shower cap on my head; Charles and Andrew help me onto the gurney, and they wave goodbye.

In the operating theater, the anesthesiologist wraps a blood pressure cuff around my arm and starts a second IV. "You'll begin to feel drowsy." She smiles as she pushes the plunger of a syringe stuck into the tubing. "I'll be inserting the NG tube after you fall asleep." Relieved to hear that news, I smile.

"You're done, Mom, the operation's over." I feel Andrew's warm hand on my cheek. It seems just seconds ago that I was wheeled into the OR.

"We took out a good-size tumor, Eliza . . ." Dr. Kinjo pauses, and I open my eyes to see him standing next to Andrew. "It was well-encapsulated," he continues, "and that's good!" Noticing the positive lilt in his voice, I smile. "We'll know more about it shortly—when the preliminary pathology report comes back." Unable to stay awake, I relax into the anesthesia.

"We're going up to the floor now, Mom." I feel Andrew's warm hand on my shoulder as he walks alongside me.

I am startled awake again when we jog around the corner into my room and see Charles and Luke perched on the wide windowsill. Luke jumps down and whispers to me, "You're doing great—it's all over!" Charles follows and asks, "You doing OK, honey?"

Three men surround me: my brother, my son, and my husband. Their love enfolding me is a tactile presence. With them holding me, I am able to yield to the thread of destiny, recognizing that there may be small choices I can make but that in large part, I am in the sway of universal forces with which I cannot, or choose not, to battle.

Charles and Andrew go out to forage for edibles, and Luke sits nearby, reading the paper. I feel a light touch on my arm and awaken to see a smiling Dr. Feng standing by the bed. "This is not the final word, but right now, the preliminary report suggests that this tumor is benign."

Luke whoops, "Did you hear that?" The relief in his voice spills out into the room. "Can you hear what the doctor is telling you?"

"Um-hmm," I mumble and smile. *But if the tumor is benign*, I wonder, *what made the CEA go up?* Too drowsy to be concerned beyond noting the inconsistency, I am soon asleep again.

Jostled awake by Luke's touch, I hear him rejoice, "It's benign! You're healthy! And as soon as you get out of here and get a little better, we'll go kayaking!" Envisaging bright-eyed otters careening around our craft, splashing their tails on the swaying kelp, I drift back to sleep.

The drone of low voices awakens me to find Andrew and Charles sitting by the bed, speaking quietly with Luke. "But she's OK," Luke insists. "And with that Dr. Kou on board, she's going to be even better!"

"But remember, that's not the final report," Andrew cautions, wary of putting a damper on the celebration. Perhaps he also is pondering the genesis of the rising CEA: Is there another tumor somewhere that neither sophisticated machines nor skilled surgeons were able to identify?

"No, it's not the last word," agrees Charles, "but I think she's going to be fine anyway."

It's getting to be late in the afternoon, and they start home for supper and an early bedtime. We have all been up since dawn, and although I have been sleeping more often than not since then, they have been propped awake by adrenalin and caffeine.

Nurses and aides are in and out periodically during the night, checking my blood pressure, temperature, wound dressing, IV levels and rates, and amounts of drainage. Toward morning, during a wound check, I peek at the glimmering silver bars marching down my belly, a narrow stairway of staples separating left from right.

An aide helps me bathe and brush my teeth and urges me to get out of bed. After sitting in the chair an hour or so, I am exhausted and relieved when she comes back to help me into bed. I am just dozing when I hear footsteps, and open my eyes to see the stooped figure of Dr. Feng stepping quietly into the room. His stance speaks volumes.

"The news is not so good," he starts.

I know that—I see that in the way he walks, the way he can't quite look at me straight on.

**Considerations for hospital staff . . .
the power of body language . . .**

Be conscious of the power of your body language. Information can be transmitted through your facial expression, your posture, and the tone of your voice. It can pierce your patient's bubble of hope, as well as provide a visual introduction for bad news. Sympathetic body language can also help patients feel your presence with them in their grief.

"The final pathology report just came in," he continues, looking slightly past my gaze. "The tumor is actually cancer: colon cancer."

Although seconds ago I thought I already knew, I realize I didn't; until the words came out of his mouth, it was not real. I want him to pull those words back, to grab them from the air where they hang so heavily and shove them into the land of unspoken possibilities.

"I'm very sorry," he adds, and I see in his face the sorrow of being the bearer of unbearable news. "The colon cancer has metastasized to your ovary."

I have nothing to say. I am sorry this is so hard for him.

"You can repeat the same chemotherapy you had last time." He hesitates before adding, "We have nothing else to offer you . . . that's all there is," he apologizes.

In the breast-cancer world, it seems that there are new treatments hitting the market monthly. Yet nothing new seems to occur in the treatment of colon cancer. The dearth of research reflects the common focus, not on organs that rid our bodies of poisons and remove waste, but on breasts, prostates, and lungs—the body parts of birth, nurturing, passion, and air.

**For your information . . . reason to hope . . .**

Just in the past couple of years, there has been an increased focus on research in the area of colon cancer, and new drugs and protocols have been introduced. This renewed interest in the "cancer of shame" has been sparked by the work of Katie Couric and others to bring this disease into the light of public awareness.[2]

"Will it increase my chances?" I ask.

"We don't know . . . there aren't studies that show it helps people with your type of cancer." (Translation: cancer that is as advanced as yours.) "But we have nothing else to offer," he pleads, "and it might help."

This feels like more of a decision than it did the first time.

"I don't know what I want." The NG tube is still in, making speaking uncomfortable, but I also don't know what to say. I need to think about this.

"You don't have to decide anything yet," he offers.

Dr. Feng is not gone long before Dr. Kinjo comes in, still in his scrubs from the day's surgeries. "You've heard, haven't you, that the . . ."

"Yes, I heard," I interrupt, wanting to save him from the awkwardness of having to announce this bleak news again. "What do you think?"

"Well, I think you should do the chemo . . . after all, it might do you some good."

"And what about the tumors? Will more . . . ?"

"We would expect them to recur in different places, and when they do, we'll take them out," he says reasonably.

"And then . . . ?"

"Well, we'll just take them out as they appear, for as long as we can . . ." I know the rest of the sentence . . . *until we can't keep up with them, and there'll be nothing more we can do.* I'm not sure if I actually hear him say that or if I simply understand it to be true.

Andrew comes in shortly for a visit before he leaves for the airport. I ask him what he thinks.

"I don't know, Mom. If there's a chance the chemo might help, perhaps it's worth it. Both your doctors are urging you to go ahead with it." He stares out the window at wisps of cloud gliding across the plate of blue sky. "But I don't know. I'll do some research when I get home and see what I can find out."

Minutes pass in silence, and he turns suddenly to me. "You know, Mom, I am *glad* this pathology report came back positive . . . because if it didn't, what was causing the CEA to rise?"

"Yeah, I thought about that, too . . ."

"Because if this tumor they took out *had been* benign, where is the bad tumor hiding? That was bothering me yesterday when that preliminary information suggested 'benign.'" Without saying so, we both realize the irony in being relieved that the final pathology report came back *positive for malignant disease.*

"At least now we know what caused the CEA to go up," Andrew continues, "and further confirmation will come with the results of the repeat labs they drew this morning."

Feeling his warm hand on my arm, I resist falling back to sleep, wanting to commit to memory the last minutes of his visit. Not sure when I might see him again, I drink in his gentle wisdom, his presence emanating peace. Wishing he would make the coming decisions for me, I also appreciate his insight in knowing that I need to assume that responsibility myself.

When Luke and Charles return from their cappuccino break, Andrew gets up, grabs his carry-on, and kisses me goodbye. "If you need me to come back, Mom, I will," he reminds me before disappearing through the door.

As Charles leaves with Andrew, Luke turns to me and insists, "You're going to be OK, I know you are!" If aspects of this disease have disheartened him, he has disclosed neither fear nor doubt to me: Whatever monstrous setback occurs, he is my cheering squad. "You're going to be OK! You're doing great!" He is my energetic force, infusing me with a steady and exuberant belief in possibility.

"I hope so," I say lamely.

"Hope so? I know so!" He pauses before launching the salvo I know is coming. "And you don't need anymore of that toxic chemo to get better! Don't let them do that to you again," he pleads. I know that, like Charles, he watched the chemo transform my body and was stunned by the devastating changes. Although they both were unflaggingly supportive, when the side effects were most difficult for me to bear, he would suggest casually, "Maybe you don't need any more . . ."

"Your body is strong." His voice interrupts my reverie. "Dr. Kou's medicine is powerful. You can heal without that chemotherapy poison." Since the chemo ended over a year ago, both he and Charles have been more vocal in their disapproval of it.

**For your information . . . Chinese herbal medicine . . .**

Although most Westerners think of acupuncture as the basis of Asian medicine, herbal formulas made expressly for the ill person are the foundation of classical Chinese medicine.[3]

When Charles returns from the airport, he sits down next to Luke and, after asking how I feel, begins abruptly, "I hope you don't decide to do any more of that chemo, honey. It nearly killed you last time!" His eyes are intent. "And we know another way now . . . Dr. Kou, and his herbs . . ."

**For your information . . . promising a cure . . .**

Typical of many doctors of Chinese medicine, Dr. Kou has made no promises to cure. If an alternative healthcare provider promises a cure, be suspicious!

When I am silent, Luke tells him, "I've been at her about that since you left . . . I think she knows how we feel about it!"

Relieved that the topic is dropped, I drift off and sleep soundly while they go out for supper. In the days that follow, I wonder about the chemo: *Will it help me live? Or will it hasten my death?* A few days after discharge from the hospital, I make an appointment for a consult with the chief of gastrointestinal oncology at UCSF.

Home for only a few days, I find the relentless noise and dust of the construction disturbing and am unable to relax. If the hammers and saws aren't keeping me on edge with their clamor, I am worrying about the silence, wondering whether the men have gone off fishing or hiking for the afternoon. It is three months since this project began, and it doesn't seem close to being finished within the four-month time frame they estimated last spring.

Since the appointment for the consult is still ten days away, we drive to Oregon to see Dr. Kou. It has just rained as we drive through the Trinity Alps, and the moisture on the pine needles glistens. Diamond shards spring from the branches. The gold of aspens and alders shimmers in the autumn sunlight. The cry of a great blue heron lifting from Shasta Lake echoes over the water. The mountain suddenly looms to our right, patches of gray rock burnished bronze by the extraordinary light of the day. The world itself is intensely alive, every ordinary aspect touched by an indescribable beauty that leaves me breathless and excited. There is a sense of just being born, the ecstasy of seeing all this wonderment for the first time. Arriving at the edges of the city, urban sounds and sights plant my feet on the ground.

Dr. Kou, after a lengthy examination, adjusts my herbs and teaches me more Qi Gong. On this first visit after surgery, he ascertains that I am still too weak for acupuncture. At least that's what I surmise: The language barrier prevents any but the most essential communication. The following week, just before our return home, I see him again, and this time, after his assessment, he places a few needles. I make appointments to return every three weeks for treatments.

I also see Dr. Krueger, recently returned from China. He explains some of the philosophy behind Chinese medicine, concepts that Dr. Kou is unable to articulate clearly. When I tell him that I am flummoxed by the choice of whether or not to repeat chemotherapy, he emphasizes that the crucial factor is that I make the decision based on what *I* believe will heal me—that I need to gather pertinent information, and then make this choice without the influence of opinions, experiences, and decisions of others.

The doctor at UCSF has read my chart and asks me a few questions,

**Hints to help you beat the odds . . . no wrong choices . . .**

When you are diagnosed with cancer, you are confronted with choices. Choosing conventional therapies, and if so, which ones? Choosing complementary or alternative therapies, and if so, which ones? Choosing how to respond to pain. Choosing how to live and how to die. Each person living with cancer responds to these choices in different ways; there is no single right way to respond.[4]

specifically about my experience with chemotherapy. "Most people tolerate 5FU very well. And because that's true of the majority, an assumption is made that it is a fairly benign drug. To the contrary, for those who do not tolerate it, such as yourself, the outcome can be grave."

In the course of our discussion, he tells me not only that I would not benefit from another round of this chemotherapy, but also that it may prove disastrous were I to attempt it. I am realizing now, with full awareness, how precarious was my condition because of the impact of those drugs. Once again skating on the thinnest of ice, I realize, with renewed intensity, just how fragile is my hold on this life.

"So you don't recommend anymore chemo?" Charles asks hopefully.

"No, I don't." His response is unequivocal. "It did her no good the first time, and there's no reason to believe it would help her this time." He hesitates before adding, "It would be dangerous to repeat it."

Leaving the clinic, Charles takes my arm. "Oh, honey, I am so relieved." There is a new buoyancy in his voice.

"I know you are."

"I just couldn't bear to see you take that stuff again." Again, I am reminded that his *watching me* suffer during that time was probably more difficult than my *being me* suffering.

At home, Charles brews herbs for the decoction while I rest, weary from the trip. I am also still depleted from the surgery and anesthesia, which, I am learning, stays with me far longer than is commonly assumed. When Abby, the facilitator of my support group calls, Charles brings me the telephone.

"I hear from Julie that your . . ."

When she hesitates, I help her out. "Yes, the cancer has spread."

She says how sorry she is and that the group is sending healing energies my way. Then she hesitates before adding, almost cheerily, "Well . . . now you can join the metastatic group!"

"Well, I'm not sure I want to do that," I demure.

"Well," she says hopefully, "the people in the metastatic group are going to know what you're going through . . . they'll understand your situation better."

"That may be true, in a way," I agree, "but I'd rather just stick with my own group . . . with the women I know."

"But . . ." I can hear the discomfort in her voice. "The thing is," she continues, "WomenCARE's policies dictate that when someone becomes metastatic, they leave their core group and join the metastatic group."

"But that's crazy! Now is when I need my group most of all—not the company of strangers." I am astounded by the logic, or lack thereof.

With this diagnosis of metastatic disease, the group has become more crucial than ever—through this past week, I have been longing to be with them again. At the same time that I am feeling nourished and buoyed by this circle of women, I am learning that I am being exiled from their company, that my new diagnosis disqualifies me from continued membership.

Blurting out, "I am appalled!" I feel a growing inner strength as I speak. My sense of justice is being threatened, and I am rising to the battle call.

"Well," she says reluctantly, "you're right. I agree with you. I think you need to be with the rest of us, and I'll tell you, the group members want you to come back!"

"So . . . we all agree then!" It sounds pretty simple to me.

"But it's the policies as written . . ." She pauses and, afraid I'll say something in anger that I'll regret, I wait.

"Tell you what," she starts enthusiastically. "You come to the meeting tomorrow, and meantime I'll get back to the director and tell her about this conversation. The policy makes no sense . . . you are absolutely right! We'll all fight it with you."

This is a strange conversation, but I like the turn it's taking. "I'll be there," I reassure her, "with bells on." Relaxing my body, I let go of my ire in the recognition that I will not be fighting this alone, that Abby and the rest of the group are joining me.

I arrive at the meeting room a little early the next morning, and Abby is there meeting with the director, whom I recognize but have never met. She jumps up from her desk and apologizes profusely.

"This is a new policy, set by the board, and we've never actually tested it. And I am so very, very sorry that you are having to go through this." Looking at me directly, with clear eyes, she continues. "The best of intentions led to this policy, but I can see now that they were misplaced. The thinking was that the person with metastatic disease might hesitate to bring things up that would upset the group members, and also that the group participants might feel uncomfortable hearing about cancers advancing. It sounds pretty absurd as I describe it to you, but . . ." She smiles and continues, "I managed to contact each board member last night, and that particular policy is being suspended for the time being. It will probably be abolished at the next board meeting!"

Abby apologizes, "I just wish we'd managed to figure this out without your having to lead the way . . ."

"It doesn't matter," I interrupt. "I just need to stay with my group, and now that can happen. Thank you."

They both apologize again, but I am too busy celebrating my triumph in resisting graduation to the metastatic group. Friends start to arrive and are equally elated to hear that the policy of banishment is being rescinded.

**Hints to help you beat the odds . . . support with Stage IV . . .**

Agencies and institutions offering support groups may have a variety of different formats: groups for men only, women only, teenagers only, people in treatment, people after the completion of treatment, people with certain types of cancer, people at certain stages of cancer, and so on. Which kind of group you choose is an individual matter. The important thing is that you are given a *choice* as to what group to attend should you be diagnosed with metastatic disease.

Soon after the surgery, I meet with Judith. Although I am experiencing a tranquil stillness deep within me, there seems to be no end to my need to explore what is happening with me now, in the light of this new diagnosis.

Recognizing that I have been graced with existing in this state of profound acceptance, Judith comments, "Living in this kind of serenity, your cells have a better chance to live."

She lets me absorb that concept before continuing, "This kind of peace is perhaps the deepest 'fighting' you can make against the cancer—this yielding and serenity may be what really helps the cells change into healthy ones."

Being there, in her presence, clears my eyes and opens my heart toward understanding the impenetrable mysteries intrinsic to this holy path. Continuing to live in the reality of the human condition, I put one foot in front of the other according to the demands of this physical life. At the same time, however, I am seeing this world through the lenses of a spiritual reality that flowered two years ago, when I stepped into that space between the worlds. And now, by this diagnosis of metastatic disease, I am further grounded in that "in-between" landscape, led further along the path of exploration into my inner world.

# *Chapter 17*
# Breathing the Pain

## DREAMING DESERTION

### *April 1999*

> *Charles is driving us to a house that he has chosen for our new home. The street is treeless, the sidewalks narrow. There is an absence of life in this area: no children playing, no people walking by, and no traffic of any kind. He stops the car in front of a small, dilapidated house on an untidy lot that is bare of any vegetation whatsoever. I notice that he leaves the car engine running while he leads me in, pushing open the front door. As I step into the hall, he backs down the steps to leave, saying he will return later. I stand in the kitchen, feeling utterly abandoned. In the eerie silence, I begin to hear the sinister echoes of an imagined fiend. Afraid, I turn to lock the door. But there is no door handle, no lock, and no hardware of any kind. There is no way to keep the door closed: It makes light squeaking sounds as the breeze pushes it slightly one way and then the other. Feeling utterly helpless and exposed, I am horrified and terribly frightened to have been left in this situation.*

Slipping out of my dream, the panic and anxiety it generated continues to tense my muscles and preoccupy my thoughts. The extent of this illness has left me totally dependent upon my family, especially upon Charles. I am reminded of my vulnerability, my frightening powerlessness. Remembering that we have houseguests arriving this afternoon, I pull myself forward into the day, pushing dream fragments to the back of my mind.

Arranging butter-colored lilies in a tall glass vase, I am aware of an undercurrent of unease in my body, a sense of something more than simple fatigue. It is six months since the surgery to remove the tangerine tumor, and during that time, I have had four bowel obstructions, all four of which were intensely painful and scary, and two of which sent me to the hospital. Recognizing that a vague sense of "something's wrong" is a more likely harbinger of an obstruction than any specific symptom, I am disheartened when the disquiet persists.

Elena and Fred arrive in the late afternoon, and joyful greetings cannot distract me from what is by now a palpable discomfort in my abdomen. With Elena's help, I manage to make dinner but leave the mealtime conversation to the others. Unable to rally for company, even those I dearly love, I can feel myself turning inward, physically and emotionally, yet I'm not sure enough of what's happening to say anything. Feeling an urgency to get upstairs and try to deflect this approaching storm, I apologize, "I need to go to bed early . . . I just can't stay up any longer."

Elena looks up and asks, "You OK?"

"I'm not sure yet," I tell her, expecting that she, a psychic, would know better than I. "I feel . . . I don't know exactly . . . not right."

"Hmm," she offers, and I wish she would make a diagnosis. *Can't she see right into my body?* I wonder.

Bed feels like a comforting friend, and I want to believe that exhaustion is the root of this unease, that tomorrow I'll wake up feeling like myself again. Their low voices drifting up the stairs lull me to sleep. When Charles comes to bed later, I feel his warm, strong body curling around mine, and even in my drowsiness I am comforted.

When I awaken the next morning, I feel somewhat rested, but still "not right." Elena and Fred are brewing their morning tea when I come down, and Charles is setting the table for breakfast.

"We want to go see those Monarchs!" Fred exclaims between sips of tea.

"They're really intriguing to watch," Charles joins in. "They just dangle there in these long, orange loops until the sun warms them, and then the sky is full of fluttering ginger stars."

"Against a deep-blue sky," I add, trying to get into the spirit of the conversation.

"Well, we really want to see them," Elena says. "We've heard about 'em for a long time."

As they collect themselves to go after breakfast, I venture, "I am going to sit this one out and let you three go on the excursion without me."

Before I finish my sentence, Elena cries, "But we want you to come with us!" Hesitating, she asks, "Why don't you want to go?"

Though touched by her genuine wish to be together, I still feel that even this brief excursion would require energy that I don't have. "I'm really tired, and . . . I'm not feeling well somehow . . ." My sentence hangs in midair as I wonder again, *Can't she see that something is really wrong?*

"Well, we'll wait for you!" she exclaims. "Have a little rest . . . we can all have a little rest, and then we'll go! It'll be good for you."

*Good for me?* I wonder.

"OK," I agree, caving in. Arguing seems to drain more energy than would the trip itself. "I'll just take a little rest . . . half an hour maybe." Now that I am committed to going, I want to get it over with so that I can come home and lie down without any pressure to engage in activity.

I need to focus on my inner turmoil, to discover what is going on in my gut. There are clues here, and although it seems like an approaching obstruction, perhaps it is something else entirely, something I need to decipher. Through these last two years, I have come to an understanding that listening to my body, reading its needs, requires a certain solitude and privacy in which I can become centered.

I stare at the ceiling, at the patterns of sunlight sliding through the wooden slats of the blinds, and recall the first obstruction that occurred about eight weeks after the surgery to remove the tumor. That night, I was awakened from sleep by intense abdominal cramps, which were reminiscent of the pain leading up to my first hospital admission two years ago. I was admitted for a blockage in the small intestine, and an NG tube was inserted to drain and rest my GI system.

The day after my admission, I remember ruefully, Charles came to see me, and I noticed that his words were slurred, his mouth slackened, his eye

**For your information . . . relieving a bowel obstruction . . .**

Fluids and gas may build up because they are unable to move past a blockage. When this occurs, a nasogastric, or NG, tube is passed through the nose and down into the stomach to remove fluids and gas, thus helping to relieve pain and pressure.

drooping. Stunned, I sat there propped up on the hospital bed, a tube up my nose, an IV pumping fluid into my veins, watching this transformation of my husband's face. *What will become of us?* I wondered. *Who will care for whom?* It was one of those moments that was so awful it became darkly comic as we stared at each other and shrugged. It turned out to be an isolated event that resolved spontaneously but was frightening at the time. I am reminded once again of the precarious nature of our lives.

When Charles comes upstairs, I tell him, "I need your help . . . I feel really awful, as if I might be getting an obstruction, and . . ."

"Now? When we have houseguests?" he asks, unbelieving. "You're getting an obstruction now?"

"I don't know for sure, but it feels as if that might be happening . . . and it's hard to be a good hostess when I feel so . . ."

"Are you having cramps?" he asks.

"No, it's just . . . it feels like that space leading up to the cramps . . . I don't know . . ."

"Well, you're probably just tired, honey," he tries to reassure me. "We've had a busy week traveling. Have a little rest and then come down." I can feel his disappointment and sense that there is little room for me to back away from my duties as hostess.

"Elena just really wants to do things with you when they're here," he adds. "Doesn't that make you happy?" he asks eagerly.

"Well, yes, except when I am feeling like this." I am beginning to sound like a complainer.

Making our way down the raised wooden footpath to the butterfly trees, I am realizing that this mild physical activity does feel good. Social exchange, however, requires energy and concentration that drains me.

"We want to take you guys out to that Thai restaurant for dinner." I am pulled from my musings by Fred's invitation. We are lying under the trees watching the orange butterflies trembling against a cobalt dish of sky. Dismissing my observations of moments ago and noting a mild but distinct nausea, I nonetheless chastise myself, *Just rally for tonight . . . stop being a baby!*

"That would be fun," Charles responds.

*Fun for you three*, I tell myself ruefully. *But I really don't feel well . . . things are shifting in my belly. I'm not being a baby. Isn't it OK to be sick?* I ask myself.

*No, it's not, not right now.* I continue my internal dialogue, challenging my body to override signals of distress. *I need to gather my resources and make this next twenty-four hours pleasant until our guests leave, and then I can be sick without distraction!*

*But no,* I argue. *How have I arrived at this place of acquiescence? Isn't this one of the lessons learned? To listen to my body? To pay attention to its inner workings and give it what it needs?*

*Well, I* am *listening to my body,* I remind myself. *I* am *putting into practice what I've been learning. I am* not *in denial. But* they *are all in denial! And worse yet, invalidating what I know to be true.*

Even recognizing what I need, the resistance is too much: Charles wants to see that Elena and Fred, who urge my participation, have the visit they expect. But I need to go to bed and curl up into sleep. Yet, in the face of opposition from people I love, I have neither the strength nor the conviction to be truly assertive or even direct.

By late afternoon, I am starting to have mild but unmistakable cramping in my upper abdomen. Leaning over the counter, swaying to the surges of pain, I wonder whether to go out to dinner, to please my guests, or whether to stay at home, to take care of my battered body.

The isolation of the dream returns and parallels my present sense of being alone. Even though there are three people in this house who love and care for me, I am being left to manage this crisis on my own.

As I rock from side to side to the rhythm of the cramps, I am astonished to hear Fred's voice. "Who knows—some good Thai food may make her feel better."

But why am I astonished? Fred has insisted many times that being sick at all is a sign of weakness, that he even feels ashamed when he himself feels the slightest bit ill.

"Sometimes these cramps just go away," Charles ventures.

*Yes, that is true,* I agree silently. *That happens when I rest and do Qi Gong and yoga.*

"Well, I take care of my body," Fred announces to Charles. "I take care of my mind, and I don't get sick! It's that simple!" The self-righteous tone of his decree recalls the ER doc announcing in triumph, "She's dehydrated because she's not drinking!" as if it were a matter of my willfulness causing the problem.

Not for the first time, I wish that Charles would say something in my defense, since I cannot. For me to respond would require a presence of mind, an energy that I don't have right now. Knowing that my staying home will cause consternation and worry, if not an actual argument, I take the path of least resistance, throw a sweater over my shoulders, and go.

In the dream, I felt abandoned and frightened when Charles left me in the ominously silent little house. Now, I want to be left alone, in the comfort of a silence that demands nothing. It was the bleak *feeling* of that dreamscape that was so scary. This house is my refuge, and I watch it get smaller as we drive down the street.

Sitting in the back of the car with Elena, I hear Fred continue to theorize. "When I get sick, I am embarrassed!" When he gets no response, he adds, "It's all in the mind anyway."

Charles concentrates on parking, and we get out of the car without having responded. This is not a topic of discussion, but rather Fred's granite Truth.

By seven thirty, sitting in the Thai restaurant amid the aromas of steaming rice, sweet chili sauce, and lemongrass, the cramps are more persistent. I try to follow the conversation while pushing food around my plate. The thought of eating anything at all is repulsive, a response I recognize as a precursor to an obstruction. The genesis of this blockage may be a new tumor, or it may arise from constrictions caused by adhesions. Remembering one of the surgeons describing adhesions like "sticky chewing gum," I imagine a logjam triggered by the knots and tangles in my gut.

When we get home, I push my shoes off and turn toward the three. "I really need to go to bed now. I can't be conversational even for a minute."

"I hope you feel better," they call after me as I climb up the stairs.

Slipping into a warm flannel nightdress, I start a routine of massaging my belly, then yoga breathing, and then getting into yoga postures that stretch the abdominal area. An hour later, Charles joins me, bringing me peppermint tea. I try a sip but am repelled. He stands behind me and rubs my abdomen, and although the pressure actually causes more pain, I say nothing, afraid to hurt his feelings. I am so glad to have him near me that I don't want to risk a retreat. So I remain silent but wince sometimes at the vigor of his touch.

I can sense his conflict and am sorry that I cannot help him. He very much wants this visit to be a good one for Elena and Fred, but he also sees that making it so has taken a toll on me. His tenderness reminds me that he does care, that it is only his intense engagement with guests that has turned him away from what I need.

As the pains increase in frequency and intensity, I am aware of the probability that I will end up in the hospital. Aware that these obstructions are potentially life threatening, I nonetheless hope each time that they will resolve with conservative measures at home. Knowing my resistance to seek medical attention could prove fatal, why do I oppose Charles's suggestions to go to the ER? Dread of the NG tube? Of the unknown procedures that might be in store?

I get into a hot bath, but find it too confining, so I get out and lean over the counter, swaying and groaning. I try more yoga, Qi Gong, and massage, but still the cramps continue, getting stronger and longer. At about four in the morning, realizing that this will not be one of the times that the obstruction will resolve spontaneously, I confess, "I think I need to go to the hospital." It seems that I can surrender only when the physical anguish in my gut outweighs the knot of fear.

"I think so, too," he agrees. He brings me clean sweatpants and a top, and helps me into them. In addition to colicky pains, my entire abdomen is exquisitely tender to the touch, and even these loose sweats hurt.

Charles writes a note to Elena and Fred explaining our absence, and we leave for the hospital.

When we get to the ER, it is empty except for a young mother with a crying baby, and a man in his twenties with an injured foot. I go to the window and when asked what is wrong, I reply, "I have a bowel obstruction."

"Don't go away—a nurse will be right out to get you," the clerk urges.

And indeed, in a minute or two, a nurse comes out and takes me to her cubicle to get vitals and ask a few more questions about my symptoms and history.

"Wait right here; we'll get you in quickly."

I am ushered back to an ER exam room and told to undress. Charles helps me pull off my clothes and tucks them into a neat pile. "Hopefully you'll be able to put these back on soon, and I'll take you home." He sits down next to the gurney and lays a hand gently on my arm.

When the nurse starts an IV, I convince myself that if I just get hydrated, I will be fine. With the inflow of fluids, I am starting to feel better. That sensation is short lived, however, and not long thereafter, I am writhing in pain, doubled over trying to find relief in a change of position.

Attentive and sympathetic, the nurse leaves and comes back with morphine. I ask her if she will give me the minimum dose, and she agrees, giving me two miligrams IV. The relief is negligible, barely taking the edge off, but I am afraid to have more, afraid the narcotic will halt peristalsis, and I imagine an obstruction expanding, all just because I can't stand the pain.

The doctor, a slender young woman with straight black hair cascading down her back, seems a bit puzzled as to what to do with me. I say I don't want to be admitted yet, and she agrees that I can be discharged to monitor my symptoms on my own. "If necessary, you can come back and be admitted to the medical floor."

**For your information . . .**
**the medical unit versus the surgical unit . . .**

Generally, people admitted to a general medical floor are *sick*, whether with heart disease, diabetes, gout, phlebitis, pneumonia, or a host of other illnesses. Patients on a surgical ward, in contrast, are more likely to be essentially healthy and hospitalized, usually briefly, for surgical procedures such as hernia repair, repair of herniated discs, gynecologic surgery, orthopedic surgery, and plastic surgery. (Cardiac and oncology patients on the surgical units are an exception.)

I am shocked: This is technically a complication of surgery. All my other admissions have been to the surgical oncology service. I never considered the possibility of being admitted to a medical floor, where staff is exhausted by caring for too many patients who need too many things. On the surgical floor, patients tend to be sturdier, healthier. If I am sent to the medical unit, I fear being misplaced or forgotten in that sea of need.

Yet although I do not want to be formally admitted, I also want to be further evaluated. I am afraid to be on my own right now. I need an ally.

Suddenly, I remember Dr. Kinjo's offer the last time I had an obstruction and turn to the nurse. "Dr. Kinjo, the one who did the surgery last September . . . he said that he would admit me to his surgical

**Hints to help you beat the odds . . . identifying an ally . . .**

The allies who spontaneously come to mind tend to be those who come from your circle of close friends and family. However, there is another pool of potential allies in hospital personnel, people with whom you have been able to communicate clearly and who you feel can empathize with your situation. Recall who has been especially helpful and understanding in the past, and call on them to come to your assistance when the occasion arises.

service if I had another episode like this." How quickly I have moved from not wanting to be admitted to agreeing to whatever it takes to stay off the medical floor!

"Oh, OK," she says cheerfully. "I'll go call him."

Charles is holding my hand and listening quietly. His body leaning toward mine, radiating warmth even in this chilly cell, is comforting. Knowing he is pressed to return to minister to Elena and Fred, I am especially appreciative that he stays with me, patiently, without monitoring the clock.

The doctor returns to say that Dr. Kinjo will admit me, that I am to have abdominal films, and that I am to have an NG tube inserted right away.

"Oh," I wince, hearing the news. "Can you put in a small one? Please?" I beg.

The doctor agrees and leaves the room as the nurse is positioning me for the insertion. From deep wells, although I am not aware of crying, tears start to spill down my cheeks. They just keep coming, marching silently, seeping salt into the corners of my mouth, and gathering momentum as they reach the sharper angles of my facial contours. Embarrassed, I peer through the watery lens and see puzzled and sympathetic eyes looking at me. Yet I am as perplexed as they: For what are these tears shed? Fear of the pain of the tube? Fear of these obstructions happening again and again? Fear of the one that will not be resolved by the NG tube? I don't know.

"Hold this cup of water, and start drinking fast when I tell you to," the nurse instructs me. "Oh, I didn't have to tell you that," she apologizes. "You must have this routine memorized."

"That's OK," I tell her as she pulls on her surgical gloves. "Besides, it seems to me that each of you has subtle variations in the details." The nurse who inserted the NG tube last time handed the cup of water to Charles and directed *him* to push me to drink on her command.

"That's true," she says, swabbing the end of the tube in gel.

My usual panic feeling the tube go up my nose and back down my throat is kept at bay as I try to sit tall to let it pass quickly. "Drink! Drink! Drink!" she orders me, " 'til there's nothing left."

Expecting the swoosh and gurgle of fluid as the tube finds my stomach, I hear only silence. Glancing toward the wall, an inspection of the two-liter container's pristine state confirms my observation. I worry that they will have to replace that rather small tube with a bigger one; the gods are punishing me for asking for favors. Then I throw up, chunks of

**Hints to help you beat the odds . . .
getting the NG tube down . . .**

Sipping water through a straw or directly from a cup helps advance the NG tube toward the stomach. The nurse or doctor inserting the tube will give you the signal when to start drinking. Each time you swallow, the tube will move forward from 3 to 5 inches. Focus on sipping as rapidly as you can until the nurse tells you to stop.[1]

totally undigested food from the day before: Thai food, carrot bits, and red pepper pieces. When I mention my fears of needing a larger NG tube, the nurse says, "That stuff wouldn't have gone through *any* size tube!" As the suction apparatus gradually begins to fill, my stomach settles slightly. I am tired from the vomiting and the unremitting pain.

When I am wheeled up to the seventh floor, I am greeted warmly by several of the nurses and aides I know from past admissions. One of the nurses empties a small syringe of morphine into my IV, and I sleep dreamlessly.

"Good morning, Eliza." A doctor who has done many of the colonoscopies stands by the bed. "The CEA, the tumor marker, that was done yesterday is 0.9."

I am so happy to hear that. I can't wait to tell Charles.

"I suggest we do a colonoscopy, just to make sure that the anastamosis site has not closed down again. With that CEA being so low, it's unlikely that you have another tumor, but maybe that area where the colon was stapled together has constricted."

When I leave for x-ray at about nine thirty, Charles still has not arrived, and I ask the nurses to tell him where I will be. I am gone about half an hour, and as I am being wheeled by the nurses' station, I ask, "Did my husband come?"

"No, not yet," one of them responds. "We've been looking out for him."

Shortly thereafter, I leave again by gurney for the procedure room on the fourth floor, where I have a colonoscopy. Waking from the light anesthesia, I hear, "There is no stricture, and not even one polyp!"

Still dreamy and lulled by the hangover of anesthesia, I am rolled back upstairs, where I expect to see Charles. This time the nurses call out as I pass by, "He's not here yet! We'll send him in as soon as he gets here!"

I sleep on and off for the rest of the day, and at about six o'clock, Charles calls and says he is about to leave home.

"Why not just come tomorrow?" I ask. "It's getting late for making the trip tonight." Disappointed that the whole day has gone by without seeing him, I am also tired and suspect that very soon I'll be asleep.

When he says, "OK," though, a twinge of disappointment grabs me, but I recover and ask him to bring me some shampoo tomorrow. My hair is standing straight up on end, fanning out to resemble an exotic bird, startled and perhaps in molt.

**Hints to help you beat the odds . . .**
**an understudy for your primary ally . . .**

If your significant other, your ally who is with you most of the time, is unable to continue supporting you, either temporarily or long term, it is important that you seek help elsewhere. Even if you convince yourself that you are reasonably well and shouldn't need any assistance, being on your own in the hospital is difficult. Ask for help! The potential for burnout is another reason to identify several allies so that they can give each other breaks and have time to tend to their own lives.

In the morning, I take a shower, wishing I had shampoo but figuring I will bathe again when I get it. The nurse disconnects the IV and tapes it to my arm, but when she reconnects it after the shower, the needle has slipped out of place, and the site has become infiltrated, swollen with fluid leaking into the surrounding tissues. So, with great difficulty, she starts another IV. My veins are riddled with scars.

Dinah comes by, having worked the night shift. She and I go on long walks, around the lanais, and up and down the corridors. By the time she leaves, I am tired and ready to sleep. Talking or even whispering takes a lot of effort, and sometimes it makes me cough. The NG tube seems to be getting more uncomfortable, actually painful—it feels raw, as if skin has been pulled off my throat. The cetacaine topical spray does not help.

I keep thinking Charles will be here and listening for his footsteps coming down the hall. He breezes in at two o'clock, drops off my shampoo, and then leaves in haste for a three o'clock massage appointment. His "visit" happens so quickly that I only nod hello and then watch

**For your information. . . . topical anesthetic spray. . . .**

A topical anaesthetic spray can be used to soothe the irritation of mucous membranes in the back of your throat. Sprayed on the target site for one second or less, it acts within seconds and lasts up to thirty minutes.[2]

him disappear down the hall. I can't understand what has happened between us. He seems so utterly self-involved. The dream returns, the panic when Charles leaves me alone in the bleak little house.

I am feeling that I have offended and inconvenienced him by being ill. What a dramatic shift from the days of his tenderly and patiently caring for me. I can feel the tears stinging my eyes and am relieved that no one is here to see. No one will ask what's the matter; I won't have to be sorry later for having admitted my misery.

I want to wash my hair, but I am afraid to have another shower: There are no veins left if the IV infiltrates again! So, I doze, watch TV, and doze some more. Clara comes at around five, and then Charles arrives not too long after. He looks at me briefly as he sits down without touching me or even approaching the bed. I am relieved that he and Clara chat together, leaving me to witness without participating.

**Suggestions for allies . . . admitting burnout . . .**

When you are exhausted and even bored with the entire sick scenario, take time off! Say you need a break, find someone else to take over, and be on your way. When you simply withdraw emotionally, without any explanation, it can be very scary and confusing for the person you have been trying to help. As on so many occasions, imagining what might account for sudden behavior changes is invariably more frightening than the truth.

By the time Dr. Kinjo comes on his nightly rounds, both Clara and Charles have departed. The NG tube continues to drain a lot, and although Dr. Kinjo decides it would be premature to remove it, he orders it to be clamped shut. If I have no problems during the night, it is possible that the tube will be removed tomorrow.

The night is torture. Just when I am tired and ready to sleep, I think I can't tolerate that tube anymore. My throat feels as if it is lined with glass shards. I seem to have no skin, just raw flesh. It feels tight and swollen—a feeling of being strangled. Swallowing is so painful that I avoid it if at all possible and spit into tissues instead. Finally, at about three a.m., I start peeling off the tape that holds the tubing to my nose. I feel desperate, actually crazed with pain. Just then, a nurse comes in, a gentle, dark-haired woman with a mellifluous voice. I gesture to her what torment this has become.

"I will take it out for you . . . I'll just say 'Patient refuses.'" She speaks matter-of-factly, and then adds, "You know, they might put it back again."

**Hints to help you beat the odds . . .**
**allies among hospital staff . . .**

As nurses are the "glue that holds it all together" in a hospital, an ally on the nursing staff can make your stay safer and more comfortable. Be sure you let them know how much you appreciate their kindness and advocacy.

I nod, assuring her that I know that, that it doesn't matter. She pulls it slowly out, and instead of the instant relief I expected, the pain in my throat is unchanged. This is very different from all the other times I have had NG tubes, when there was fabulous euphoria when they were finally removed, and I could swallow and talk without pain and impediment. But this time, it is hard to detect its absence. I am relieved to get it out, but the searing pain persists, and I am unable to sleep. Since my bowels are still inactive, I am afraid to ask for morphine, reluctant to do anything that might impede their recovery. I pass a miserable night, spitting secretions into tissues every few minutes to avoid swallowing.

The next morning, it hurts a bit less when I swallow, but increasingly, it feels as if something is pressing against my trachea. Although I realize that it is swelling that is causing this pressure, I instinctively keep changing position and loosening my gown in an attempt to find relief.

Charles comes in the late afternoon and, avoiding eye contact, settles into the reclining chair to watch TV. As he seeks refuge in the TV screen, I am conveniently distracted by the appearance of my first "meal" of red Jell-O and cranberry juice. He seems to have no interest in communi-

> **For your information . . . problems with the NG tube . . .**
>
> It is possible that repeated insertions of NG tubes over time can traumatize the pharynx, causing pain and edema (swelling). As well, the overuse of topical anesthetic spray can irritate the throat, leading to increased discomfort.

cating, and neither have I. My throat hurts too much to speak, and even if it did not, I am not sure what I would say. He has become a stranger again.

When Dr. Kinjo comes in around seven, he hears bowel sounds through his stethoscope, and Charles asks brightly, "You going to let her come home tonight?"

"I don't see why not," he turns to me. "Your bowels seem to be waking up, and you've managed OK without the NG tube."

Still unable to speak with the swelling and bruising in my throat, I nod in agreement.

"When this happens again, though," he continues, " you will have to be seen by the general surgery group." *I don't know anyone in surgery anymore*, I think to myself, *and I don't want there to be a next time.*

He leaves, and we start getting stuff ready to go. There isn't much to do, as I brought little with me, and there are no flowers, cards, or trinkets. We drive home, the silence spreading a chasm between us. Charles seems to have reached his limit of caring for me. It has become boring, perhaps annoying. When we pull into the driveway, I am shocked when he gets out of the car and walks up to the front door. He has neither come around to help me, nor even to see whether I am OK. I can't talk at all now, so I can't call for help. My throat feels not only sore but also tight, as if it is closing up. I hobble slowly to the door and make my way upstairs, where I fall gratefully into bed. I can hear Charles in the kitchen, and then the clamor of the TV as he surfs the channels. Perhaps he is angry that I could not make myself more available for our houseguests, now departed.

"Do you want something to eat?" He stands in the doorway, TV remote in his hand, waiting for an answer.

"Um-umm," I answer. Noticing from his expression that he has not heard me, I muster my strength and steel myself for the pain, as I say clearly, "No. No, thank you." Not sure what might taste good to me, I also am unable to utter any words other than that simple response. How different it would have been had he appeared with a cup of tea, a glass of water, a bowl of miso. Anything, any offering, would have made me feel cared for and safe.

**Suggestions for primary allies . . . getting help . . .**

If you feel a distance growing between you and the person you love, you are probably not getting the support that you need for yourself. The weight of the responsibility you have assumed can be overwhelming, leaving you neither time nor energy for meeting your own needs, leading to resentment, frustration, and anxiety. Get ongoing support from other allies, consider joining a support group for friends and family of people with cancer, or see a therapist for some individual counseling to get you through this.

Charles goes to the gym in the morning, and then plays golf in the afternoon. Again, I am astonished at his intense self-absorption. My utter dependence on him makes me afraid to object, to question his behavior, lest doing so invites his anger. The risk of incurring his wrath silences me. I spend a quiet day in bed, sleeping and reading, but mostly wondering what is going through his mind. I feel as if we are living the dream, as if he has left me in a place that is neither safe nor secure, and I am alone to cope without him. Although we share a physical space, we are otherwise as separate as in the dream. He does not seem particularly happy to have me home and more often than not ignores me.

"Do you want anything?" he asks from the doorway of the bedroom. He never seems to think of what might be helpful. As I cannot talk, it seems too much work to communicate what I might want, and anyway, I would like to feel as if he could figure out what might be helpful, like a glass of water.

Max and Pat, my uncle and aunt, call to invite us to dinner.

**For your information . . . more about role confusion . . .**

Roles change when somebody in the household is sick, and initially the expectation is that the illness will resolve itself and life will resume as before. However, when the illness becomes chronic, requiring repeated and extended role changes, burnout is not only possible but likely. Resentment can build when the roles of cook, nurse, housekeeper, and companion are vacated, or when the roles of breadwinner and protector are abandoned because of illness. When one person moves out of a role or roles, every other person in that household has to readjust to compensate.

**Suggestions for allies . . . preventing burnout . . .**

Bringing more people into the circle of support will reduce the possibility of burnout, especially for the primary ally (the partner or significant other), who is assuming the most constant responsibility for caretaking. Facilitating connections with more family and close friends can reduce the intensity of the dependency connection with the primary ally.

"Yes," I nod vigorously. I will not be able to talk, but I need to get out from what has become an oppressive household, just the two of us, stretching further and further apart.

Several days later, when I am able to talk again, I think of asking him what is happening. Now I can care for myself without his help, yet during those earlier days, I was feeling utterly abandoned, and furthermore, unable to seek help from family and friends, as doing so would involve disclosing this gap in our relationship.

"What happened when I was in the hospital?" I begin. We are sitting at the breakfast table, the morning paper spread out in front of us.

"What do you mean?" he breaks in, a palpable edge in his voice.

"You seemed so far away . . . you were so busy . . ."

"That's not true!"

"Well, I felt so alone." I speak slowly. "I felt far, far away from you."

"I was right there!" I can see his skin redden with agitation.

"Even when we got home from the hospital," I persist, "you left me to shuffle from the car to the house on my own, and by the time I got there, you were in the kitchen doing something, and then watching TV . . . I felt almost as if I didn't exist."

"What do you mean?" He stands up and starts for the door. Pausing, he puts his hands in his pockets and turns to me. "I drove back and forth to the hospital, bringing you shampoo and then bringing you home . . .

**Hints to help you beat the odds . . .**
**communication, communication . . .**

Keeping your communication open, during stressful times especially, is essential. One way to assure that it remain open and free of prejudice is to try to listen to each other without judgment, respecting one another's feelings as valid, even if they differ.

and while you were there, I entertained Elena and Fred on my own!" His voice rises in frustration.

"I know that was hard for you." I retreat. "I'm sorry."

"It *was* hard!" He turns to go, and then stops himself. "Do you want me to get you anything now?"

"No, thanks."

The door closes behind him, and I am relieved that I didn't push any harder. I regret bringing it up at all, as he clearly remembers those days differently and is only angered by my questioning his conduct. *Are my expectations too high?* I wonder. *Am I asking something of him that he cannot give? But he gave so much when I was critically ill*, I remind myself. *Are his capacities for kindness and compassion drained?*

I wish we might have been able to talk about it without his feeling attacked, without my feeling afraid that, in his anger, he would truly abandon me. I can understand his not *wanting* to do any more, and I could even accept that, were he able to articulate it. Had that been the case, someone else would been able to come to help me during this time, leaving him free and unencumbered, and I would have felt safer and cared for. It was the shock of his disregard that made it so hard, his inaccessibility that was frightening.

Dream fragments loop into my awareness. In the dream, he not only became unavailable himself but also took me to an isolated and barren place apart from all I knew. And now, living the dream, I am cut off from him and aching for the love and careful ministrations that he once gave so generously.

In the days that follow, the tension softens, and the chasm narrows, not because our discussion led to resolution, but because I am beginning to ponder his experience as caretaker, which, in turn, generates my compassion.

**Hints to help you beat the odds . . .**
**taking care of the caretaker . . .**

In the crisis of acute illness, attention is understandably focused on the patient. The primary ally, who may be assuming several new roles as well as maintaining some semblance of his old roles, is at risk of becoming overwhelmed by his added responsibilities. The circle of allies can be helpful in offering specific help to allow time off. And it's important that you recognize the limitations of his strength and endurance, and encourage frequent breaks.

For the last two years, the structure of Charles's days has been determined by my needs. He has driven me hundreds of miles to appointments with the surgeons and the oncologists, for CT scans and chemotherapy, for ceramic studio and singing lessons. During the time I had the colostomy, he helped me with every aspect of care, including those I could barely tolerate myself. Every other day, making my decoctions according to Dr. Kou's instructions, he has carefully weighed the herbs, boiled them, strained off the water, and boiled them again. During my various operations, he has dozed in front of TV screens in bleak waiting rooms, and afterward, he has slept by my bed on a hard, narrow cot under fraying blankets. He has spent untold days sitting quietly in the back of the hospital room, listening to the wheeze of some machines and the beeps of others, and watching the mysterious ministrations to a body that responded only occasionally.

Charles has gone to nearly every chemo session with me and tenderly cared for me afterward. He never complained, never expressed exhaustion, and rarely expressed frustration. Although there were times I urged him to take a break and allow someone else to relieve him, he declined. Perhaps the fear of something happening to me in his absence kept him from leaving my side, from taking the break he so needed. Perhaps he felt that leaving me would indicate a lack of caring.

The days, weeks, and months of caretaking are only now displaying their toll, a toll that is made more difficult by Charles being unable to discuss his feelings about what this long siege has meant for him. Unable to articulate the extent of his exhaustion, he likely cannot acknowledge it even to himself.

Why was I not able to see this crisis coming? His response of turning away when he felt utterly used up is not atypical. Books and articles are written about "caretaker burnout," a growing problem given the rise in chronic disease. Yet I was unable to anticipate it. All my resources were exhausted by meeting the tasks of healing, requiring a focus on myself that left me unable to imagine, in any detail, how this experience might

**Hints to help you beat the odds . . .**
**expressing gratitude to your primary ally . . .**

A simple thank you will be heard less clearly than an actual naming of the many things that your primary ally has done for you. Thoughtfully listing the many things he or she did for which you are thankful provides witness to the gift you have been given.

be affecting Charles. There have been times when I have thought to myself, *Surely* watching *me in this pain, and being unable to make it better, is harder than* being *the me that's suffering.*

This perusal of the last few weeks is leading me to realize that my journey henceforth may be to go on more independently. As strength and resilience are returning to me, I understand and can accept Charles's limitations. I welcome his involvement, yet know I can ask for help elsewhere when he is otherwise engaged. I realize now that when he turned from me at a time of intense need, by so doing, he pushed me to discover my own resilience, my own capabilities, and my own astonishing strengths that brought me to understand the complexities underlying his behavior.

## *Chapter 18*

# Redefining Normal

### DREAMING WISDOM

#### *September 1999*

*I am standing on a solid porch with a cement floor that curves up to form low walls. The form reminds me of the roundish boat in the nursery rhyme "Three Men in a Tub." On an identical adjacent porch, three older women sit and quietly talk among themselves. They apparently have the key that I need to gain entry to this house. One of the women hands me the key, with the understanding that I will return it as soon as I have opened the door. After turning the lock in the door, I hand the key back to them and nod in appreciation. They tell me that I no longer need it, that it has already opened the door to the wisdom I seek. Going into the house, I am startled to hear the rush of water. I follow the sound down to the basement, where there are two spigots, both dripping water onto the gray cement floor, which is swirling and rippling with the collected water of . . . how many hours? Days? I understand that I am going on a journey that requires a deep cleansing prior to departure. The faucets continue to drip while I carefully load a pile of white laundry into the washing machine. I finally turn my attention to them and turn the spigots off with a quick twist to the right. Once the sound of dripping stops, I am astonished that I didn't stop the flow as soon as I discovered it.*

As I awake, the night's images bleed into my day, and I am already pondering preparations for the dream journey. Who are these dream crones who gave me their key? If only I could pull myself back into the boat to learn more. The sun splashes across the ceiling, yet I continue to mull over the imagery. Are these apparitions the Three Fates: Klotho, Atropos, and Lachesis? Still tethered to my dream, I can hear, over the drone of Charles's shower, the purr of Klotho's spinning wheel beginning the thread of existence, the thump of Atropos's wooden shuttle weaving stories into lives, and the sharp snip of Lachesis's scissors marking endings. The old woman's key not only opened my physical house but perhaps also accessing an expanded view of my interior world.

I think of the gates that this illness has opened to me and those that it has softly but irrevocably closed. A door has firmly closed on the possibility of reclaiming the "normal" that I once knew. Each day during this long year after the completion of chemo, I have peered hopefully into the mirror, wondering, *Is this the day that "normal" will return?* Feeling the ache in my joints persisting though months and now years, I have wondered when I'll be able to move again as I once did.

It is only now that I am beginning to understand that I will not be returning to that normal. The aging that leaped into fast-forward during chemo has slowed to a more acceptable pace, but there is sadly no reversal of the processes already completed. Chemo, and perhaps the disease itself, has sped up the momentum of aging, and I am left with stiff joints, dry hair and skin, and a sometimes unreliable memory, which is perhaps the most frustrating of all. The normal I once knew has vanished, an unattainable and misty province of my past.

So my gaze reverses. No longer looking back in anticipation of my return to what *was*, I now look ahead to define the structures and context of my new way of being: *How will I be in the world? How will I be with myself? What does my new normal look like?*

Judith, my Jungian therapist, continues to help me find my place in that space between the worlds. She coaxes me to bring into the light the shadows that I have not heretofore recognized, helps me articulate the dramatic shifts in my worldview, and helps me integrate the mysteries in which I have partaken.

Physically aware of the power of life and death, I set aside intimate times with myself during which I can deeply focus on living the lessons learned. When I look at a crowded calendar in the morning and tell myself, *You can get through this; you can do all these things and then fall apart tonight,* I realize that the simple lesson to slow down, take time to breathe deeply, and savor the richness of my days is a teaching that I have not yet integrated. Lessons that I thought at one time were imbedded in my mind forever have become elusive and shoved into the background of too many busy days.

I am challenged to stay awake in a world that conspires to hypnotize with a crushing abundance of seductive possibilities and a profusion of sensory demands that beg response. The possibilities for overprogramming my days are endless and compelling. During the acute phases of my illness, supported by Charles's generous spirit, I was bound to live with myself in a holy solitude, the only interruptions being the manifestations and demands of my disease. Now, however, I can no longer rely on signs and symptoms to remind me of the value of stillness, to force me to move slowly, to encourage me to set aside time for simply being. It is up to me to disengage, if necessary, from the frenzy of a hurried life. Yoga, walking, and being deliberately still are helpful tools for slowing down. And within me are the resources to support living consciously. Images of the dream come to me, images of the key that unlocks the door to wisdom. Learning the lessons are one thing. Taking them into my being, integrating them thoroughly, is a commitment I have made but not yet fulfilled.

The covenants I am working to abandon include *I am always strong, I will always nourish, I will rely on myself,* and *I will be what you want me to be.* As is common to many women, especially so to those in the helping professions, those old vows lead to unhealthy responses, including feelings of being overwhelmed with trying to meet people's needs for my time, attention, and services.

Although requests and expectations were for worthy and important causes, I not infrequently felt exploited and resentful. Identifying what *I* truly want can be rapidly obscured by consideration of what *others* need of me. I am asked to do many things that have unquestionable significance and value, yet if I agree to all of them, I begin to lose the me with whom I am only now getting acquainted.

Because I have a type of cancer that can be difficult to discuss, and because it is known through word of mouth and through public speaking engagements that I am willing to talk about it, I receive many phone calls and e-mails from the newly diagnosed, some of whom I know, most of whom I do not. I receive requests from newly diagnosed people who want a referral to Dr. Kou, and I gladly connect them. I also hear from people with other kinds of cancer, usually those who want to talk about the more spiritual and energetic aspects of living with terminal illness. Although these dialogues are nourishing to me in many ways, they also consume substantial energy. Yet I find it difficult when asked to help someone dealing with this terrifying diagnosis to turn him or her down in order to restore my own energies and reinvigorate my own life force.

These seekers have been catalysts in my writing this book, which I hope, will be a source of information for those eager to benefit from my experience both in living with this disease and in acknowledging how different life is when you step outside the world as we know it. That I am grateful for the lessons brought to me by this experience is often what people want to hear and understand.

I am learning to create new vows that are consistent with my redefined reality. They include a commitment to spend time in nourishing relationships, a commitment to ongoing attempts to state my needs clearly and then negotiate to get them met, and a commitment to value "downtime." My extended family members are energetic and tireless, their days packed with tasks and activities that contribute to each other's welfare and also to our community. I see them painting someone's first house, cleaning out a rental unit, serving on the city council and various nonprofit boards, patiently teaching our youngest citizens, working with wounded inner-city kids, and I am exhausted. Within this context, it requires great effort to claim downtime and to unapologetically respond, "Nothing" when asked, "What did you do today?"

My new normal is being constructed on the foundation of these new vows. I wrestle with deciding in what way I will use my time. There are limitless opportunities for helping people individually or through community organizations. When asked to participate, I remind myself that I need to carefully assess my own needs and available resources before responding.

Without cancer's overwhelming assault on my life, I would undoubtedly be continuing to live with a certain assumption of immortality, an unspoken understanding that the spool of time rolls into infinity, that there will always be time to "do what I want to do." And a parallel delusion is that there is always more energy, more time. I am learning to accept not only the limits of my body but also the rigidity of every hour having sixty minutes, and no more, and every day having twenty-four hours, not twenty-five. It is incumbent upon me to choose, and to choose well, in what way I will apportion my resources.

The changes occurring in these vows are opening the way to more peaceful and satisfying days. Aware now of the potency of life and death, my tolerance for frittering away time in humdrum activities diminishes. I am less inclined to see a movie or attend a function that doesn't really interest me. My time is finite, and I want to spend it well. This is not to devalue time for relaxation and renewal. "Doing nothing" is a noble pursuit and very different from spending time doing what is meaningless or depleting.

During the active phase of illness, I was able to focus deeply on the lessons being offered. As I work now to remember and honor the profound teachings of this experience, I am also challenged to stay awake. The dream returns, the image of precious resources being wasted because of my inattention. Stepping out from my spiritual hermitage to reenter the turmoil and restless vigor of humanity, my challenge now, amid the rush of distractions, is to hold onto what I have learned and to stay alert to the subtleties and nuances of lessons yet to come.

# *Epilogue*
# Letting Go

***September 2004***

It is just over six years since I heard the diagnosis of metastatic colon cancer. And I have yet to hear the snap of Lachesis's scissors. Astonishingly, I am well, and diagnostic tests continue to suggest that whatever cancer may be milling about in my body is imperceptible to current measuring devices. Despite my overall good health, there have been the occasional scares—once a suspicious lump in my breast; another time, one near my lower rib. Each time a lab value deviates from normal, each time I feel an irregularity in the contours of my body, I realize how deeply I hunger for a healthy future. Although I acknowledge the resumption of good health to be precarious, I nonetheless, in some deep way, have faith that it will be ongoing.

For over three years, the bowel obstructions that plagued me subsequent to the 1998 surgery continued to recur every two to three months, and about half required hospitalization. Because dehydration appeared to be the crucial contributory factor, I aimed for a state of "superhydration," my goal being to drink one gallon of water a day. In an effort to further reduce the risk of blockages, I adhered to a strict diet limiting dairy, wheat, and refined foods. The obstructions often occurred when I had been too busy to drink adequate fluids or had deviated from the diet while traveling or visiting friends. Aside from the physical pain, there was also the anxiety of never knowing when the next blockage might occur. However, the surgeons were reluctant to open me up again to excise the adhesions, as an additional operation would risk creating additional scars, negating the benefit of surgery or even exacerbating an already troublesome condition.

In February of 2002, I was taken by ambulance to the local hospital for a severe obstruction. As this hospital is not a participant in my health plan, for the first time I received care at a facility with which I had no prior history. With a new team of doctors taking a fresh look, the routine of the NG tube and taking nothing by mouth was not followed by the expected discharge home a few days later.

When the surgeon came into the hospital room on the third day after admission, I assumed he would be discussing the removal of the NG tube and then my discharge.

"Not at all!" he said firmly. "We need to resolve these blockages and to do that we need to go in there and take out what's causing them."

"Surgery?" I asked dumbly.

"Of course," he replied solemnly.

"I thought you were going to say I could go home soon." I smiled at my error in judgment.

"Well, you'll go home before too long, but not before we take care of what's causing these obstructions." He smiled and then said decisively, "It doesn't make sense to just send you home, only to have you come back with another one in a couple of months, and then another . . ."

My surgeons had heretofore discussed the options many times with me and were reluctant, for good reason, to risk further exacerbation of the adhesions by operating.

Although I agreed with their counsel, at this point I am so exhausted by the pain of this latest bowel obstruction that I willingly comply with the new surgeon's plan.

A few hours later, drowsy from anesthesia, I was wheeled out of the OR and into the recovery room. The surgeon told me that my abdomen had been rife with sticky adhesions and that he had removed one fist-sized clump of tangled tissue.

"How anything at all got through that narrow passage . . ." He shook his head. "It's amazing!"

Now, two-and-a-half years later, I am obstruction free. The relief is hard to describe. I am able to plan and to travel, without the constraints of being near a hospital "just in case." I no longer have to carry huge water bottles wherever I go and am free to eat a wider range of foods.

I continue to see Dr. Kou every eight to ten weeks for acupuncture and Qi Gong, and I take my daily herbs as he prescribes. Outliving my prognosis, I believe, is in large part due to Dr. Kou's ministrations. The tumors, which were expected to multiply and eventually overwhelm my body, have not shown up!

I also see my family-practice physician every six months and have regular CEA levels drawn. Of course, I hope that I won't have to call upon the skills of oncologists and surgeons again, but if it should become necessary, I'll have already had several rehearsals!

Although the particular WomenCARE support group of which I was a member has ended, I served on their board of directors until 2004, when I found myself spending more and more time in British Columbia. When I am in town, I continue to meet with the women in my "Cancer Club," a couple of whom are veterans of the support group at WomenCARE. In the company of these women who also live in that space between worlds, I can disclose the terrors of recurrence, the exhilaration of healing, the anguish of waiting for test results, and the triumph of one more round dancing with NED: No Evidence of Disease.

On three occasions, I have read selections from *Living with Colon Cancer: Beating the Odds* on the radio, and each time, the responses have been poignant. People have called the station, sometimes moved to tears by what they have heard, sometimes frustrated that the book was, at the time, unavailable. I have also participated in public forums, such as conferences on cancer, classes on death and dying, and a speaker series on living with cancer. Telling my story has been healing for me, and hearing the responses and stories of the audience has been both inspiring and heart wrenching.

Questions range from the concrete, such as details of signs and symptoms, to the practical, such as how to find support and information. A number of people have asked, *Why did you, a healthcare professional, tolerate the shoddy care you received from the ER personnel when you were first sick?* The answer is simple: I was stunned into submission by the potent triad of pain, exhaustion, and dehydration. The distress occurring on a physical level deeply affected my capacity to think clearly and diminished my ability to forcefully respond to the physicians' easy dismissal of my crisis. And, with the passing of hours and days and increasing debility, I became further immobilized, physically and mentally. Difficult as this was for me, an "insider" familiar with the language and culture peculiar to the institution, I shudder to think of the barriers faced by one for whom the hospital is an alien world.

Through the crisis of this illness, and through the treatments I endured, I felt that I was taking religious vows, vows in blood and body and bone. During the long siege by the disease and its treatment, the daily reminders of pain, discomfort, and physical changes kept me alert to living the lessons learned. Remembering the crones of my dream, perhaps they appeared to underscore my need to continue taking in new information, to keep seeking the well of wisdom to which they are giving me access.

That sharp edge of teetering on the abyss has dulled. In this time of stability, I risk being lulled into complacency by the comfortable routine that is shaping my days. The fundamental promise of my new covenant with myself is to stay awake, to recall the awesome terrain of terminal disease even when robust health has dulled my memory.

# Glossary

The following definitions have been compiled by the nursing advisory board of Pharmacia and Upjohn Company to provide you with a better understanding of words frequently used in cancer care. If you have any questions related to the content, please consult your health-care provider.[1]

**Acute**: A sudden onset of symptoms or disease.

**Adjuvant chemotherapy**: Chemotherapy given to kill any remaining cancer cells, usually after all detectable tumor are removed by surgery or radiotherapy.

**Analgesic**: Any drug that relieves pain. Aspirin and acetaminophen are mild analgesics.

**Anemia**: A condition in which a decreased number of red blood cells may cause symptoms that include tiredness, shortness of breath, and weakness.

**Anorexia**: The loss of appetite.

**Antibody**: A substance formed by the body to help defend it against infection.

**Antigen**: Any substance that causes the body to produce natural antibodies.

**Antineoplastic agent**: A drug that prevents, kills, or blocks the growth and spread of cancer cells.

**Autoimmunity**: A condition in which the body's immune system mistakenly fights and rejects the body's own tissues.

**Barium enema**: The use of a milky solution (barium sulfate) given by an enema to allow x-ray examination of the lower intestinal tract.

**Barium swallow**: The use of a milky solution (barium sulfate) given orally to allow x-ray examination of the upper intestinal tract.

**Benign growth**: A swelling or growth that is not cancerous and does not spread from one part of the body to another.

**Biopsy**: The surgical removal of tissue for microscopic examination to aid in diagnosis.

**Blood cells**: Minute structures produced in the bone marrow; they consist of red blood cells, white blood cells, and platelets.

**Blood count**: The number of red blood cells, white blood cells, and platelets in a sample of blood.

**Bone marrow**: The spongy material found inside the bones. Most blood cells are made in the bone marrow.

**Bone marrow suppression**: A decrease in the production of blood cells.

**Cancer**: A group of diseases in which malignant cells grow out of control and spread to other parts of the body.

**Cancer in situ**: The stage where the cancer is still confined to the tissue in which it started.

**Carcinoembryonic antigen (CEA)**: A blood tumor marker.

**Carcinogen**: A substance that causes cancer.

**Carcinoma**: A type of cancer that starts in the skin or the lining of organs.

**CAT scan (CT scan)**: A test using computers and x-rays to create images of various parts of the body.

**Cellulitis**: The inflammation of an area of the skin (epithelial layer).

**Central venous catheter**: A special intravenous tubing that is surgically inserted into a large vein near the heart and exits from the chest or abdomen. The catheter allows medications, fluids, or blood products to be given and blood samples to be taken.

**Cervical nodes**: Lymph nodes in the neck.

**Chemotherapy**: The treatment of cancer with drugs.

**Chronic**: Persisting over a long period of time.

**Colonoscopy**: A procedure to look at the colon or large bowel through a lighted, flexible tube.

**Colostomy**: A surgical procedure by which an opening is created between the colon and the outside of the abdomen to allow stool to be emptied into a collection bag.

**Combination chemotherapy**: The use of more than one drug during cancer treatment.

**CSF (colony-stimulating factor)**: An injectable substance used to stimulate the bone marrow to produce more cells.

**Drug resistance**: The result of cells' ability to resist the effects of a specific drug.

**Edema**: The accumulation of fluid in part of the body.

**Erythema**: Redness of the skin.

**Erythrocyte**: The red blood cell that carries oxygen to body cells and carbon dioxide away from body cells.

**Estrogen**: A female hormone produced primarily by the ovaries.

**Excision**: Surgical removal.

**Extravasation**: The leaking of intravenous fluids or medications into tissue surrounding the infusion site. Extravasation may cause tissue damage.

**Fine-needle aspirate**: A procedure in which a needle is inserted, under local anesthesia, to obtain a sample for the evaluation of suspicious tissue.

**Frozen section**: A technique in which tissue is removed and then quick-frozen and examined under a microscope by a pathologist.

**Granulocyte**: A type of white blood cell that kills bacteria.

**Guaiac test**: A test that checks for hidden blood in the stool.

**Hematocrit (Hct)**: The percentage of red blood cells in the blood. A low hematocrit measurement indicates anemia.

**Hematologist**: A doctor who specializes in the problems of blood and bone marrow.

**Hematology**: The science that studies the blood.

**Hematuria**: Blood in the urine.

**Hemoccult (Guaiac) test**: A test that checks for hidden blood in the stool.

**Herpes simplex**: The most common virus that causes sores often seen around the mouth, commonly called cold sores.

**Herpes zoster**: A virus that settles around certain nerves, causing blisters, swelling, and pain. This condition is also called shingles.

**Hickman catheter**: A special intravenous tubing that is surgically inserted into a large vein near the heart. *See* central venous catheter.

**Hodgkin's disease**: A cancer that affects the lymph nodes. *See* lymphoma.

**Hormones**: Substances secreted by various organs of the body that regulate growth, metabolism, and reproduction.

**Hospice**: A concept of supportive care to meet the special needs of patients and family during the terminal stages of illness. The care may be delivered in the home or hospital by a specially trained team of professionals.

**Human immunodeficiency virus (HIV)**: The virus that causes AIDS.

**Human leukocyte antigen test (HLA)**: A special blood test used to match a blood or bone marrow donor to a recipient for transfusion or transplant.

**Hyperalimentation**: The intravenous administration of a highly nutritious solution.

**Ileostomy**: A surgical opening in the abdomen connected to the small intestine to allow stool to be emptied into a collection bag.

**Immunity (immune system)**: The body's ability to fight infection and disease.

**Immunosuppression**: A weakening of the immune system that causes a lowered ability to fight infection and disease.

**Immunotherapy**: The artificial stimulation of the body's immune system to treat or fight disease.

**Infiltration**: The leaking of fluid or medicines into tissues, which can cause swelling.

**Infusion**: Delivering fluids or medications into the bloodstream over a period of time.

**Infusion pump**: A device that delivers measured amounts of fluids or medications into the bloodstream over a period of time.

**Injection**: Pushing a medication into the body with the use of a syringe and needle.

- **Intramuscular (IM)**: Into the muscle.
- **Intravenous (IV)**: Into the vein.
- **Subcutaneous**: Into the fatty tissue under the skin.

**Lesion**: A lump or abscess that may be caused by injury or disease, such as cancer.

**Leukemia**: Cancer of the blood. White blood cells may be produced in excessive amounts and are unable to work properly.

**Leukocyte**: *See* white blood cell.

**Leukopenia**: A low number of white blood cells.

**Lymphatic system**: A network that includes lymph nodes, lymph, and lymph vessels that serves as a filtering system for the blood.

**Lymph nodes**: Hundreds of small, oval bodies that contain lymph. Lymph nodes act as our first line of defense against infections and cancer.

**Lymphocytes**: White blood cells that kill viruses and defend against the invasion of foreign material.

**Magnetic resonance imaging (MRI)**: A sophisticated test that provides in-depth images of organs and structures in the body.

**Malignant tumor**: A tumor made up of cancer cells of the type that can spread to other parts of the body.

**Metastasize**: To spread from the first cancer site, for example, breast cancer that spreads to the bone.

**Monoclonal antibodies**: Artificially manufactured antibodies specifically designed to find targets on cancer cells for diagnostic or treatment purposes.

**Mucosa (mucous membranes)**: The lining of the mouth and gastrointestinal tract.

**Mucositis**: Inflammation of the lining of the mouth or gastrointestinal tract.

**Myeloma**: A malignant tumor of the bone marrow associated with the production of abnormal proteins.

**Myelosuppression**: A decrease in the production of red blood cells, platelets, and some white blood cells by the bone marrow.

**Neoplasm**: A new growth of tissue or cells; a tumor that is generally malignant.

**Neutropenia**: A decreased number of neutrophils, a type of white blood cell.

**Non-Hodgkin's lymphoma**: A cancer of the lymphatic system. Non-Hodgkin's lymphoma is related to Hodgkin's disease but is made up of different cell types. *See* lymphoma.

**Oncologist**: A doctor who specializes in oncology.

**Oncology**: The study and treatment of cancer.

**Oncology clinical nurse specialist**: A registered nurse with a master's degree who specializes in the education and treatment of cancer patients.

**Palliative treatment**: Treatment aimed at the relief of pain and symptoms of disease but not intended to cure the disease.

**Pap (Papanicolaou) smear**: A test to detect cancer of the cervix.

**Pathology**: The study of disease by the examination of tissues and body fluids under the microscope. A doctor who specializes in pathology is called a pathologist.

**Petechiae**: Tiny areas of bleeding under the skin, usually caused by a low platelet count.

**Photosensitivity**: Extreme sensitivity to the sun, leaving the patient prone to sunburns. This can be a side effect of some cancer drugs and radiation.

**Placebo**: An inert substance often used in clinical trials for comparison.

**Platelet (plt)**: Cells in the blood that are responsible for clotting.

**Platelet count**: The number of platelets in a blood sample.

**Polyp**: A growth of tissue protruding into a body cavity. Polyps may be benign or malignant.

**Port-implanted**: A catheter connected to a quarter-sized disc that is surgically placed just below the skin in the chest or abdomen. The tube is inserted into a large vein or artery directly into the bloodstream. Fluids, drugs, or blood products can be infused, and blood can be drawn through a needle that is stuck into the disc.

**Primary tumor**: The original cancer site. For example, breast cancer that has spread to the bone is still called breast cancer.

**Prognosis**: The projected outcome of a disease; the life expectancy.

**Protocol**: A treatment plan.

**Radiation therapy**: X-ray treatment that damages or kills cancer cells.

**Radiologist**: A doctor who specializes in the use of x-rays to diagnose and treat disease.

**Recurrence**: The reappearance of a disease after a period of remission.

**Red blood cells (erythrocytes)**: Cells in the blood that deliver oxygen to tissues and take carbon dioxide from them.

**Red blood count (RBC)**: The number of red blood cells seen in a blood sample.

**Regression**: The shrinkage of cancer growth.

**Relapse**: The reappearance of a disease after its apparent cessation.

**Remission**: Complete or partial disappearance of the signs and symptoms of disease.

**Risk factor**: Anything that increases a person's chances of developing cancer.

**Sarcoma**: A malignant tumor of muscles or connective tissue such as bone and cartilage.

**Side effects**: Secondary effects of drugs used for disease treatment.

**Sigmoidoscopy**: The visual examination of the rectum and lower colon using a tubular instrument called a sigmoidoscope.

**Staging**: The determination of the extent of cancer in the body.

**Steroids**: A type of hormone.

**Stoma**: An artificial opening between two cavities or between a cavity and the surface of the body.

**Stomatitis**: Temporary inflammation and soreness of the mouth.

**Systemic disease**: A disease that affects the entire body instead of a specific organ.

**Taste alteration**: A temporary change in taste perception.

**Thrombocytopenia**: An abnormally low number of platelets (thrombocytes). If the platelet count is too low, bleeding could occur.

**Tumor**: An abnormal overgrowth of cells. Tumors can be either benign or malignant.

**Ultrasound examination**: The use of high frequency sound waves to aid in diagnosis.

**Ureterostomy**: A surgical procedure consisting of cutting the ureters from the bladder and connecting them to an opening (stoma) on the abdomen, allowing urine to flow into a collection bag.

**Venipuncture**: Puncturing a vein in order to obtain blood samples, to start an intravenous drip, or to give medication.

**Virus**: Tiny infectious agents that are smaller than bacteria. The common cold is caused by a virus, and the herpes simplex virus causes cold sores.

**White blood cells (WBC)**: General term for a variety of cells responsible for fighting invading germs, infection, and allergy-causing agents. Specific white blood cells include granulocytes and lymphocytes.

**White blood count (WBC)**: The actual number of white blood cells seen in a blood sample.

**X-ray**: High-energy electromagnetic radiation used to diagnose and treat disease. Also a diagnostic test that uses high energy to visualize internal body organs.

# Notes

## INTRODUCTION

1. "Prevalence and Incidence of Colorectal Cancer," Wrong Diagnosis, http://www.wrongdiagnosis.com/c/colorectal/prevalence.htm (accessed June 25, 2005).

2. "Colorectal Cancer Stats," Canadian Cancer Society, 2005, http://www.cancer.ca/ccs/internet/standard/0,3182,3172_14447_langId-en,00.html (accessed June 22, 2005).

3. "Prevalence and Incidence of Colorectal Cancer."

4. "Colorectal Cancer Screening," National Cancer Institute, US National Institutes of Health, February 24, 2005, http://www.nci.nih.gov/cancertopics/pdq/screening/colorectal/Patient/page3 (accessed June 23, 2005).

## CHAPTER 1

1. Wendy Johnson, "Juggling Patients and Priorities: Life in the Emergency Department," May 7, 2002, http://www.cvh.on.ca/community/articles/actyh200201c.htm (accessed June 27, 2005).

2. "Constipation," Ask the Nurse, http://www.med-help.net/Constipation.html (accessed June 25, 2005).

3. Jacqueline A. Hart, "Dehydration," Medline Plus Medical Encyclopedia, May 28, 2004, http://www.nlm.nih.gov/medlineplus/ency/article/000982.htm (accessed June 22, 2005).

4. Ibid.

5. "Flexible Sigmoidoscopy," National Digestive Diseases Information Clearinghouse, November 2004, http://digestive.niddk.nih.gov/ddiseases/pubs/sigmoidoscopy/ (accessed June 22, 2005).

6. Jan Nissl, "Digital Rectal Exam (DRE)," WebMD, December 16, 2004, http://my.webmd.com/hw/colorectal_cancer/hw4404.asp (accessed June 22, 2005).

## CHAPTER 2

1. Mark Bennett Pochapin, *What Your Doctor May Not Tell You about Colorectal Cancer* (New York: Warner Books, 2004), pp. 15–16.

2. Ibid., pp. 145–48.

3. Ibid., pp. 150–51.

4. "Colon Cancer Treatment: Stages of Colon Cancer," National Cancer Institute, May 20, 2005, http://www.nci.nih.gov/cancertopics/pdq/treatment/colon/Patient/page2 (accessed June 22, 2005).

5. Pochapin, *What Your Doctor May Not Tell You*, pp. 191–92.

6. "Phlebitis," Columbia Electronic Encyclopedia, InfoPlease, 2005, http://www.infoplease.com/ce6/sci/A0838820.html (accessed June 22, 2005).

## CHAPTER 3

1. "Colostomy: A Patient's Perspective," MedicineNet.com, April 17, 2002, http://www.medicinenet.com/colostomy_a_patients_perspective/page4.htm (accessed June 28, 2005).

2. "Clinical Trials: Questions and Answers," National Cancer Institute, January 14, 2004, http://cis.nci.nih.gov/fact/2_11.htm (accessed June 28, 2005).

3. "Colostomy: A Patient's Perspective."

## CHAPTER 4

1. "Colon Cancer Treatment: Treatment Option Overview," National Cancer Institute, May 20, 2005, http://www.cancer.gov/cancertopics/pdq/treatment/colon/Patient/page4#Keypoint16 (accessed June 20, 2005).

2. Norman Cousins, *The Anatomy of an Illness as Perceived by the Patient* (New York: Norton, 1979).

3. Norman Cousins, *The Healing Heart* (New York: Norton, 1979).

4. "Communicating with Your Oncologist: Tips from Physicians," Cancer Treatment Information, OncoLink, http://www.oncolink.upenn.edu/treatment/article.cfm?c=7&s=42&id=49 (accessed June 22, 2005).

## CHAPTER 5

1. George Rowland, personal letter, July 1996.
2. John D. Potter et al., "Food Nutrition and the Prevention of Cancer: A Global Perspective," American Institute for Cancer Research, July 1997, http://www.aicr.org/research/report_summary.lasso#dietaryrecommendations (accessed June 22, 2005).
3. "Fluorouracil (5FU)," Cancer Research UK: Cancer Help, April 8, 2004, http://www.cancerhelp.org.uk/help/default.asp?page=4007 (accessed June 22, 2005).
4. "Managing Mouth Sores Resulting from Chemotherapy," Cancer Consultants Oncology Research Center, 2005, http://patient.cancerconsultants.com/cancer_tips.aspx?id=187 (accessed June 20, 2005).

## CHAPTER 6

1. "Your Mouth," Cancer Research UK, March 23, 2004, http://www.cancerhelp.org.uk/help/default.asp?page=312 (accessed June 20, 2005).
2. "Mouth Sores Due to Chemotherapy," Chemocare.com, 2005, Cleveland Clinic Foundation, http://www.chemocare.com/managing/fullstory.sps?iNewsid=24406&itype=1875 (accessed June 29, 2005).
3. Richard Woodman, "Study Confirms Red Meat Link with Bowel Cancer," Reuters Health, MedLine Plus, June 14, 2005, http://www.nlm.nih.gov/medlineplus/news/fullstory_25215.html (accessed June 20, 2005).
4. "Nutrition Action Healthletter: Colon Cancer and Carbs," *Journal of the National Cancer Institute* 96 (April 2004): 229.
5. "Fatigue," Cancer Research UK, May 2004, http://www.cancerhelp.org.uk/help/default.asp?page=8390 (accessed June 22, 2005).
6. Robert Buckman, *What You Really Need to Know about Cancer* (Toronto, Ontario: Key Porter Books, 1995), p. 248.
7. "Colon Cancer Treatment: Stages of Colon Cancer," National Cancer Institute, May 20, 2005, http://www.nci.nih.gov/cancertopics/pdq/treatment/colon/Patient/page2 (accesses June 20, 2005).

## CHAPTER 7

1. "Power of Art to Heal," Arts and Healing Network, 2003, http://www.artheals.org/power.html (accessed June 23, 2005).

2. "Guided Imagery or Visualization," Holistic Online, http://www.holistic-online.com/guided-imagery.htm (accessed June 29, 2005).

3. "Chemotherapy," Inside Medicine.Net, July 4, 2002, http://www.medicinenet.com/chemotherapy/article.htm (accessed June 22, 2005).

4. "Hair Loss (Alopecia)," CancerCare, http://www.cancercare.org/SymptomManagement/SymptomManagementList.cfm?c=524 (accessed June 23, 2005).

5. "Fluorouracil (5FU)," Cancer BACUP, June 6, 2005, http://www.cancerbacup.org.uk/Treatments/Chemotherapy/Individualdrugs/Fluorouracil (accessed June 25, 2005).

6. Patty Fawkes and Rebecca Rosser, "Review of Blood Collection Equipment," California Association for Medical Laboratory Technology, Distance Learning Program, http://www.camlt.org/DL_web/954_blood_col.html (accessed June 22, 2005).

7. "Management of a Central Line," Cancer BACUP March 1, 2004, http://www.cancerbacup.org.uk/Treatments/Chemotherapy/Managingacentralline (accessed June 22, 2005).

8. "What Is a Vascular Access Device?" Cancer Consultants Oncology Resource Center, http://patient.cancerconsultants.com/cancer_tips.aspx?id=196 (accessed June 23, 2005).

9. Mark Bennett Pochapin, *What Your Doctor May Not Tell You about Colorectal Cancer* (New York: Warner Books, 2004), p. 191.

10. Katrina Claghorn and Ellen Sweeney, "Winter 2001–2002 Nutrition Nuggets Newsletter," Abramson Cancer Center of the University of Pennsylvania, OncoLink, December 30, 2001, http://oncolink.com/coping/article.cfm?c=3&s=40&ss=87&id=532 (accessed June 22, 2005).

## CHAPTER 8

1. Frieda Fordham, *An Introduction to Jung's Psychology* (New York: Penguin Books, 1953), chap. 6: "Dreams and Their Interpretation."

2. "Symbolism of Eyes and Hair," September 7, 2001, http://www.three-musketeers.net/mike/eyes.html (accessed June 22, 2005).

3. American Cancer Society, "Look Good, Feel Better: For Women in Cancer Treatment and in Charge of Their Lives," 2004, http://www.lookgoodfeelbetter.org/women/explore/qa.htm (accessed June 22, 2005).

4. "Fluorouracil (5FU)," Cancer Research UK, April 8, 2004, http://www.cancerhelp.org.uk/help/default.asp?page=4007 (accessed June 22, 2005).

5. A. R. Fleischauer et al., "Garlic Consumption and Cancer Prevention: Meta-analyses of Colorectal and Stomach Cancers, *American Journal of Clinical Nutrition* 72 (2000): 1047–52, http://www.ncbi.nlm.nih.gov/entrez/query.fcgi?cmd=Retrieve&db=Pub Med&list_uids=11010950&dopt=Abstract (accessed June 22, 2005).

6. "Chemotherapy and You: A Guide to Self-Help during Cancer Treatments; How Can I Help Prevent Infections?" National Cancer Institute, National Institutes of Health, June 1, 1999, http://www.nci.nih.gov/cancertopics/chemotherapy-and-you/page4#C9 (accessed June 29, 2005).

7. Joel W. Goldwein, "Chemotherapy for Patients: Introductory Information," Abramson Cancer Center of the University of Pennsylvania, OncoLink, November 1, 2001, http://www.oncolink.upenn.edu/treatment/article.cfm?c=2&s=9&id=72 (accessed June 22, 2005).

8. Ibid.

9. Ibid.

## CHAPTER 9

1. "Fluorouracil (Adrucil, 5-FU)," Abramson Cancer Center of the University of Pennsylvania, OncoLink, February 10, 2004, http://www.oncolink.upenn.edu/treatment/article.cfm?c=2&s=10&id=172 (accessed June 22, 2005).

2. "Gallstones," National Digestive Diseases Clearing House (a service of the National Institute of Diabetes and Digestive and Kidney Diseases), Novermber 2004, http://digestive.niddk.nih.gov/ddiseases/pubs/gallstones/index.htm#treated (accessed June 22, 2005).

3. "Gallstones," National Digestive Diseases Clearing House, November 2004, http://digestive.niddk.nih.gov/ddiseases/pubs/gallstones/index.htm (accessed June 22, 2005).

4. Joseph Campbell, "Follow Your Bliss—Exerpts from *The Power of Myth* PBS Interviews with Bill Moyers," Joseph Campbell Foundation, 1987, http://www.jcf.org/bliss.php (accessed June 22, 2005).

5. "Sparta," *Compton's Encyclopedia*, http://www.crystalinks.com/sparta.html (accessed June 22, 2005).

## CHAPTER 10

1. "Chemotherapy and You: A Guide to Self-Help during Cancer Treatments; How Can I Help Control Diarrhea?" National Cancer Institute, National Institutes of Health, June 1, 1999, http://www.nci.nih.gov/cancertopics/chemotherapy-and-you/page4#C14 (accessed June 29, 2005).

2. Ibid.
3. Ibid.
4. "Orthostatic Hypotension Information Page: What Is Orthostatic Hypotension?" NINDS (National Institute of Neurological Disorders and Stroke), February 9, 2005, http://www.ninds.nih.gov/health_and_medical/disorders/orthosta_doc.htm (accessed June 22, 2005).
5. Mayo Clinic Staff, "Water: How Much Should You Drink Every Day?" MayoClinic.com, April 22, 2005, http://www.mayoclinic.com/invoke.cfm?objectid=1488D60D-E694-4EE6-A0DFA79E4CEF5FD3 (accessed June 22, 2005).
6. Michael Lerner, *Choices in Healing* (Cambridge, MA: MIT Press, 1994), pp. 13–14.

## CHAPTER 11

1. X-Plain.com Patient Education Institute, http://www.nlm.nih.gov/medlineplus/tutorials/coloncancersurgery/gs039101.html (accessed June 22, 2005).
2. "Necrosis," MedLine Plus Medical Encyclopedia, October 1, 2004, http://www.nlm.nih.gov/medlineplus/ency/article/002266.htm (accessed June 22, 2005).
3. Noel Elliott, "Care of the Patient Requiring a Nasogastric Tube," Nursewise, January 2, 2002, http://nursing.about.com/gi/dynamic/offsite.htm?site=http://www.nursewise.com/courses/ng_hour.htm (accessed June 20, 2005).

## CHAPTER 12

1. "Colon Cancer," About Colon Cancer, http://coloncancer.about.com/od/caregivers/ (accessed June 20, 2005).
2. Christian Stone, "Intestinal Obstruction," MedLine Plus Medical Encyclopedia, July 16, 2004, http://www.nlm.nih.gov/medlineplus/ency/article/000260.htm (accessed June 25, 2005).
3. "Colonoscopy," National Digestive Diseases Clearinghouse, November 2004, http://digestive.niddk.nih.gov/ddiseases/pubs/colonoscopy/ (accessed June 22, 2005).
4. Ibid.
5. "CEA: Glossary of Cancer Terms," Cancer Network, 2005, http://www.cancerhub.info/reference/glossary.aspx?find=C (accessed June 29, 2005).

## CHAPTER 13

1. Jan Nissl, "How to Prepare: Colonoscopy Test Overview," WebMD, September 20, 2004, http://my.webmd.com/hw/colorectal_cancer/hw209694.asp#hw209701 (accessed June 30, 2005).

## CHAPTER 14

1. Mark Bennett Pochapin, *What Your Doctor May Not Tell You about Colorectal Cancer* (New York: Warner Books, 2004), p. 189.

## CHAPTER 15

1. "Breathing for Relaxation," Army Physical Fitness Research Institute, http://carlisle-www.army.mil/apfri/breathing_for_relaxation.htm (accessed June 23, 2005).
2. "Ultrasound—Abdomen," Radiology Info, June 14, 2005, http://www.radiologyinfo.org/content/ultrasound-abdomen.htm (accessed June 20, 2005).
3. "Metastatic Cancer: Questions and Answers," National Cancer Institute, September 1, 2004, http://cis.nci.nih.gov/fact/6_20.htm (accessed June 29, 2005).
4. "Frequently Asked Questions about Traditional Chinese Medicine (TCM) and Acupuncture," Healing People Network, http://www.healingpeople.com/index.php?option=content&task=view&id=557&Itemid=143 (accessed June 20, 2005).
5. "What Is Qi Gong?" QiGong Institute, 2004, http://www.qigonginstitute.org/main_page/main_page.php (accessed June 20, 2005).

## CHAPTER 16

1. Lawrence LeShan, *Cancer as a Turning Point: A Handbook for People with Cancer, Their Families, and Health Professionals* (New York: Dutton, 1989).
2. Katie Couric, "About NCCRA: A Message from Katie Couric," 2005, http://www.eifoundation.org/national/nccra/vision/message_from_katie.html (accessed June 29, 2005).
3. Michael Lerner, *Choices in Healing* (Cambridge, MA: MIT Press, 1994), p. 372.
4. Ibid., p. 25.

## CHAPTER 17

1. "Nasogastric (Ryles) Tubes," Patients Plus, September 7, 2004, http://www.patient.co.uk/showdoc/40000186/ (accessed June 29, 2005).

2. "PDR Drug Information for Cetacaine Topical Anesthetic," Drugs.com, November 11, 1999, http://www.drugs.com/PDR/Cetacaine_Topical_Anesthetic.html (accessed June 25, 2005).

## GLOSSARY

1. "Cancer Glossary," Medicine Online, http://www.meds.com/glossary.html (accessed June 22, 2005); "Glossary," Colon Cancer Alliance, http://www.ccalliance.org/about/disease/glossary.html (accessed June 22, 2005).

# Bibliography

Achterberg, Jeanne et al. *Cancer as a Turning Point: From Surviving to Thriving.* Louisville, CO: Sounds True Audiobooks, 2000.

Barrie, Barbara. *Don't Die of Embarrassment.* New York: Scribner, 1999.

Bartlow, Bruce G. *Medical Care of the Soul.* Boulder, CO: Johnson Books, 2000.

Boucher, Sandy. *Hidden Spring: A Buddhist Woman Confronts Cancer.* Somerville, MA: Wisdom Publications, 2000.

"Breathing for Relaxation." Army Physical Fitness Research Institute. http://carlisle-www.army.mil/apfri/breathing_for_relaxation.htm (accessed June 23, 2005).

Buckman, Robert. *What You Really Need to Know About Cancer.* Toronto, ON: Key Porter, 1995.

Campbell, Joseph. "Follow Your Bliss" (excerpts from *The Power of Myth* PBS interviews with Bill Moyers). Joseph Campbell Foundation, 1987. http://www.jcf.org/bliss.php (accessed June 22, 2005).

"CEA: Glossary of Cancer Terms." Cancer Network, 2005. http://www.cancerhub.info/reference/glossary.aspx?find=C (accessed June 29, 2005).

"Chemotherapy." Inside Medicine.Net, July 4, 2002. http://www.medicinenet.com/chemotherapy/article.htm (accessed June 22, 2005)

"Chemotherapy and You: A Guide to Self-Help During Cancer Treatments; How Can I Help Control Diarrhea?" National Cancer Institute—National Institutes of Health, June 1, 1999. http://www.nci.nih.gov/cancertopics/chemotherapy-and-you/page4#C14 (accessed June 29, 2005).

"Chemotherapy and You: A Guide to Self-Help During Cancer Treatments; How Can I Help Prevent Infections?" National Cancer Institute—National

Institutes of Health, June 1, 1999. http://www.nci.nih.gov/cancertopics/chemotherapy-and-you/page4#C9 (accessed June 29, 2005).

Claghorn, Katrina, and Ellen Sweeney. "Winter 2001–2002 Nutrition Nuggets Newsletter." Abramson Cancer Center of the University of Pennsylvania—OncoLink, December 30, 2001. http://oncolink.com/coping/article.cfm?c=3&s=40&ss=87&id=532 (accessed June 22, 2005).

"Clinical Trials: Questions and Answers." National Cancer Institute, January 14, 2004. http://cis.nci.nih.gov/fact/2_11.htm (accessed June 28, 2005).

Cohen, Richard M. *Blindsided: A Reluctant Memoir.* New York: HarperCollins, 2004.

"Colon Cancer." About Colon Cancer. http://coloncancer.about.com/od/caregivers/ (accessed June 20, 2005).

"Colon Cancer and Carbs." *Journal of the National Cancer Institute* 96 (June 20, 2005): 229.

"Colon Cancer Treatment: Stages of Colon Cancer." National Cancer Institute, May 20, 2005. http://www.nci.nih.gov/cancertopics/pdq/treatment/colon/Patient/page2 (accessed June 22, 2005).

"Colon Cancer Treatment: Treatment Option Overview." National Cancer Institute, May 20, 2005. http://www.cancer.gov/cancertopics/pdq/treatment/colon/Patient/page4#Keypoint16 (accessed June 20, 2005).

"Colostomy: A Patient's Perspective." MedicineNet.com, April 17, 2002. http://www.medicinenet.com/colostomy_a_patients_perspective/page4.htm (accessed June 28, 2005).

"Communicating with Your Oncologist: Tips from Physicians." Cancer Treatment Information—OncoLink. http://www.oncolink.upenn.edu/treatment/article.cfm?c=7&s=42&id=49. (accessed June 22, 2005).

"Constipation." Ask the Nurse. http://www.med-help.net/Constipation.html (accessed June 25, 2005).

Couric, Katie. "About NCCRA: A Message From Katie Couric." 2005. http://www.eifoundation.org/national/nccra/vision/message_from_katie.html (accessed June 29, 2005).

Cousins, Norman. *The Anatomy of an Illness as Perceived by the Patient.* New York: Norton, 1979.

———. *The Healing Heart.* New York: Norton, 1983.

"Dehydration." Medline Plus Medical Encyclopedia, May 28, 2004. http://www.nlm.nih.gov/medlineplus/ency/article/000982.htm (accessed June 22, 2005).

Elliott, Noel. "Care of the Patient Requiring a Nasogastric Tube." Nursewise, January 2, 2002. http://nursing.about.com/gi/dynamic/offsite.htm?site=http://www.nursewise.com/courses/ng_hour.htm (accessed June 20, 2005).

Esko, Wendy. *Aveline Kushi's Introducing Macrobiotic Cooking.* New York: Japan Publications, 1987.

"Fatigue." Cancer Research UK, May 2004. http://www.cancerhelp.org.uk/help/default.asp?page=8390. (accessed June 22, 2005).

Fawkes, Patty, and Rebecca Rosser. "Review of Blood Collection Equipment." California Association for Medical Laboratory Technology—Distance Learning Program. http://www.camlt.org/DL_web/954_blood_col.html (accessed June 22, 2005).

Feste, Catherine. *The Physician Within: Taking Charge of Your Well-Being.* Minneapolis: Wellness Series, 1987.

Fleischauer, A. R. et al. "Garlic Consumption and Cancer Prevention: Meta-analyses of Colorectal and Stomach Cancers." *American Journal of Clinical Nutrition* 72 (2000):1047–52. http://www.ncbi.nlm.nih.gov/entrez/query.fcgi?cmd=Retrieve&db=PubMed&list_uids=11010950&dopt=Abstract (accessed June 22, 2005).

"Flexible Sigmoidoscopy." National Digestive Diseases Information Clearinghouse, November 2004. http://digestive.niddk.nih.gov/ddiseases/pubs/sigmoidoscopy/ (accessed June 22, 2005).

"Fluorouracil (5FU)." Cancer BACUP, June 6, 2005. http://www.cancerbacup.org.uk/Treatments/Chemotherapy/Individualdrugs/Fluorouracil (accessed 25 June 2005).

"Fluorouracil (5-FU)." Cancer Research UK, April 8, 2004. http://www.cancerhelp.org.uk/help/default.asp?page=4007. (accessed June 22, 2005).

"Fluorouracil (Adrucil, 5-FU)." Abramson Cancer Center of the University of Pennsylvania—OncoLink, February 10, 2004. http://www.oncolink.upenn.edu/treatment/article.cfm?c=2&s=10&id=172 (accessed June 22, 2005).

Fordham, Frieda. *An Introduction to Jung's Psychology.* New York and London: Penguin Books, 1953.

"Frequently Asked Questions About Traditional Chinese Medicine (TCM) and Acupuncture." Healing People Network. http://www.healingpeople.com/index.php?option=content&task=view&id=557&Itemid=143 (accessed June 20, 2005).

"Gallstones." National Digestive Diseases Clearing House, Novermber 2004. http://digestive.niddk.nih.gov/ddiseases/pubs/gallstones/index.htm (accessed June 22, 2005).

Gaynor, Mitchell L., and Jerry Hickey. *Dr. Gaynor's Cancer Prevention Program.* New York: Kensington Books, 1999.

Goldwein, Joel W. "Chemotherapy for Patients: Introductory Information." Abramson Cancer Center of the University of Pennsylvania—OncoLink, November 1, 2001. http://www.oncolink.upenn.edu/treatment/article.cfm?c=2&s=9&id=72 (accessed June 22, 2005).

Grof, Stan, and Christina Grof. *Beyond Death: The Gates of Consciousness.* London: Thames and Hudson, 1980.

Groopman, Jerome. *The Anatomy of Hope: How People Prevail in the Face of Illness.* New York: Random House, 2003.

———. *The Measure of Our Days: New Beginnings at Life's End.* New York: Penguin Books, 1998.

"Guided Imagery or Visualization." Holistic Online. http://www.holistic-online.com/guided-imagery.htm (accessed June 29, 2005).

Guterson, David. *East of the Mountains*. New York: Harcourt, 1999.

"Hair Loss (Alopecia)." CancerCare. http://www.cancercare.org/SymptomManagement/SymptomManagementList.cfm?c=524 (accessed June 23, 2005).

Handler, Evan. *Time on Fire: My Comedy of Terrors*. New York: Henry Holt, 1996.

Hirschberg, Caryle, and Marc Ian Barasch. *Remarkable Recovery*. New York: Riverhead, 1995.

"Intestinal Obstruction." MedLine Plus Medical Encyclopedia July 16, 2004. http://www.nlm.nih.gov/medlineplus/ency/article/000260.htm (accessed June 25 2005).

Johnson, Wendy. "Juggling Patients and Priorities: Life in the Emergency Department." May 7, 2002. http://www.cvh.on.ca/community/articles/actyh200201c.htm (accessed June 27, 2005).

Kabat-Zinn, Jon. *Full Catastrophe Living: Using the Wisdom of Your Body and Mind to Face Stress, Pain, and Illness*. New York: Delta, 1990.

Kornfield, Jack. *After the Ecstasy, the Laundry: How the Heart Grows Wise on the Spiritual Path*. New York: Bantam, 2000.

Kuner, Susan, Carol Matzkin Orsborn, Linda Quigley, and Karen Leigh Stroup. *Speak the Language of Healing*. Berkeley, CA: Conari, 2001.

Lad, Usha, and Vasant Lad. *Ayurvedic Cooking for Self Healing*. Albuquerque: Ayurvedic Press, 1997.

Lerner, Max. *Wrestling With the Angel: A Memoir of My Triumph over Illness*. New York: Norton, 1991.

Lerner, Michael. *Choices in Healing*. Cambridge, MA: MIT Press, 1994.

LeShan, Lawrence. *Cancer as a Turning Point: A Handbook for People with Cancer, Their Families, and Health Professionals*. New York: Plume, 1994.

Levine, Stephen. *Healing into Life and Death*. New York: Anchor, 1989.

———, and Ondrea Levine. *Who Dies?: An Investigation of Conscious Living and Conscious Dying*. New York: Anchor, 1989.

"Look Good Feel Better: For Women in Cancer Treatment and in Charge of Their Lives." American Cancer Society, 2004. http://www.lookgoodfeelbetter.org/women/explore/qa.htm (accessed June 22, 2005).

Mackey, Francis. *Why Die of Colon Cancer?* Bethel, CT: Rutledge Books, 2000.

"Management of a Central Line." Cancer BACUP, March 1, 2004. http://www.cancerbacup.org.uk/Treatments/Chemotherapy/Managingacentralline (accessed June 22, 2005).

"Managing Mouth Sores Resulting from Chemotherapy." Cancer Consultants Oncology Research Center, 2005. http://patient.cancerconsultants.com/cancer_tips.aspx?id=187. (accessed June 20, 2005).

Markova, Dawna. *I Will Not Die an Unlived Life: Reclaiming Purpose and Passion*. Berkeley, CA: Conari, 2000.

Mayo Clinic Staff. "Water: How Much Should You Drink Every Day?" Mayo Clinic.com, April 22, 2005. http://www.mayoclinic.com/invoke.cfm?objectid=1488D60D-E694-4EE6-A0DFA79E4CEF5FD3 (accessed June 22, 2005).

"Metastatic Cancer: Questions and Answers." National Cancer Institute. http://cis.nci.nih.gov/fact/6_20.htm (accessed June 29, 2005).

Miskovitz, Paul, and Marian Betancourt. *What To Do If You Get Colon Cancer : A Specialist Helps You Take Charge and Make Informed Choices.* Hoboken, NJ: Wiley, 1997.

Moody, Raymond. *Life After Life : The Investigation of a Phenomenon—Survival of Bodily Death.* San Francisco: Harper, 2001.

Morningstar, Amadea, and Urmila Desai. *The Ayurvedic Cookbook.* Twin Lakes, WI: Lotus Press, 1990.

"Mouth Sores due to Chemotherapy." Chemocare.com, 2005. http://www.chemocare.com/managing/fullstory.sps?iNewsid=24406&itype=1875 (accessed June 29, 2005).

"Nasogastric (Ryles) Tubes." Patients Plus, September 7, 2004. http://www.patient.co.uk/showdoc/40000186/ (accessed June 29, 2005).

"Necrosis." MedLine Plus Medical Encyclopedia, October 1, 2004. http://www.nlm.nih.gov/medlineplus/ency/article/002266.htm (accessed October 2, 2004).

Nissl, Jan. "Digital Rectal Exam (DRE)." Web MD, December 16, 2004. http://my.webmd.com/hw/colorectal_cancer/hw4404.asp (accessed June 24, 2005).

"Orthostatic Hypotension Information Page: What Is Orthostatic Hypotension?" National Institute of Neurological Disorders and Stroke (NINDS), February 9, 2005. http://www.ninds.nih.gov/health_and_medical/disorders/orthosta_doc.htm (accessed June 22, 2005).

"Phlebitis." Columbia Electronic Encyclopedia—InfoPlease, 2005. http://www.infoplease.com/ce6/sci/A0838820.html (accessed June 22, 2005).

Pochapin, Mark Bennett. *What Your Doctor May Not Tell You About Colorectal Cancer.* New York: Warner Books, 2004.

Potter, John D. et al. "Food Nutrition and the Prevention of Cancer: A Global Perspective." American Institute for Cancer Research, July 1997. http://www.aicr.org/research/report_summary.lasso#dietaryrecommendations (accessed June 22, 2005).

"Power of Art to Heal." Arts and Healing Network, 2003. http://www.artheals.org/power.html (accessed June 23,2005).

Remen, Rachel Naomi. *Kitchen Table Wisdom: Stories that Heal.* New York: Riverhead, 1997.

———. *My Grandfathers Blessings: Stories of Strength, Refuge, and Belonging.* New York: Riverhead, 2001.

Richards, Victor. *Cancer: The Wayward Cell.* Berkeley and Los Angeles: University of California Press: 1972.

Rinpoche, Sogyal, *The Tibetan Book of Living and Dying*. San Francisco: Harper, 1994.

Rodgers, Joni. *Bald in the Land of Big Hair*. New York: Harper Collins, 2001.

Rossman, Martin L. *Fighting Cancer from Within: How to Use the Power of Your Mind for Healing*. New York: Owl Books, 2003.

———. *Guided Imagery for Self-Healing: An Essential Resource for Anyone Seeking Wellness*. Oakland: Kramer, 2000.

Shapiro, Dan. *Mom's Marijuana: Life, Love, and Beating the Odds*. New York: Vintage Books, 2001.

Simonton, O. Carl, James Creighton, and Stephanie Matthews Simonton. *Getting Well Again : The Bestselling Classic About the Simontons' Revolutionary Lifesaving Self-Awareness Techniques*. New York: Bantam, 1992.

"Sparta." Compton's Encyclopedia. http://www.crystalinks.com/sparta.html (accessed June 22, 2005).

"Symbolism of Eyes and Hair." September 7, 2001. http://www.three-musketeers.net/mike/eyes.html (accessed June 25, 2005).

Todd, Alexandra Dundas. *Double Vision: An East–West Collaboration for Coping with Cancer*. Hanover, NH: University of New England Press, 1994.

"Ultrasound—Abdomen." Radiology Info, June 14, 2005. http://www.radiologyinfo.org/content/ultrasound-abdomen.htm (accessed June 20, 2005).

Weil, Andrew. *Spontaneous Healing: How to Discover and Embrace Your Body's Natural Ability to Maintain and Heal Itself.* New York: Ballantine Books, 1996.

"What is Qi Gong?" National Qigong Association. http://www.nqa.org/qigong.html (accessed June 29, 2005).

Woodman, Richard. "Study Confirms Red Meat Link with Bowel Cancer." Reuters Health, June 14, 2005. MedLine Plus. http://www.nlm.nih.gov/medlineplus/news/fullstory_25215.html (accessed June 20, 2005).

X-Plain.com Patient Education Institute. http://www.nlm.nih.gov/medlineplus/tutorials/colon cancersurgery/gs039101.html (accessed June 22, 2005).

"Your Mouth." Cancer Research UK, March 23, 2004. http://www.cancerhelp.org.uk/help/default.asp?page=312 (accessed June 20, 2005).

# Web Site Resources

**Abramson Cancer Center of the University of Pennsylvania**—"OncoLink was founded in 1994 by Penn cancer specialists with a mission to help cancer patients, families, health care professionals and the general public get accurate cancer-related information at no charge."
http://www.oncolink.org/types/article.cfm?c=5&s=11&ss=605&id=9458

**The American Cancer Society**—"The American Cancer Society is the nationwide community-based voluntary health organization dedicated to eliminating cancer as a major health problem by preventing cancer, saving lives, and diminishing suffering from cancer, through research, education, advocacy, and service."
http://www.cancer.org/docroot/home/index.asp?level=0

**The American Society of Colon and Rectal Surgeons**—"The American Society of Colon and Rectal Surgeons is an association of surgeons and other professionals dedicated to assuring high quality patient care by advancing the science through research and education for prevention and management of disorders and diseases of the colon, rectum and anus."
http://www.fascrs.org/index.cfm

**BC Cancer Agency**—"The BC Cancer Agency provides a cancer care program for the people of British Columbia, including prevention,

screening and early detection, diagnosis and treatment services, support programs, community programs, research and education."
http://www.bccancer.bc.ca/default.htm

**Canadian Cancer Resources Directory**—"The aim of 'Guide to Internet Resources for Cancer' is to make it easier to find more specific information quickly. This is achieved by providing a directory of some of the key cancer-related sites and pages. Links are sorted into categories (by disease-type, medical speciality, country, etc.), and where possible, annotation is provided to give the reader a brief description of each site / organisation. As well as links the site presents basic information about cancer-related topics."
http://www.cancerindex.org/clinks5c.htm

**The Canadian Cancer Society**—"The Canadian Cancer Society is a national, community-based organization of volunteers whose mission is the eradication of cancer and the enhancement of the quality of life of people living with cancer."
http://www.cancer.ca/ccs/internet/frontdoor/0,,3172,00.html

**Cancer Advocacy Coalition of Canada**—"The CACC mission is to make comprehensive and patient-centred cancer care a national priority in Canada."
http://www.canceradvocacy.ca/ourmission.htm

**The Collaborative on Health and the Environment**—"The Collaborative on Health and the Environment (CHE) is a nonpartisan partnership of individuals and organizations concerned with the role of the environment in human and ecosystem health. CHE seeks to raise the level of scientific and public dialogue about the role of environmental contaminants and other environmental factors in many of the common diseases, disorders and conditions of our time."
http://www.cheforhealth.org/

**Colon Cancer Alliance**—"The Colon Cancer Alliance (CCA) is an organization of colon and rectal cancer survivors, their families, caregivers, people genetically predisposed to the disease and the medical community. [They] began as a group of people participating in an online discussion list for colorectal cancer patients. In 1999, the CCA was for-

mally incorporated as a non-profit organization dedicated to patient support, advocacy and education."
http://www.ccalliance.org/

**Colon Cancer Concern**—"Colon Cancer Concern (CCC) is the UK's leading charity dedicated to reducing deaths from bowel cancer and improving the quality of life of those affected by the disease. CCC has taken a lead in assisting people to make fully informed decisions and choices about their treatment, management, care and support."
http://www.coloncancer.org.uk/

**Colorectal Cancer Association of Canada**—"The Colorectal Cancer Association of Canada (CCAC) is the first non-profit organization dedicated to supporting people with colorectal cancer, their families and caregivers. Its mission is to improve the quality of life of patients and increase awareness of the disease."
http://www.ccac-accc.ca/

**Colorectal Cancer Network**—Their mission is to "eliminate colon cancer and support patients."
http://www.colorectal-cancer.net/

**Commonweal Cancer Help Program**—"The Commonweal Cancer Help Program (CCHP) is a week-long retreat for people with cancer. [Their] goal is to help participants live better and, where possible, longer lives. The Cancer Help Program addresses the unmet needs of people with cancer. These include finding balanced information on choices in healing, mainstream and complementary therapies; exploring emotional and spiritual dimensions of cancer; discovering that illness can sometimes lead to a richer and fuller life; and experiencing genuine community with others facing a cancer diagnosis."
http://www.commonweal.org/programs/cancer-help.html

**Entertainment Industry Foundation**—The Entertainment Industry Foundation's mission is "to raise awareness and funds for important causes such as childhood hunger, cancer research, creative arts, education, cardiovascular research, and much more."
http://www.eifoundation.org/about/

**Harvard Center for Cancer Prevention**—"Colorectal cancer is the second leading cause of cancer death in the United States, but it doesn't need to be. More than half of all colorectal cancers could be prevented with routine screening and a healthy lifestyle. To help address this issue, the Harvard Center for Cancer Prevention has partnered with the Massachusetts Colorectal Cancer Working Group" to develop information and resources, including an interactive risk assessment guide.
http://www.yourdiseaserisk.harvard.edu/

**Healing Journeys Cancer as a Turning Point, From Surviving to Thriving Conferences**—"[Their] mission at Healing Journeys is to promote and support healing by assisting people with cancer or other life-altering illnesses to access their own healing potential and their ability to thrive."
http://www.healingjourneys.org/

**Health Care Without Harm**—"Health Care Without Harm is an international coalition of hospitals and health care systems, medical professionals, community groups, health-affected constituencies, labor unions, environmental and environmental health organizations and religious groups. . . . Mission: To transform the health care industry worldwide, without compromising patient safety or care, so that it is ecologically sustainable and no longer a source of harm to public health and the environment."
http://www.noharm.org

**Health Services/Technology Assessment Text (HSTAT)**—"The Health Services Technology/Assessment Texts (HSTAT) is a free, Web-based resource of full-text documents that provide health information and support health care decision making. HSTAT's audience includes health care providers, health service researchers, policy makers, payers, consumers and the information professionals who serve these groups."
http://www.ncbi.nlm.nih.gov/books/bv.fcgi?rid=hstat

**The Institute for the Study of Health and Illness**—"The Institute for the Study of Health and Illness (ISHI) at Commonweal is an education and training center for physicians who wish to renew their commitment to service and to live by the values that have motivated physicians through the ages. Since 1991, ISHI has offered a series of innovative Cat-

egory 1 CME retreat workshops that enable physicians to find deeper satisfaction and meaning in the day-to-day practice of medicine."
http://www.commonweal.org/ishi/

**The International Ostomy Association**—An association of ostomy associations, is committed to the improvement of the quality of life of ostomates and those with related surgeries, worldwide.
http://www.ostomyinternational.org/

**The Johns Hopkins Medical Institutions Colon Cancer Home Page**—"The Johns Hopkins Medical Institutions has become the leading center for the treatment and study of colorectal cancer. [They] created this Web page to detail the research and clinical developments, as well as the members of the multidisciplinary team of clinicians and scientists assembled here at Johns Hopkins to fight colon cancer."
http://pathology.jhu.edu/COLON_CA/

**MD Anderson Cancer Center**—"The mission of The University of Texas M. D. Anderson Cancer Center is to eliminate cancer in Texas, the nation, and the world through outstanding programs that integrate patient care, research and prevention, and through education for undergraduate and graduate students, trainees, professionals, employees and the public."
http://www3.mdanderson.org/depts/hcc/

**Memorial Sloan Kettering Cancer Institute**—"Memorial Sloan-Kettering Cancer Center, composed of Memorial Hospital for Cancer and Allied Diseases and Sloan-Kettering Institute, is dedicated to excellence in the prevention, treatment, and cure of cancer through patient care, research, and education. Memorial Hospital for Cancer and Allied Diseases provides patient care. Early detection, precise diagnosis, individually tailored treatment, and concern for a patient's needs are the hallmarks of the care provided."
http://www.mskcc.org/mskcc/html/311.cfm

**National Cancer Institute**—"The National Cancer Institute (NCI) is a component of the National Institutes of Health (NIH), one of eight agencies that compose the Public Health Service (PHS) in the Department of Health and Human Services (DHHS). The NCI, established under the

National Cancer Act of 1937, is the Federal Government's principal agency for cancer research and training. . . . The National Cancer Institute coordinates the National Cancer Program, which conducts and supports research, training, health information dissemination, and other programs with respect to the cause, diagnosis, prevention, and treatment of cancer, rehabilitation from cancer, and the continuing care of cancer patients and the families of cancer patients."
http://www.nci.nih.gov/

**National Cancer Institute, Colon Cancer Treatment**—Excellent and detailed information about colon cancer and the treatments available.
http://www.cancer.gov/cancerinfo/pdq/treatment/colon/patient/

**National Cancer Institute of Canada (NCIC)**—"To undertake and support cancer research and related programs in Canada that will lead to the reduction of the incidence, morbidity and mortality from cancer."
http://www.ncic.cancer.ca/ncic/internet/home/0%2C%2C84658243_langId-en%2C00.html

**National Center for Complementary and Alternative Medicine**—"The National Center for Complementary and Alternative Medicine (NCCAM) is 1 of the 27 institutes and centers that make up the National Institutes of Health (NIH). NCCAM is dedicated to exploring complementary and alternative healing practices in the context of rigorous science, training complementary and alternative medicine (CAM) researchers, and disseminating authoritative information to the public and professionals."
http://nccam.nih.gov/

**National Colorectal Cancer Research Alliance**—"The National Colorectal Cancer Research Alliance (NCCRA), a program of the Entertainment Industry Foundation, is dedicated to the eradication of colorectal cancer by promoting the importance of early medical screening and funding research to develop better tests, treatments, and ultimately a cure."
http://www.eifoundation.org/national/nccra/splash/

**National Colorectal Cancer Roundtable**—The National Colorectal Cancer Roundtable's mission is "to advance colorectal cancer control efforts by improving communication, coordination, and collaboration

among health agencies, medical-professional organizations, and the public."
http://www.nccrt.org/General/GeneralContent.aspx?article_id=1§ion_id=1

**The National Library of Medicine**—"The National Library of Medicine (NLM), on the campus of the National Institutes of Health in Bethesda, Maryland, is the world's largest medical library. The Library collects materials and provides information and research services in all areas of biomedicine and health care."
http://www.nlm.nih.gov/

**PDQ—NCI's Comprehensive Cancer Database**—"PDQ (Physician Data Query) is NCI's comprehensive cancer database. It contains peer-reviewed summaries on cancer treatment, screening, prevention, genetics, and supportive care, and complementary and alternative medicine; a registry of approximately 2,000 open and 13,000 closed cancer clinical trials from around the world; and directories of physicians, professionals who provide genetics services, and organizations that provide cancer care."
http://www.nci.nih.gov/cancertopics/pdq/cancerdatabase

**The Sidney Kimmel Cancer Center at Johns Hopkins**—"The Johns Hopkins Kimmel Cancer Center . . . One of only 41 cancer centers in the country designated by the National Cancer Institute (NCI) as a Comprehensive Cancer Center. Patients who visit the Kimmel Cancer Center have access to some of the most innovative and advanced therapies in the world. Because Center clinicians and research scientists work closely together, new drugs and treatments developed in the laboratory are quickly transferred to the clinical setting, offering patients improved therapeutic options."
http://www.hopkinskimmelcancercenter.org/cancertypes/colon-rectal-cancer.cfm?cancerid=78

**UCSF Comprehensive Cancer Center**—"The overarching goal of the UCSF Comprehensive Cancer Center is to shepherd new approaches to cancer prevention, detection, and treatment into clinical and population settings, where they can be tested and evaluated. Multidisciplinary programs—which include lab scientists, clinical investigators, providers of

patient care, epidemiologists, and sociobehavioral scientists—facilitate this process by focusing research on relevant issues to patients and persons at risk of cancer. The UCSF Cancer Resource Center, a multimedia information hub for patients, family members, caregivers, and the interested public, provides direct services to hundreds of individuals each month. Its free information services include access to a multimedia library; computer stations where visitors can access specialized databases as well as browse Internet resources; personalized assistance with online searches; and information on community events and resources. For patients who are unable to travel, staff members perform research on their behalf in response to requests by telephone, letter, and e-mail."
http://cc.ucsf.edu/

**Web MD Health Colon Cancer**—"The WebMD content staff blends award-winning expertise in medicine, journalism, health communication and content creation to bring you the best health information possible. Our esteemed colleagues at MedicineNet.com are frequent contributors to WebMD and comprise our Medical Editorial Board. Our Independent Medical Review Board continuously reviews the site for accuracy and timeliness."
http://my.webmd.com/search/search_results/?filter=mywebmd_all_filter &query=colon+cancer&go.x=14&go.y=12

**WomenCARE—Women's Cancer Advocacy Resources & Education**—"WomenCARE offers a safe haven where women who are making the cancer journey will find mutual support, shared experience and open hearts. Throughout diagnosis, healing, surviving or dying, our mission is to provide FREE cancer advocacy, resources, education and support to women with cancer, to their families and friends, and to healthcare practitioners working in the field."
http://www.womencaresantacruz.org/

**The World Health Organization**—"The World Health Organization is the United Nations specialized agency for health. It was established on 7 April 1948. WHO's objective, as set out in its Constitution, is the attainment by all peoples of the highest possible level of health. Health is defined in WHO's Constitution as a state of complete physical, mental and social well-being and not merely the absence of disease or infirmity."
http://www.who.int/en/

# Sidebar Index

## CONSIDERATIONS/ SUGGESTIONS FOR HOSPITAL STAFF



## FOR YOUR INFORMATION

## HINTS TO HELP YOU BEAT THE ODDS

## SUGGESTIONS FOR ALLIES



## SUGGESTIONS FOR FAMILY AND FRIENDS

# Subject Index